T0296791

Prospects of Blockchain Technology for Accelerating Scientific Advancement in Healthcare

Malaya Dutta Borah
National Institute of Technology (NIT), India

Peng Zhang
Belmont University, USA

Ganesh Chandra Deka
Ministry of Skill Development and Entrepreneurship, Government of India, India

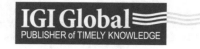

A volume in the Advances in Healthcare Information Systems and Administration (AHISA) Book Series

Published in the United States of America by
IGI Global
Medical Information Science Reference (an imprint of IGI Global)
701 E. Chocolate Avenue
Hershey PA, USA 17033
Tel: 717-533-8845
Fax: 717-533-8661
E-mail: cust@igi-global.com
Web site: http://www.igi-global.com

Library of Congress Cataloging-in-Publication Data

Names: Dutta Borah, Malaya, 1976- editor. | Zhang, Peng, 1992- editor. |
  Deka, Ganesh Chandra, 1969- editor.
Title: Prospects of blockchain technology for accelerating scientific
  advancement in healthcare / Malaya Dutta Borah, Peng Zhang, Ganesh
  Chandra Deka, editor.
Description: Hershey, PA : Medical Information Science Reference, 2021. |
  Includes bibliographical references and index. | Summary: "This edited
  book brings forth the prospects and research trends of blockchain in
  healthcare, including recent research findings of various authors on
  blockchain in healthcare, current state-of-the-art blockchain in
  application in healthcare and various challenges faced by the healthcare
  community in securing healthcare data"-- Provided by publisher.
Identifiers: LCCN 2021042592 (print) | LCCN 2021042593 (ebook) | ISBN
  9781799896067 (hardcover) | ISBN 9781799896074 (ebook)
Subjects: LCSH: Medical care--Data processing. | Blockchains (Databases)
Classification: LCC R858 .P797 2022 (print) | LCC R858 (ebook) | DDC
  610.285--dc23/eng/20211004
LC record available at https://lccn.loc.gov/2021042592
LC ebook record available at https://lccn.loc.gov/2021042593

This book is published in the IGI Global book series Advances in Healthcare Information Systems and Administration (AHISA) (ISSN: 2328-1243; eISSN: 2328-126X)

British Cataloguing in Publication Data
A Cataloguing in Publication record for this book is available from the British Library.

All work contributed to this book is new, previously-unpublished material.
The views expressed in this book are those of the authors, but not necessarily of the publisher.

For electronic access to this publication, please contact: eresources@igi-global.com.

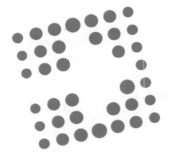

Advances in Healthcare Information Systems and Administration (AHISA) Book Series

ISSN:2328-1243
EISSN:2328-126X

Editor-in-Chief: Anastasius Moumtzoglou Hellenic Society for Quality & Safety in Healthcare and P. & A. Kyriakou Children's Hospital, Greece

MISSION

The **Advances in Healthcare Information Systems and Administration (AHISA) Book Series** aims to provide a channel for international researchers to progress the field of study on technology and its implications on healthcare and health information systems. With the growing focus on healthcare and the importance of enhancing this industry to tend to the expanding population, the book series seeks to accelerate the awareness of technological advancements of health information systems and expand awareness and implementation.

Driven by advancing technologies and their clinical applications, the emerging field of health information systems and informatics is still searching for coherent directing frameworks to advance health care and clinical practices and research. Conducting research in these areas is both promising and challenging due to a host of factors, including rapidly evolving technologies and their application complexity. At the same time, organizational issues, including technology adoption, diffusion and acceptance as well as cost benefits and cost effectiveness of advancing health information systems and informatics applications as innovative forms of investment in healthcare are gaining attention as well. **AHISA** addresses these concepts and critical issues.

COVERAGE

- Clinical Decision Support Design, Development and Implementation
- Telemedicine
- IT Applications in Physical Therapeutic Treatments
- Management of Emerging Health Care Technologies
- Measurements and Impact of HISA on Public and Social Policy
- Role of informatics specialists
- E-Health and M-Health
- IS in Healthcare
- Pharmaceutical and Home Healthcare Informatics
- Virtual health technologies

IGI Global is currently accepting manuscripts for publication within this series. To submit a proposal for a volume in this series, please contact our Acquisition Editors at Acquisitions@igi-global.com or visit: http://www.igi-global.com/publish/.

Titles in this Series

For a list of additional titles in this series, please visit:
www.igi-global.com/book-series/advances-healthcare-information-systems-administration/37156

Quality of Healthcare in the Aftermath of the COVID-19 Pandemic
Anastasius Moumtzoglou (P&A Kyriakou Children's Hospital, Greece)
Medical Information Science Reference • © 2022 • 403pp • H/C (ISBN: 9781799891987)
• US $325.00

Handbook of Research on Applied Intelligence for Health and Clinical Informatics
Anuradha Dheeraj Thakare (Pimpri Chinchwad College of Engineering, Savitribai Phule Pune University, India) Sanjeev J. Wagh (Shivaji University, India) Manisha Sunil Bhende (Dr. D.Y. Patil Institute of Engineering, Management, and Research Akurdi, India & Savitribai Phule Pune University, India) Ahmed M. Anter (Beni-Suef University, Egypt) and Xiao-Zhi Gao (University of Eastern Finland, Finland)
Medical Information Science Reference • © 2022 • 470pp • H/C (ISBN: 9781799877097)
• US $425.00

Developing Maternal Health Decision Support Systems in Developing Countries
Vincent Mzazi (University of South Africa, South Africa)
Medical Information Science Reference • © 2021 • 286pp • H/C (ISBN: 9781799839583)
• US $265.00

Cloud-Based M-Health Systems for Vein Image Enhancement and Feature Extraction Emerging Research and Opportunities
Kamta Nath Mishra (Birla Institute of Technology, India) and Subhash Chandra Pandey (Birla Institute of Technology, India)
Medical Information Science Reference • © 2021 • 246pp • H/C (ISBN: 9781799845379)
• US $195.00

The NHS and Contemporary Health Challenges From a Multilevel Perspective
Louise Dalingwater (Sorbonne Université, France)
Medical Information Science Reference • © 2020 • 261pp • H/C (ISBN: 9781799839286)
• US $265.00

For an entire list of titles in this series, please visit:
www.igi-global.com/book-series/advances-healthcare-information-systems-administration/37156

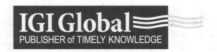

701 East Chocolate Avenue, Hershey, PA 17033, USA
Tel: 717-533-8845 x100 • Fax: 717-533-8661
E-Mail: cust@igi-global.com • www.igi-global.com

EDITORIAL ADVISORY BOARD

Table of Contents

Detailed Table of Contents

Chapter 1

With the technological sector booming combined with the internet revolutionizing the 21st century, along with the current coronavirus pandemic, more and more hands are getting virtually connected. Today, cyber criminals are not only behind money but are also designed to access, delete, or extort a user's sensitive data. These attacks range from DoS (denial of service) attacks and phishing to eavesdropping attacks. Blockchain is a technology that aims to keep data safe from being corrupted or accidentally deleted while maintaining its history. This technology has an impact on various industries, but the healthcare industry is impacted significantly. This chapter presents a systematic review of different use cases and applications of blockchain in healthcare. This chapter further discusses issues, solutions, and the future scope in blockchain applications in healthcare industries. An idea is to give a complete state of the art and challenges to better understand its utility in the healthcare sector.

Chapter 2

Many sectors, including finance, government, energy, health, and others, have found interest in blockchain technology over the last decade. It's no exaggeration to state that blockchain is pervasive in the healthcare industry. According to industry insiders, its application in healthcare has yet to achieve its full potential, but the implications might be substantial as it matures. This chapter presents the ongoing research trends, the existing issues and challenges, and presents future research opportunities to understand blockchain better. This chapter also throws light on the concepts of blockchain. This chapter also presents some examples of the uses of blockchain in healthcare. The authors hope that this chapter provides insight to the readers on the present and future research opportunities of blockchain in healthcare.

Chapter 3

With blockchain technology, the healthcare sector can have data efficiency, data access flexibility, interconnection, transparency, and security. This chapter reviews the development of blockchain technology usage, current implementation challenges of blockchain technology, and includes references for the applications of blockchain technology in healthcare. A systematic review of current status, desired status called ideal status, and the research gap of use of blockchain technology in application areas of the healthcare industry are included along with identification of possible research agendas for future research.

Chapter 4

Healthcare service providers are dependent on accurate information systems. Some crucial challenges are (1) improvement of patient caring services, (2) containing the deployment cost of information systems, and (3) avoiding any disturbances in its business processes at the time of data gathering and processing activities. Technological advancements are a significant driver of efficient healthcare information systems and services. By creating a rich healthcare-related data foundation and integrating technologies like the internet of things (IoT), blockchain technology, artificial intelligence (AI) techniques, and big data analytics, the digital transformation in healthcare is recognized as a pivotal component to tackle these challenges. For example, it can improve diagnostics, prevention, and patient therapy, ultimately empowering caregivers to use an evidence-based method to enhance clinical decision-making. Real-time interactions permit a physician to monitor a patient 'live' instead of interaction regularly (e.g., weekly, monthly). This way, healthcare operation can provide better services. However, the IoT system creates the risk of a sensitive data breach without a highly secure infrastructure. Blockchain technology improves the reliance on a centralized authority to certify information integrity and ownership and mediate transactions and exchange of digital assets. As a result, the mining process in the blockchain is very resource-intensive; hence, miners create coalition groups to cross-check each block of transactions in return for a reward. In addition, it creates enormous competition among miners, and consequently, dishonest mining strategies (e.g., block withholding attack, selfish mining, eclipse attack) need to be controlled. Consequently, it is necessary to regulate the mining process to make miners accountable for any dishonest mining behaviours; game theory can help regulate it. Finally, this chapter presents a survey of game theory used to address the common issues in the blockchain network.

Supply chain has been the main process of sustainable products/services flow from supplier to customer in various industries. Blockchain has been a revolution in cryptocurrency, and it is the tamperproof, timestamp, consensus-based algorithm with the decentralized ledger. There are emerging applications of blockchain from financials to healthcare and creating various jobs in service industries. Big data and Industry 4.0 with the blockchain ecosystems can bring efficiencies and real-time transactions in the pharmaceutical industry from origin to distribution in the healthcare supply chain. This chapter shall explain the physical aspects of the integration of blockchain and supply chain management in pharmaceutical industries.

This chapter introduces a blockchain-based infrastructure to support the traceability of medical products and implementation of unique device identification. Therefore, in the next pages, the characteristics of blockchain technology as well as benefits and challenges in supply chain management are described. After that, regulations for medical supply chains are gathered with a focus on American and European regulations and interlinked with the current concepts of the labling medical products.

Finally, a technical blockchain-based solution is conceptualized with regard to full and light node system in medical supply chains before the chapter is concluded with an outlook and further scientific and technical research possibilities.

Chapter 7

This chapter shows that blockchain has a lot of potential for revolutionizing the traditional healthcare industry. When attempting to completely integrate blockchain technology with existing EHR systems, however, a number of research and operational hurdles remain. The authors evaluated and discussed some of these issues in this chapter. After that, they discovered a variety of possible research topics, such as IoT, big data, machine learning, and edge computing. They offer a methodology for implementing blockchain technology in the healthcare industry for electronic health records (EHR). The goal of the proposed structure is to first integrate blockchain technology for EHR and then to enable safe storage of electronic data for users of the framework by setting access controls. They hope that this review will help us gain a better understanding of the development and deployment of future generation EHR systems that will benefit humankind.

Healthcare industry operation needs resources and information sharing between business partners. Internet of things (IoT) aims to simplify distributing data collection in the healthcare business, sharing and processing information across collaborative business partners using appropriate information system architecture. However, a large portion of existing IoT-based healthcare systems leveraged for managing data is centralized, posing potential risks of a single point of failure in natural disasters. The medical data privacy and security problems could result from a delay in treatment progress, even endangering the patient's life. This chapter describes the use of blockchain-enabled secure management of healthcare systems. Blockchain technology contributes to transactional data's intelligent and flexible handling through appropriate convergence with IoT technology in supporting data integration, processing, and providing data privacy and security-related issues. Finally, the chapter presents challenges and solutions on blockchain-based electronic healthcare record (EHR) systems.

Prachurjya Kashyap, National Institute of Technology, Silchar, India
Syed Tafreed Numan, National Institute of Technology, Silchar, India
Amit Kumar, National Institute of Technology, Silchar, India
Rohit Paul, National Institute of Technology, Silchar, India
Boddu Venkateswarlu, National Institute of Technology, Silchar, India
Naresh Babu Muppalaneni, National Institute of Technology, Silchar,
India
Malaya Dutta Borah, National Institute of Technology, Silchar, India

Supply chain is one of critical components of vaccination drive. A robust and efficient supply chain of vaccines would help increase the speed and efficiency of vaccination, therefore reducing vaccine wastage. This system uses centralised algorithms. They are prone to single point of failure in terms of transparency, trackability and traceability, immutability, audit, and trust. These issues stymie and slow the distribution of COVID-19 vaccinations, and they make it impossible to provide a safe, secure, transparent, and reliable distribution and delivery process of COVID-19 vaccines. The authors propose a blockchain-based approach to manage data linked to COVID-19 vaccines. To automate vaccination tracing, a smart contract for vaccine distribution is being created. The authors discuss and implement the proposed solution, as well as their implementation testing and validation; they evaluate the proposed solution by performing cost and security analyses and comparing them to existing solutions, and they evaluate the proposed solution by performing cost and security analyses and comparing them to existing solutions.

Amulya Murthy Aku, KAHER's KLE SBMK Ayurveda Mahavidyalaya,
India

In a variety of ways, blockchain technology has the potential to enhance healthcare and well-being in the future. Products of high value but low volume such as pharmaceuticals, health food, cosmetics, and other things can all benefit from the potential applications of this technology in these niche sectors. In this chapter, the authors examine the breadth and applications of blockchain technology in the ancient Indian medical system, as well as the challenges and opportunities it presents. Ayurvedic science has been around for 5000 years and contains all of the principles, techniques, and treatments necessary to not only prevent and promote health but also to cure any underlying health concerns that may exist. This will improve the statistical reliability of clinical data in Ayurvedic medicine, as well as make it simpler to distinguish between false and accurate data while analyzing clinical data.

Chapter 11

Blockchain technology is paving its way from novel technology to leveraging its exclusive proficiencies. This technology refers to a platform that chronologically accounts and tracks the transactions and assets via distributed ledgers in a network. In today's scenario, the blockchain technology is gaining traction to completely revolutionize the healthcare services. This chapter discusses different competitive advantages offered by the healthcare sector on inclusion of blockchain technology in their strategic decisions and models. One of the key focus areas of the chapter includes market determinants impacting blockchain technology in the healthcare industry along with the market sizing and forecast analysis. Further, this chapter emphasizes how the blockchain concepts help in simplifying healthcare businesses amidst different challenges being faced by these industries in today's competitive scenario.

Foreword

Without an iota of doubt, it is doubly clear that the technological sector is booming across industry verticals. With the penetrative, persuasive and pervasive Internet, the world is deeply connected. Such an extreme connectivity has opened fresh opportunities and possibilities for innovators, individuals and institutions. However, in such an open environment, cybercriminals are becoming hyperactive to steal confidential, customer and corporate information to achieve financial gains. The cyber-attackers are not only behind money but also Access, Delete, or Extort users' sensitive data for fun. These range from DoS (Denial of Service), phishing to eavesdropping attacks. Blockchain is a technology being widely popularized to have the wherewithal to keep data safe from being corrupted or accidentally deleted. This technology has impacted on various industries such as finance, government, energy, healthcare.

Blockchain is widely leveraged in the healthcare industry. With blockchain technology, the healthcare sector can have data efficiency, data access flexibility, interconnection, transparency, and security. Some of the potential applications of blockchain in healthcare services are data security, Clinical Trials & Precision Medicine, Personalizing the Healthcare Services, Healthcare Data Management, Strengthening Public Health Surveillance, e-Healthcare to Customers, Healthcare Administration & Medicine Management, Telehealth & Telemedicine, Managing Medical Imaging, Developing Smart Healthcare System, and Healthcare Information System.

Another important feature of this book is about the deliberations in pharmaceutical industry. Blockchain also can bring efficiencies and real-time transactions in the pharmaceutical industry from the origin to distribution in the healthcare supply chain management.

This edited book titled *Prospects of Blockchain Technology for Accelerating Scientific Advancement in Healthcare* has 11 chapters contributed by renowned authors from various reputed Universities, Institutions and Research organizations. The chapters discuss issues, solutions and future scope in blockchain applications in healthcare industries. This book will be beneficial for Academia, Researcher and Practitioners of Healthcare and Blockchain technology,

Pethuru Raj
Reliance Jio Platforms Ltd., India

Preface

Blockchain is a technology that aims to keep data safe from being corrupted or accidentally deleted while maintaining its history. This technology has impact on various industries, but Healthcare industry is impacted significantly. Chapter 1 presents a systematic review of different use cases and applications of blockchain in healthcare. Chapter 2 presents an insight to the readers on the present and future research opportunities of blockchain in healthcare.

Chapter 3 is a systematic review of identification of possible research agendas for blockchain in healthcare. Chapter 4 presents a review of game theory models used to address common issues in the blockchain network. It includes different security issues (e.g., selfish mining, Denial of Service (DoS) attack, regarding mining management). Chapter 5 explains the aspects of Integration of Blockchain and supply chain management in Pharmaceutical Industries.

Chapter 6 introduces a blockchain-based infrastructure to support the traceability of medical products and implementation of unique device identification. A technical blockchain-based solution is conceptualized with regard to full and light node system in medical supply chains, Also, an outlook and further scientific and technical research possibilities are deliberated upon.

Chapter 7 first integrates blockchain technology for HER (Electronic Health Record) and then to enable safe storage of electronic data for users of the framework by setting access controls.

Chapter 8 describes the use of blockchain-enabled secure management and analysis of the healthcare system. Finally, the chapter reviews recent research challenges and solutions on blockchain-based electronic health record (EHR) systems.

In Chapter 9, supply chain is one of critical components of COVID-19 vaccination drive, a robust and efficient supply chain of vaccines would help increase speed and efficiency of vaccination therefore reducing vaccine wastage. This chapter proposes a blockchain-based approach to manage data linked to covid-19 Vaccines.

Chapter 10 explores the prospects of applications of blockchain technology in the 5000 years old Ancient Indian medical system called Ayurvedic science to improve the statistical reliability of clinical data by analyzing the data. Finally, Chapter 11 explores the advantages of inclusion of blockchain technology in strategic decisions making. The chapter also emphasizes on how the blockchain concepts helps in simplifying healthcare businesses, amidst different challenges being faced by these industries in today's competitive scenario.

This book can be a good reference book for researchers, academia, and practitioners.

Malaya Dutta Borah

Peng Zhang

Ganesh Chandra Deka

Acknowledgment

We, the Editorial team sincerely thank all the Chapter contributors, Reviewers and Friends for their wholehearted support.

Malaya Dutta Borah

Peng Zhang

Ganesh Chandra Deka

Chapter 1
Blockchain in Smart Healthcare Systems:
Hope or Despair?

Shilpa Mahajan
The NorthCap University, India

ABSTRACT

With the technological sector booming combined with the internet revolutionizing the 21st century, along with the current coronavirus pandemic, more and more hands are getting virtually connected. Today, cyber criminals are not only behind money but are also designed to access, delete, or extort a user's sensitive data. These attacks range from DoS (denial of service) attacks and phishing to eavesdropping attacks. Blockchain is a technology that aims to keep data safe from being corrupted or accidentally deleted while maintaining its history. This technology has an impact on various industries, but the healthcare industry is impacted significantly. This chapter presents a systematic review of different use cases and applications of blockchain in healthcare. This chapter further discusses issues, solutions, and the future scope in blockchain applications in healthcare industries. An idea is to give a complete state of the art and challenges to better understand its utility in the healthcare sector.

1. SMART HEALTHCARE AND ITS CHALLENGES

Smart Healthcare system make use of digital technology such as IOT, wearable devices, cloud services, internet, AI/ML to access information dynamically, connecting people and organisations related to healthcare. This allow fast sharing

DOI: 10.4018/978-1-7998-9606-7.ch001

of data, maintaining of patient history, standardization of data and quick service to the patient. There are certain challenges associated with smart healthcare systems.

Figure 1. Chain of Blocks of a Blockchain

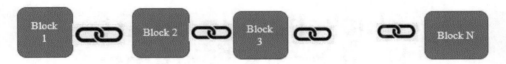

- Data Accuracy: The accuracy of data plays a significant role in deciding the quality and kind of treatment for the patient. The health provider will always refer to the data shared by the devices. If the data collected is inaccurate and unauthenticated, this will impact the treatment of the patient.
- Interoperability of data: Data stored using different data structures can result in storing data in varied formats. This will create a hindrance in data sharing among hospitals. Thus, standardization of data using standard data format will allow sharing of data among hospitals and easy for service providers to understand.
- Security of Data: The historical healthcare data should be preserved for malicious attack so that this data may not get altered or deleted. The patient records should remain intact so that right treatment can be given by health providers.
- Data Handling: The healthcare data should be stored, shared, managed and maintained properly so that this data may not get altered or lost.

2. BLOCKCHAIN BASICS

Blockchain is a decentralized method of storing data on to blocks. These blocks are linked with one another through a chain. The purpose is to overcome double record problem of a centralized systems. The records in blockchain are timestamped to keep them as a reference during disputes. This technique was developed for secure transmission of data, money, contracts without the involvement of third party. The data stored on a blockchain is difficult to change. It is a software based technology that require internet for running. It comprises of several parts like database, computers and application software.

Blocks are uniquely identified using a hash. A change in block results in creation of new hash. Each block contains data, hash and hash of previous block. This will not only link blocks together but will also ensure security since change in one block results in change in hash which makes the block invalid in a chain as shown in Figure 1.

2.1 Types of blockchain

There are different types of blockchains possible in the ecosystem.

Public

In a public blockchain any user can participate by creating a block, making any transaction in a block or by mining a block. Bitcoin is an examples of public blockchain.

Private

In a private blockchain, only selected member of an organisation can be a part of this type of blockchain. Hyperledger project is an examples of private blockchain.

Consortium

A consortium blockchain is said partially-decentralised or semi-decentralised which is controlled by a group of organisations. The member organisations can participate by running as a full node. R3 is an example of consortium blockchain

Consensus Algorithm

Blockchain is decentralized where all nodes are connected and share data with their peers. To maintain secure, reliable trust relationship among the nodes consensus algorithm is used. Using this algorithm, all peers reach to an common agreement with respect to present state of the ledger.

This algorithm aims to develop trust relationship among unknown peers and creates a reliable network. It also ensures that the new block added to the block is the one which was agreed upon by all nodes in the Blockchain. The objectives of this algorithm is giving equal rights to each node, ensure mandatory participation of nodes, a sense of commitment and collaboration among nodes.

Proof of Work (PoW)

PoW is consensus algorithm used in a blockchain that is used to confirm transaction and creates and add new block to the chain. Bitcoin is the first application that uses

Figure 2. Benefits of Using Smart Contracts

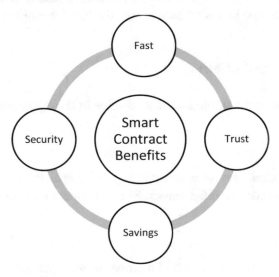

the concept of PoW. Bitcoin uses lot of cryptocurrencies. The block creation time in a bitcoin is approximately 10 mins. Another project that uses POW is Ethereum. The purpose of using PoW concept is to avoid attacks as lot of computations is required to create and execute block.

Smart contracts

Smart contracts are self-executing contracts that executed when some pre-determined conditions are met. These programs are stored in the blockchain. These contracts allows to build a trust relationship among parties without the involvement of any third party. The contract involves simple "If/When … then…" conditions that are written as code in a blockchain. This also enables fast transfer of crypto currency as per the conditions agreed by the parties.

List of attributes used by blockchain to build trust relationship among entities.

- Distributed: No central server is controlling the sharing of data. All nodes can view, share and update transaction in real time in a blockchain
- Secure: All transactions are encrypted using strong crypto algorithms. Users are authenticated and various permissions rights can be set on data.
- Transparent: All nodes have a copy of data with them. Any user can view and access transaction data without involvement of third party.

- Consensus based: All nodes must agree to make a transaction valid. This can be achieved using consensus algorithms.
- Flexible: Smart contracts can be utilized to apply certain conditions. This can be used to achieve standardization of Processes.

3. NEED OF BLOCKCHAIN IN SMART HEALTHCARE SYSTEMS

3.1 Counterfeit drugs

Counterfeit drugs are problem of national concern. As per WHO reports one out of 10 medical products in the market is a falsified product. It is really shocking to find that India is the largest producer of these falsified products, according to the outsourcing pharma report 2012. Medical practitioner sells these products to the innocent patients at cheap prizes. These drugs may contain original ingredients in wrong quantities, inferior ingredients, expired products or wrong ingredients. Counterfeit drugs are often confused with generic drugs which in turn act as an obstacle and affects the pharmaceutical market where generic products are sold and used (Williams,2014).

There are various factors like easy access to internet, illegal distribution of pharmaceutical drugs that has led to growth of Illegal drug market. It has become a challenging task for regulatory bodies to keep check on them. Expensive drugs used for the treatment of life-threatening diseases like cancer are counterfeit, alluring consumers to buy them at low priced. Also, patients that buy medicines from online sites are often fall prey to these falsified drugs. Thus, it is always advised to buy medicines from an authorized pharmacy. Thousands of people die every year after consuming these counterfeit drugs. Number of technologies have been developed to ensure that original drug should reach from the manufacture to the pharmacy. Consumers who wish to buy medicines online should ensure that they should buy drug only from a verified pharmaceutical site.

Blockchain is considered to be the technology that can break the chain of distribution of counterfeit drugs. It is a distributed ledger consist of blocks of transactions of data. The data is encrypted using specialized algorithms and is authenticated by others. It is a peer to peer model that is fast, transparent, secure and organized. Number of papers have been proposed on the usage of blockchain in healthcare sector.

A Hyperledger project was introduced in 2019 to limit drug counterfeit (Arsene,2019). Some of the big brands like CISCO, Block stream, Accenture are involved in this research-based project. This project aims to issue a timestamp on

Figure 3. Relationship of Blockchain and Supply Chain

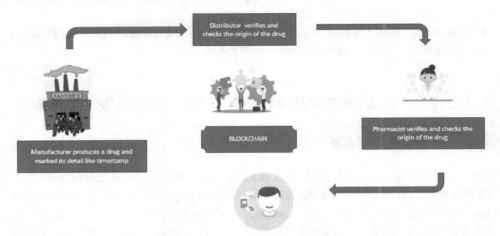

every manufactured drug. Thus, every drug is traceable with its manufacturing details [2].

In this paper [Sony,2020], author proposed a decentralized architecture with the shared ledger system. To avoid drug counterfeit, a model is proposed that will track the drug from its manufacturing, distribution until it reaches to the consumer.

3.2 Block Chain and Supply Chain

Blockchain is reliable in context each user can write as well as view transactions. All transitions a linked in a chain. Thus in supply chain, A manufacture can create a transaction by adding its detail, Timestamp and digital certificate (Edwin,2017). The details will be authenticated and then only added in a block. The details cannot be altered but can be updated based on consensus. This will make harder for the thieves to stole medicines as all details can be viewed and monitored by all parties.

Data collection plays a vital role in healthcare sector. Proper data maintenance ensures effective communication between patient and doctor, easy referral to lab reports and treatment history which will lead to health outcomes [5]. There are devices exist in the market that are used for the collection of patient data. Some of the methods used are discussed below.

3.3 Customer Relationship Manager (CRM)

A CRM healthcare system works by collecting Patient information from all aspects like clinic data, websites, social and behavioural reference. This will provide a holistic view of the patient habits. This data a be later used by doctors for studying the patient properly and provide him best possible treatment. This data can also be used by the hospital to identify their target consumers by initiating different market campaign for more projection.

3.4 Electronic Health Record (EHR)

Electronic Health Record (EHR) is an electronic way of storing patient details. This device will enable easy maintenance of patient medical history, its clinic transcripts, lab reports and medication List. The core Features functions of EHR are

- Minimizing medical errors
- Safe care
- Maintenance of patient record
- Decision support
- Reporting and Analysis
- Effective exchange and coordination

3.5 Wearable medical devices

Now days, number of wearable devices exist in the market in the form of smart watch, Fitness tracker, wearable camera etc. These devices contain embedded sensors which will keep track of activities of the bodies. These devices not only gather information but also transfer gathered information to health workers for monitoring of Plus rate, Oxygen level, temperature and other activities. Everyday tons of data got collected by these devices and transmitted to their server that can also be used by data analyst enthusiastic for research purposes. These data can further be used to find out the dependencies between collected data and diseases as shown in figure 4.

Healthcare industry task is not only to manage data but to organize and analyse data in order to obtain some useful information which can be used for treating patient illnesses. It is becoming a challenging task to manage large volume of data.

There are many reasons behind poor management of data. The transition from paper-based tracking to digitization is not easily acceptable. Even today, large volume of data has been left unattended which is not digitized thus not integrated in current Health Care Management System. This data includes not only medical prescriptions but also Lab reports, MRI Scans, images and videos. To convert this data into a single format becomes a challenging task. Also, the format of data required by the hospital may not be the desired format. The conversion of data leads to duplicacy and sometime discrepancy in data.

Figure 4. Data collection using wearable devices

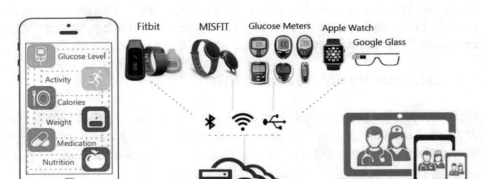

Medical data constantly keep on changing. Patient during the course of his treatment undergoes various test. With time, new test and scans came up which leads to creating of new type of data.

Every person has medical history. With time this data keeps on evolving. It becomes essential to maintain and manage this data. Mis organization of data leads to slow down of the treatment of the patient. Medical data also follows certain rules and regulations. Poor data quality makes it difficult to meet all regulatory requirements and thus to pass required audits.

Blockchain for managing healthcare data has numerous benefits in comparison to traditional data management techniques. Blockchain decentralization management concept gives different stake holders like hospital, patient, Doctors etc equal rights where they can collaborate independently. This technique do not allow data to be appended by any stake holder once uploaded, which results in preserving critical information. It also preserves reports from origin and saves them digitally in a chain like all history like patient clinical receipts, reports which can be later refereed by the doctor in treatment. All data in a blockchain are encrypted using some cryptographic algorithms. This increases security and privacy of data. Only the owner will have a private key to decrypt the data.

In (Michael J.,2017) Author defined one of the pilot projects of USA for storing Food and Drug data of Translational Sciences. Tis project uses Ethereum to manage data access using Virtual Private Network as shown in figure 5. This Project also uses strong cryptographic algorithms for securing data.

Amount of personal data collected through wearable devices can be stored efficiently by Blockchain service providers. These service provider uses numerous

Figure 5. Use of Ethereum for storing data

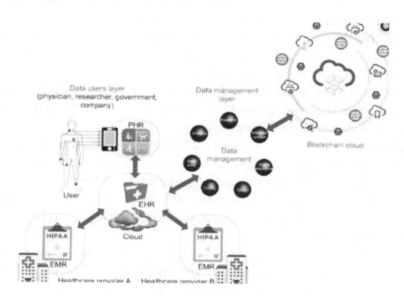

distributed applications that enable patient and health practioners to independently participate in telemedicine avoiding middleman as shown in figure 6.

Block not only offers more control of the patient to their own but also ensures data integrity by adopting distributed ledger methodology to promote privacy, security for stake holders. When any stake holder wants to make change in any data the said member is first authenticated through series of steps and the every must authorize

Figure 6. Use of Blockchain by Health practitioner for storing data

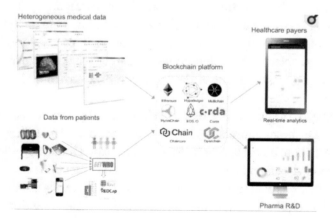

to confirm change in the data and then only the data can be amended. Conflicts can be resolved using timestamps of the requested edits.

Patients can receive automated alerts when any other wants to access or change individual heath record. Block chain offers patient single holistic view of their medical history giving full access control.

Providers can also collaborate with one another sharing patient records the patient no longer required to keep files which move back and forth for reference among different heath providers.

Medication reconciliation is another difficult task in managing patient data. Counselling two or more health practitioners for treatment results in taking same medicine more than once. This can result fatal for a patient. Block chain can be used to avoid such discrepancies. If one provider writes a prescription that is identical to the another. The flag cab be raised of duplication and thus prevent patient to take same medicine doubling it.

Maintaining patient records like name, Location, Insurance plans through his lifelong up to date is a challenging task. Mis identification of patient could results in wrong treatment due to lack of access of correct healthcare information. This issue can be taken by blockchain which maintain the ledger of patient record which is not append able and all patient history is maintained in a chain.

3.6 Data Privacy and Security

Large amount of health care data collected on day to day basis must be safe from data breaches. This patient data is kept confidential so that it cannot be stolen by hackers. With the emergence of new technologies, new apps are used for collecting user data using wearable sensors. Patient must be confident that his medical data is safe and apps are following privacy laws maintaining secrecy.

Advancement in technology promotes shifting to digital health records maintenance. This era brought a new revolution in healthcare industry (Dimitrov,2019). The volume data is converted to value data and is used by data analytics company for analysing .and obtaining some useful information. This revolution also invites various types of attacks on these data centres. Scarcity of skilled professionals, use of old technologies, vast amount of data and complex environment all make this data vulnerable.

In (Kupwade,2014) author discussed various security and privacy issues of big data life cycle. Different approaches have been discussed like Hiding a needle in a haystack 47, Attribute based encryption Access control, Homomorphic encryption, Storage path encryption and so on. to safe guard data from attack.

There are numerous data security issues faced by Health care sectors. The transition of paper records to digital has undoubtedly increase the efficiency and quality of record maintenance but it also increased the attack surface of these healthcare providers. Moving to electronic health care maintenance of system enhanced performance but it also increased attacks on these systems.

Many providers us outdated hardware which no longer support new sophisticated software. Since the medical equipment are costly and providers are little reluctant in spending money on these equipment. WannaCry ransomware was able to infect NHS and many other organisations because their system was not updated and contains older versions of Window.

The organisations were not aware about the data breaches that can infect systems and they are not prepared to handle these attacks. Lack of awareness leads to cyber-attacks. Small Healthcare related organisations do not have resources and skilled security professions to keep data safe from attacks. These organisations have limited resources to prevent cyber-attacks.

Healthcare providers maintain centralized data so that it can be used by any provider when required but this also makes data resilience to attack. Hackers attack this data through small providers who are more vulnerable to attacks due to lack or resources. Thus hacker attack big providers through these small organisations.

Health care data is considered to be very valuable as compared to normal financial data since credit card information can be used only once but health related data can be used multiple times for retrieving multiple information. The older information can be as valuable as after 20 years. Criminals are always after these types of information. Patients can also access medical data. The login credentials data may not be protected wisely by the patient so data breach can occur and easily targeted by cyber attackers.

Health care providers are required to make decision whether to spend money on trained staff and technologies or on staff training, hiring specialised IT security staff. Lack of knowledge and risk associated with large amount of data leads healthcare data vulnerable to attacks. In order to protect data, a user roles with privileges need to be defined so that every user has limited access to the data. All users cannot view and tamper confidential data (Abouelmehdi,2017). This will enable integrity of data.

Blockchain is a decentralized and trustworthy system as trust relationships among the blocks can be obtained using cryptography technologies and mathematical models. Blockchain can even overcome limitation of single point of failure. The patient records are recorded in the distributed ledger and all these blocks have backups and this data can be access anytime from anywhere (Shi, S.,2020). This makes system transparent and results in developing trust relationship among blocks.

There are number of properties of blockchain like decentralization, harder modification of blocks, incentive mechanisms of miners, easier record updating and audibility make it suitable option for healthcare systems

3.6 Secure data storage

Blockchain can be used for EHR based systems but there are privacy issues since blockchain is a public database and it has data risk to be exposed. Some measures like encryption of data using cryptographic algorithms, access control mechanisms or hashing techniques can be used for data privacy.

Number of techniques has been proposed by authors in different papers.

In author suggested an elliptic Curve Cryptography technique to encrypt data and send data through secure channel for a healthcare based model. In another paper (Al Omar, 2017) for bio metric application a unique public and private keys for data is provided which is collected using sensors.

In smartphone based App based on blockchain is proposed which uses MPC technique (Lee S.H.,2018). This App perform computations on encrypted data and the actual data is never revealed.

To avoid attacks on these systems, the encrypted keys need to be changed frequently. This involves lot of cost in terms of storage management of large number of keys. All the historical keys are required to be saved and managed since they can be used to decrypt historical data when required. This also involves lot of additional computation.

Various ways has been proposed to address this issues. One scheme for Body Sensor Network to preserve privacy of sensor data by using an efficient recovery key management scheme is suggested. This does not require storing of encrypted keys. A fuzzy value method is suggested for generation, backup and recovery of keys.

Another important aspect for a secure HER based system is kay management. The keys must not be shared at an cost. The loss of keys results in the loss of control of the user on a data. The attackers will have a control to manipulate the data. Thus both encryption of keys and its management should be considered while designing an efficient secure system. An access control mechanism for proper authentication and authorization of user should be done to check user identity.

3.7 Data sharing

Data sharing is an important component in healthcare industry as different resources like patient, Clinic, laboratory relies on these collected data. Data is shared among different organisations and it becomes very challenging due to its heterogeneity nature. Thus interoperability is required to standardized and maintain the quality of data. The three important aspects can be considered under this are:

Some compatible format must be designed for data collection.

Exchange of data should be done accurately considering different data structures. Organizations should work together for secure and timely communication of data

Interoperability is considered to be important as lack of standards can result in data sharing failure. As per the study (Yue X.,2016) countries have adopted different standards like European Committee for Standardisation (CEN) and Digital Imaging and Communications in Medicine (DICOM).

For a Successful EHR system interoperability of data among different organisation must be followed. There must be some standardization for data sharing among different healthcare providers.

Though data sharing is considered to be a serious approach for maintaining the quality of healthcare services but many hindrances still exist like malicious attack, leakage of data, lack of trust relation among competing organisations, unauthorized access of data and so on. Thus it become necessary to ensure privacy and security of data and proper access control mechanisms must be used so that only authorized entities are able to access secure information. Also building up of trust relationship among different organisation through collaborations must be encouraged.

Access Control List allows to give controlled access to entities by permitting and deny access by managing permissions on various conditions. Usage of access control mechanism with block chain ensures creation of trustworthy system. Smart contracts can also be used for controlling access to the users. Many existing work shows the use of smart contracts on secure health care systems. In Begoyan, 2007) author discussed the applicability of smart contact on a block chain which verifies the access conditions of the data requestor. If conditions are not met, the system can abort the session.

In 2019, author proposed an access protocol wherein mobile users request are checked against the defined policies (Nguyen,2019). The smart contract will verify user transactions to prevent any malicious attempt on the data. The policies of access control defines which entity is authorized to perform which operation on the data but there are other policies also which consider other parameters like attributes, purpose etc. An author in 2016 proposed purpose centric access control model which separates a raw data from statistical data (Peterson, 2016). This allow transactions to be processed with different strategies considering different purposes.

To ensure secure data sharing and reliable access control mechanism a cryptography technology can be used for enhancing security. A symmetric encryption key generation (Dubovitskaya,2017) framework is proposed in a paper where patient can generate key to encrypt/ decrypt data while sharing it with doctors. If the key gets compromised, a new key will be generated and shared with the patient. Only the patient can share key and set my smart contract for secure data sharing.

In 2018, (Ramani V.,2018) proposed a request based method in which only the patient is authorized to modify data. No one can modify the data without patient consent. A lightweight public key cryptographic operation is used to enhance the

Figure 7. Security can be achieved using smart contract with cryptography technology

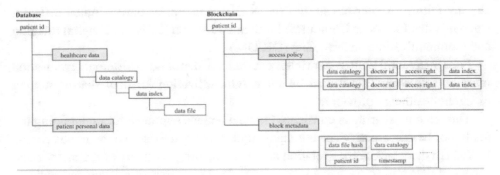

security of the system. Even no data can be written on the block without patient notification on to the blockchain.

As shown in figure 7, An amalgamation of access control mechanism using smart contract with cryptography technology on a data can achieve secure data sharing among different entities.

3.8 Data audit

Audit logs can serve as a proof if any dispute arises among entities. These logs can be used as a security mechanism to track events when some misuse access privileges or if someone back off and show dis honest behaviour. These logs can some important information like timestamp of the logged data, User ID of the requested user, Owner whose data is accessed, type of action and the result validity of the request.

In proposed a data sharing model that can track the dishonest behaviour of the user and can revoke access rights during any malicious activity (Qi X.,2017). A blockchain based system is proposed which manages all logs generates by different operations (Fernandez,2013). Smart contracts are used for creating, managing and auditing of logs. Audit logs provide an important aspect for detecting anomalies and malicious behaviour to improve the security of access control mechanisms. Thus, block chain plays a crucial role in auditing and accountability of data when any dispute occurs.

For maintaining complete patient data as audit log is expensive in terms of time and storage. The representation of audit logs is difficult to understand and interpret. Interoperability among different organisations for sharing of audit logs in standardized format is required.

3.9 Identity manager

User Authentication is the first step to grant any access rights to the user. Once user identity is verified, the specific rights are granted to the shared data. Various user authentication methods used are bio metric authentication, verification based on public key encryption and many others. In EHR system, Master Patient Index can act as a integrity indicator that can actually link user to its information. In blockchain, user private key can be used for transaction and public key can be used for user identification.

In (Omar, 2017) a registration based module is defined where any user that request for any information is required to register first and need to preserve its ID and log in details for accessing data through secured channel.

The main motive behind identity manager is to ensure that only authenticated user can access specified information but relying only on password based authentication can lead to various attacks. A man in middle attack can help attacker to intercept user account details and user account can be compromised and sensitive information may be stolen. Thus attention should be paid to use cryptographic algorithm for storing user details which can hide actual identity of the user and malicious attacks can be avoided.

4. BLOCKCHAIN CHALLENGES IN HEALTHCARE

Blockchain technology is a new and there are only few scenarios where the applicability is checked but there are certain blockchain models which are not checked yet. The generation of large amount of data comprises of medical records, documents, images and lab reports requires a significant amount of storage. This data grows with time and becomes difficult for a blockchain to accommodate this data. Blockchain also suffers from expensive computing and high bandwidth overhead makes it unsuitable for practical environment. Multiple organisations accessing data parallelly generating large volume of data, requesting frequent changes makes blockchain unstable. Few specific challenges are listed below

- There are no rules and policies developed to address the usage of blockchain in healthcare industry.
- The cost of creating and maintaining a healthcare blockchain is not known yet. These uncertainties can result in use of blockchain.
- Accommodation of healthcare records on blockchain requires lot of storage. How this storage need can be taken care by the blockchain with time.

- Access permissions, Ownership, access grants on a shared data on a blockchain is yet to be discovered.
- People are resistance to adopt to new technology like blockchain.
- There are certain issues related to the consensus algorithms. These algorithms lacks efficiency.
- Some times these technology takes lot of time to response due to some technical glitches.

5. CONCLUSION AND ITS FUTURE SCOPE

In this era of digitization, Block chain has a great potential in coming years. It can be used in various applications for maintaining security and efficient transmission of data. Though blockchain has a bright future ahead but still its impact on the healthcare industry is not much. This technology is still evolving, and its impact can be seen in the coming years on the healthcare industry. In this paper, the advantages of blockchain technology in the coming years and its full potential can be explored (Tapscott, 2019), with giant firms like Google, Amazon, and Facebook, which are ready to exploit the advantages of these upcoming technologies. Some of the achievements of the blockchain are discussed below. A recent survey was conducted by Deloitte Global (Deloitte, 2019) in 2019 that define that attitude of the business leaders are changing and they are developing interest in this technology. These leaders believe that this technology can serve as a solution to business problems across industries and use cases. A paradigm shift has occurred that enable blockchain to develop practical business solutions for mainstream applications. Blockchain guarantees trust, assures transparency and providing direct control to the user by removing intermediaries by maintaining extra security and privacy for transactions executed over the Internet. Along with these advantages, there are number of limitations discussed above like cost of its implementation, long response time, need for improvement of consensus algorithms and many more. This fact cannot be ignored that as the usage will increase, more improvements will occur, and this leads to advancement in technology on Internet. Such advancements will surely overcome the existing limitations of the blockchain. There are two aspects where the blockchain technology can be applied. The first will include all those applications that require decentralization and super secured networks like IoT (Zhang, 2019), AVs (Jenkinson's, 2018) and smart contracts. In future, to use such applications blockchain technology is a must. AI can be another area which when combined with blockchain can substantially improve its existence and value. These advances will lead to secure data as well as maintaining decentralization of the big giants who holds and owned by companies like Google and Facebook. This will give freedom to the individual to hold and control data in its own way and how much data to be shared and make available to the other parties. These two technologies can be combined to work in the area of cyber security wherein secure data transactions can be carried out and data can be protected from cyber-attacks to create a protection shield against cyberattacks by training machine learning algorithms to automate real-time threat detection and to learn continuously about the behaviour of attackers, while decentralized architecture can minimize the inherent vulnerability of centralized databases (Pollock, 2018). Highly sensitive and personal data can be used to determine patterns in sensitive cases involving the healthcare sector using blockchain's ability of storing data securely and through immutability. This technology can also be used to determine the nature of AI algorithm by tracking how output affected by changing input. Thus, AI can increase the efficiency of blockchain far better than humans. Bitcoin, viewed as blockchain's first innovative success (Huillet, 2019), can be utilized with AI applications which further leads to the popularity of both Bitcoin and AI, as well as their various applications. Various areas of amalgamation of Blockchain and AI remained unexplored which can lead to technological advancements in future. However, there is considerable potential that can raise their separate, as well as their combined, usefulness to new, high levels of value and applicability. Like any new technology there will be development and adoption fits and starts over time. But in the case of blockchain, there appears to be a concerted effort to move the technology forward. Other potential applications include informed consent management, clinical trial data management, insurance coverage, and claims adjudication. Over the next two five years we will likely see success stories that will prove that these early-stage investments were worth the effort.

In this paper, we have compared the conventional healthcare industry with smart healthcare system. This paper throws lights on how block chain can be helpful in storing data efficiently but also how data can be shared securely among various entities. Different use cases related to smart healthcare has been discussed. Block chain limitations are also discussed at the end.

REFERENCES

Abouelmehdi, K., Abderrahim, B., Khaloufi, H., & Saadi, M. (2017). Big data security and privacy in healthcare: A Review. *Procedia Computer Science, 113*, 73-80. . doi:10.1016/j.procs.2017.08.292

Al Omar, A., Rahman, M. S., Basu, A., & Kiyomoto, S. (2017). Mainchain: a blockchain based privacy preserving platform for healthcare data. In *International Conference on Security, Privacy and Anonymity in Computation, Communication and Storage* (pp. 534–543) Springer. 10.1007/978-3-319-72395-2_49

Arsene, C. (2019). *Hyperledger Project Explores Fighting Counterfeit Drugs with Blockchain.* Available online: https://healthcareweekly.com/blockchain-in-healthcare- guide/

Begoyan, A. (2007). *An overview of interoperability standards for electronic health records.* Society for Design and Process Science.

Casey & Wong. (2017). Global supply chains are about to get better, thanks to blockchain. *Harvard Business Review.* https://hbr.org/2017/03/global-supply-chains-are-about-to-get-better-thanks-to-blockchain

Deloitte. (2019). *Deloitte's 2019 Global Blockchain Survey: Blockchain Gets Down to Business.* https://www2.deloitte.com/content/dam/Deloitte/se/Documents/risk/DI_2019-global-blockchainsurvey.pdf

Dimitrov, D. V. (2019). Blockchain Applications for Healthcare Data Management. *Healthcare Informatics Research*, *25*(1), 51–56. doi:10.4258/hir.2019.25.1.51 PMID:30788182

Dubovitskaya, A., Xu, Z., Ryu, S., Schumacher, M., & Wang, F. (2017). Secure and trustable electronic medical records sharing using blockchain. *AMIA Annual Symposium Proceedings American Medical Informatics Association,* 650-659.

Fernandez-Alemán, J. L., Señor, I. C., Lozoya, P. Á. O., & Toval, A. (2013). Security and privacy in electronic health records: A systematic literature review. *Journal of Biomedical Informatics*, *246*(3), 541–562. doi:10.1016/j.jbi.2012.12.003 PMID:23305810

Huillet, M. (2019). China's State-Run Media: Bitcoin Is Blockchain's First Success. *Cointelegraph.* https://cointelegraph.com

Jenkinson, G. (2019) Can Blockchain Become an Integral Part of Autonomous Vehicles? *Cointelegraph. 2019.* https://cointelegraph.com/news/can-blockchain-become-an-integral-part-of-autonomous-vehicles

Lee, S. H., & Yang, C. S. (2018). Fingernail analysis management system using microscopy sensor and blockchain technology. *International Journal of Distributed Sensor Networks*, *14*(3), 1–13. doi:10.1177/1550147718767044

Lopez, E. (2017). *Big Pharma builds blockchain prototype to stop counterfeits.* Supply Chain Dive. https://www.supplychaindive.com/news/big-pharma-blockchain-experiment-returns/525689

Nguyen, D. C., Pathirana, P. N., Ding, M., & Seneviratne, A. (2019). A. Blockchain for secure hrs sharing of mobile cloud based e-health systems. *IEEE Access : Practical Innovations, Open Solutions*, 7, 66792–66806. doi:10.1109/ACCESS.2019.2917555

Patil, K. H., & Seshadri, R. (2014). Big Data Security and Privacy Issues in Healthcare. In Proceedings IEEE International Congress on Big Data (pp. 762-765). IEEE.

Peterson, K., Deeduvanu, R., Kanjamala, P., & Boles, K. (2016). A blockchain-based approach to health information exchange networks. *Proc. NIST Workshop Blockchain Healthcare.*

Pollock, D. (2018). The Fourth Industrial Revolution Built on Blockchain and Advanced with AI. *Forbes.* https://www.forbes.com/sites/darrynpollock/2018/11/30/the-fourth-industrial-revolutionbuilt-on-blockchain-and-advanced-with-ai/#7ce023c24242

Qi, X., Sifah, E. B., Asamoah, K. O., Gao, J., Du, X., & Guizani, M. (2017). Medshare: Trust-less medical data sharing among cloud service providers via blockchain. *IEEE Access : Practical Innovations, Open Solutions*, 5(99), 14757–14767.

Ramani, V., Kumar, T., Bracken, A., Liyanage, M., & Yliantila, M. (2018). Secure and efficient data accessibility in blockchain based healthcare systems. *IEEE Global Communications Conference*, 206–212. 10.1109/GLOCOM.2018.8647221

Sahoo, M., Samanta, S. & Sahoo, S. (2020). A Blockchain Based Model to Eliminate Drug Counterfeiting. In Machine Learning and Information Processing (pp. 213-224). Springer Publishing.

Shi, S., He, D., Li, L., Kumar, N., Khan, M. K., & Choo, K. R. (2020). Applications of blockchain in ensuring the security and privacy of electronic health record systems: A survey. *Computers & Security*, 97, 101–166. doi:10.1016/j.cose.2020.101966 PMID:32834254

Tapscott, D., & Vargas, R. V. (2019). Unleashing the Power of Blockchain in the Enterprise. *MIT Sloan Manag.* https://sloanreview.mit.edu/article/unleashing-the-power-of-blockchain-in-the-enterprise

Williams, L., & Mcknight, E. (2014). The Real impact of counterfeit Medicine. *U. S. Pharmacist*, 39(6), 44–46.

Yue, X., Wang, H., Jin, D., Li, M., & Jiang, W. (2016). Healthcare data gateways: Found healthcare intelligence on blockchain with novel privacy risk control. *Journal of Medical Systems*, *40*(10), 206–218. doi:10.100710916-016-0574-6 PMID:27565509

Zhang, L. (2019). Why Blockchain and IoT Are Perfect Partners. *DZone*. https://dzone.com/ articles/why-blockchain-and-iot-are-perfect-partners

KEY TERMS AND DEFINITIONS

Consensus: It an open decision agreed by group of people.

Contract: It is legal agreement between the two parties.

Cryptography: It is a process of hiding data using some encryption techniques.

Digitization: It is a process of sharing data such as image, audio, text using computers.

Ethereum: It is open source blockchain cryptocurrency exist today.

Healthcare: Management System: A system that manages healthcare data of patients and hospitals.

Hyperledger: It is an open source project focussed on developing tools and framework for blockchain community.

Privacy: It's a right to keep one's personal information hidden.

Security: It is state of being protected.

Wireless System: A radio channel used for transmitting data.

Chapter 2
Present and Future Prospects of Blockchain Technology in Healthcare

Muralidhar Kurni
(iD) https://orcid.org/0000-0002-3324-893X
GITAM University (Deemed), Hyderabad, India

Saritha K.
Sri Venkateswara Degree and P.G. College, Ananthapuramu, India

Mujeeb Shaik Mohammed
GITAM University (Deemed), Hyderabad, India

ABSTRACT

Many sectors, including finance, government, energy, health, and others, have found interest in blockchain technology over the last decade. It's no exaggeration to state that blockchain is pervasive in the healthcare industry. According to industry insiders, its application in healthcare has yet to achieve its full potential, but the implications might be substantial as it matures. This chapter presents the ongoing research trends, the existing issues and challenges, and presents future research opportunities to understand blockchain better. This chapter also throws light on the concepts of blockchain. This chapter also presents some examples of the uses of blockchain in healthcare. The authors hope that this chapter provides insight to the readers on the present and future research opportunities of blockchain in healthcare.

DOI: 10.4018/978-1-7998-9606-7.ch002

INTRODUCTION

Blockchain technology is ready to alter global healthcare quickly. The technology is predicted to have an annual compound rate of increase of 70 percent in healthcare over the next few years, due to increasing data breaches in the industry, according to a recent TechSci Research report (New Age TechSci Research Pvt Ltd, 2020).

For several reasons, Blockchain is essential to healthcare (IEEE, 2021):

1. Firstly, it enables the secure sharing of sensitive information without copying it and can eliminate healthcare records errors. The data is also timestamped, giving it more security. Blockchain is capable of securely streamlining health care payments. This eliminates the need to rely on costly equipment while cutting overhead costs dramatically.
2. Second, blockchain enables the worldwide sharing of research data between health professionals and researchers, providing them the opportunity to work together to resolve complicated medical problems and diseases.
3. Third, blockchain provides the capability for cryptocurrency research for scientists and health organizations. Regulations will be required to ensure fair trade worldwide, but this can contribute to access for all to healthcare.
4. Finally, blockchain will offer collaboration tools for individual health organizations, eliminating global health disparities during the fight against diseases.

This chapter examines how blockchain can transform our present infrastructure of healthcare. The industry includes several players (providers, patient payers, suppliers, research institutes, manufacturers, etc.) with varied roles and requirements. This chapter seeks to better understanding blockchain's scope and present future research guidelines for all healthcare players.

BASIC CONCEPTS OF BLOCKCHAIN

We examine in this section the key characteristics of blockchain technology to help comprehend the rest of the chapter.

Blockchain's Overview and Architecture

Blockchain is mainly an internet-level peer-to-peer network (Iansiti & Lakhani, 2017), launched in 2008 as part of a Bitcoin proposal (Nakamoto, 2008). The blockchain is a public leader consisting of a succession of blocks containing a complete history of transaction records in the network. A blockchain is a public ledger consisting of a chain of blocks in which all the transaction records are permanently stored. One block essentially consists of a body and a header. Every block's header contains the hash of the previous block. Thus, a linked list is created, where the last element is based on the block structure of the current element. A timestamp also exists in a block header that specifies when the block was created and a nonce that is typically set to an arbitrary value (which the miner would subsequently change to a specific Hash value). This nonce prevents double-spending by solving a mathematical puzzle.

Blockchain transactions are small units of work that have publicly specified characteristics. A majority of system participants agree that each transaction will be checked. This ensures that transactions are manipulated when packaged in the blockchain. All participants reproduce, host, and maintain the same ledger copy (Iansiti & Lakhani, 2017). Business logic can be encoded using intelligent contracts, a self-executing code for blockchain processing regardless of the blockchain type. Included in a blockchain, smart contracts are permanently resistant to manipulation, as nobody can modify what has been programmed, automatically verify itself and apply itself when the rules are fulfilled at any point. In the broadest sense, among the many key characteristics of blockchain, one may identify decentralization, immutability, the ability to reach all participants, censorship resistance, the availability of blockchain copies, and anonymity.

Blockchain systems taxonomy

Present blockchain systems are classified into four categories: public, private, consortium, and hybrid (Ray et al., 2020).

- *Public blockchains*: Decentralized networks are created by public blockchains where every member can read and contribute to the consensus process. (e.g., Bitcoin and Ethereum (Wood, 2014)).
- *Private blockchains*: Private blockchains are for individual solutions used to track data transactions between departments or people. The network requires the approval of each participant to be a known member once it's met.
- *Blockchain consortium*: A blockchain consortium is a privileged group with a permissible network and the public. This database keeps track of how participants interact and is therefore useful for audit and synchronization purposes.
- *Hybrid blockchains*: Hybrid blockchains integrate private and public blockchains. To make the book accessible to the public, a public blockchain is used, and a private blockchain in the background controls the access to the modifications.

BLOCKCHAIN IN HEALTHCARE

A large part of its Gross Domestic Product (GDP) in developing countries is spent on healthcare. But, with ineffective processes and violations of health data, hospital costs continue to increase. It is one area that can improve the problem with the blockchain. It can do a lot, from secure encryption to epidemic management (Thomas & Coveney, 2012).

Blockchains Are Building Blocks of Improved Healthcare

An improved health outcome requires one worldwide, a huge blockchain that effectively handles high volumes of data to serve as the sole source of information rather than multiple digital ledgers (Nguyen, 2021). Throughout 2020 and already in 2021, we had been inundated with medical headlines – endless pandemic analysis and response analysis, gaudy statistics punctuated with insight into what better could have been done – but little airtime was provided for the healthcare information infrastructure on which so many of us relied. The data systems and information technology that support it have largely failed to keep pace with all advances and innovations in the healthcare business.

Exceptionally fragmented are contemporary health information systems. While the number of personal health data is expanding, information remains, almost always, confined within silos, isolated and unavailable outside the bounds of closed and proprietary systems - from doctors to pharmacies, laboratories, and hospitals to even our mobile phones and smart devices. This is ineffective, but it restricts a healthcare provider's ability to manage the complete range of patient information in real-time to achieve the best health outcomes. Blockchain technology – and in particular – a single global blockchain offering a solution – is increasingly noticing the transformational potential of healthcare companies.

A single, global blockchain can provide the basis for a universal, worldwide electronic health record, ensuring that a safe digital environment is available to everyone in the healthcare provider's chain to store and manage patient information in a verifiable way (if authorized by the patient). An up-to-date, complete picture of patient health could be incorporated into each new information item so that doctors, pharmacists, and other providers could provide better counsel to patients. The same safeguards to prevent duplication of digital monetary expenditures may be used to avoid duplication of pharmaceutical prescriptions, while blockchain private keys could be utilized as a means of authenticating identification and validating insurance coverage. And with the blockchain, the use of its unique qualities enables us to iterate and create beyond the limits of existing systems.

While patient data are stored on the blockchain (with privacy protection) or off-chain (and managed through on-chain access rights), a blockchain-based electronic health record system will not only allow healthcare providers to get a holistic view of patient information and to deliver better health outcomes. It is probably unusual for many of us to have the year also brought a greater need to exercise control over our healthcare in a year in which physical language and population health figures have become regulars in our everyday (socially distant) conversation.

A blockchain-based recording system allows patients to retain complete control over their data and choose who and when to access their data. It might offer a physician-patient health provider permission, or it could cover commercial purposes, allowing a pharmaceutical company to have access to your data in exchange for micropayments of digital currency to perform clinical research. Controlling the patient would also facilitate moving between healthcare providers far more quickly than at present and ensure the completeness and accuracy of the information given – which could then be applied to various circumstances.

An initiative initiated by the founders of PDX, Inc., a 40-year-old U.S. medical data company with pharmaceutical software and technology solutions experience, is one of the leading companies for these visions (Nguyen, 2021). Using the Bitcoin S.V. blockchain, EHR Data is the first electronic health record globally to allow individuals to securely, control, and make money from their personal health information and provide greater real-time access to data for health care professionals and researchers. The Platform can assist several instances in which better health outcomes can be achieved, from monitoring narcotic drugs to Covid-19.

As the world's greatest public health campaign in human history starts with the Covid-19 immunization deployment, governments and health experts consider the impact of a blockchain recording system on running the initiative. A unified computerized record would ensure that the correct type and dosage are delivered at the right intervals irrespective of where each vaccine course was provided. Subsequently, this single, unchanging vaccination record might be used to validate admittance to public areas or transport for digital 'passports.'

The risk of blockchain technology impacting the health care sector goes beyond a purely patient-provider paradigm. Blockchain technologies help ensure that pharmaceutical products are honest and transparent, and often a long-lasting procedure that is subject to rigorous monitoring for the integrity of the data or 'hygiene.' If the data are not recorded properly, or worse, is purposefully manufactured or obscured, whole research together with possibly billions of dollars and years can be completely discredited. Blockchain technology facilitates convenient and auditable tracking of clinical research-generated data sets, benefiting governments with pharmaceutical approval tasks and improved patient health results.

Veridat is a new U.S. company that likewise uses Bitcoin S.V. blockchain as a platform for a system that delivers the pharmaceutical industry integrity and data hygiene (Nguyen, 2021). The field of clinical pharmaceutical research has long been subject to trust and transparency concerns, resulting in testing and large data generation that can considerably impact the prospects of corporations developing and patients receiving the ensuing medicinal products. Ensuring this data's integrity, validity, and confidence is extremely important to ensure that optimal health outcomes may be achieved as efficiently as possible. Veridat can communicate auditability and trust in the industry by using the blockchain to timely clinical research data. JuvaTech, a conduct neuroscience firm aiding researchers undertaking therapeutic composite testing and a leading pharmaceutical manufacturer, is already evaluating the Platform of Veridat.

A blockchain with a robust foundation to accommodate large data capacity is essential to achieve better health. Another requirement is a single global blockchain, which can grow large numbers of data efficiently handle to serve as the one source of information, rather than having several digital ledgers for the industry, so that everyone in all health services may at the same time access the same data.

This is a big goal for healthcare, and only with a blockchain that advances an equally large view can one be achieved.

Applications in healthcare

In five key areas, blockchains in healthcare can be envisaged (Thomas & Coveney, 2012):

- Electronic Medical Record Management (EMR)
- Health data protection
- Management of personal health records data
- Management of point-of-care genomics
- Management of data in electronic health records

The following are certain specific applications (Thomas & Coveney, 2012).

1. *Research*: Currently, electronic health records are only possible for an organization or network of organizations to automatically update and share medical information on a particular patient. This could be expanded if the information was arranged so that only PHI (Protected Health Information) or Personally Identifiable Information (PII) in the top layer of the blockchain was not available. That would enable researchers and other organizations to access this huge spectrum of data with hundreds of thousands of patients. The amount

of data available would dramatically increase the number of clinical studies, safety incidents, reports of adverse events, and public health announcements.

2. *Seamless switching between providers of patients*: The same blockchain information could enable patients to unlock their health data and exchange it easily with other organizations or providers via a shared private key. This could contribute to the interoperability and cooperation between various users in Health Information Technology (HIT).

3. *Faster, more affordable, better patient care*: Blockchain can build a single system for the safe and quick retrieval of authorized users for storing, continually updating health records. By preventing misunderstandings between different specialists participating in patient care, countless mistakes can be avoided, diagnoses and actions can be quicker, and each patient's care can be tailored.

4. *Interoperable Electronic Health Records*: As businesses increasingly want to increase the transparency of share data, blockchain technology might provide one layer of the transaction, where firms can use a secure system to submit share data by storing a specific set of standardized chain data, which contains a private chipboard link to separately stored information such as radiographic or other images. When applied to connection smoothness, the use of smart contracts and consistent approval protocols can have a dramatic impact.

5. *Data security*: Over 176 million infringements occurred in health records between 2009 and 2017. The safe features of the Blockchain are far more suited to protecting health information. Each person has a public identification or key and a secret key that can only be unlocked for the required time. In addition, the requirement to personally target each user to obtain sensitive information constrained hacking. Hacking, therefore, blockchains can provide an endless health information audit trail.

6. *Remote monitoring and mobile health apps*: Mobile applications with advanced technologies are becoming more and more relevant today. Within this context, the secure placement of EMRs (Electronic medical records) in the blockchain network allowed the transfer of medical data to healthcare providers, who can use it for home care and self-monitoring. However, the root vulnerability makes this a particularly vulnerable area for malware, and a hacker could obtain the patient's private key by exploiting the root vulnerability.

7. *Tracking and safeguarding health care*: Blockchain might make it possible to maintain complete transparency to guard against and identify pharmaceuticals' traceability. Not only can it keep track of money and energy used to produce these items, but it can also monitor labor expenses and carbon emissions as well.

8. *Health insurance claims*: The blockchain is unique in its ability to display medical events if they took place and is not likely to alter data for fraud purposes at a later point.
9. *Tracking disease and disease outbreaks*: The blockchain's unique features can help report ailments and explore disease patterns in real-time that can help to pinpoint the characteristics of its genesis and propagation.
10. *Protection of genomics*: Genomic data theft has become an essential challenge for several organizations delivering DNA sequencing to the individual. Blockchain can prevent and even offer an online market for researchers to buy genomic information. This could encourage safe sales and reduce costly intermediaries.

At this stage, there aren't that many healthcare applications using blockchain technology. Blockchain technology frameworks including Ethereum and Hyperledger Fabric are now being used on a limited scale. Blockchain services could improve the administration of healthcare data with increased security and mechanisms to promote synchronized transactions.

BLOCKCHAIN IN HEALTH 4.0

A shift to a completely automated environment using exponential technologies such as Artificial Intelligence (AI), Internet of Things (IoT), sensing networks, and concepts from blockchain is projected to be the next definite step towards the future (Mukherjee & Singh, 2020). Our way of living, working, and communicating with each other and technology is changing fundamentally; we are involved in the Fourth Industrial Revolution.

Industry 4.0, in addition to improved quality of life and sustainable outcomes, is a rising era of connection and interaction between parts, machines, and humans that can deliver massive production and efficiency dividends. The health sector is using technologies to digitize health records and automate numerous potential clinical processes. The field has undergone its development and is now available in Healthcare Version 3.0, the Web 3.0 extension, which incorporates increased transparency of personal health data to maximize its experience with the interface. To achieve the new age of health 4.0, the merger of the two revolutions could play a vital part in emerging blockchain technology. To transform health services, the need for interoperability in all clinics in the same hospital, the need for up-to-date records across multiple health care facilities, and the need for trustworthy and transparent documentation of individual health data need the use of blockchain concepts. In Health 4.0, the extent of Industry 4.0 is shown in Fig. 1.

Figure 1. Industry 4.0 healthcare extension
(Mukherjee & Singh, 2020)

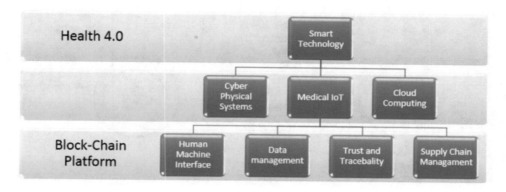

Health 4.0

A demographic and socio-economic shift has led to healthcare systems developing over the years across vast portions of the world. The field of medicine cannot be left behind by introducing fundamentally new strategies such as Industry 4.0. Health 4.0 is a strategic concept for the health field derived from the 4.0 movement of the industry (Alla et al., 2018). The concept aims at services virtualization, document decentralization, and personalization, leading to a global enhancement of services through technology for patients, professionals, and other stakeholders. Health 4.0 is geared to a full transformation of the medical business, driven by networked electronic healthcare record (EHR) systems, Artificial Intelligence (A.I.), wearable and corporate sensor network data, and better data analytics.

The recent change from conventional hospital architecture to Health 4.0 standard architecture can be seen in Fig. 2.

The traditional framework does not only serve the demands of the patient but encompasses them. The system is not patient-centered, in other words. The services are meant to serve the patient's needs and desires rather than incorporating the patient's role in the architecture. In the image, it can be seen that the Health 4.0 hospital standards differ from this type of construction. The customer of the service is the recipient and is at the center of the frame. This client also has other aspects, whose primary objective is to provide the patient with the finest medical experience. Health 4.0 aims to improve healthcare's predictivity and personality by coherently working together and converging participants and stakeholders.

Health 4.0, with its state-of-the-art concepts based on new and modernized technology, the patient-focused design opens doors for improved patient care and better health outcomes and offers significant stakeholder value.

Figure 2. Architecture transformation
(Mukherjee & Singh, 2020)

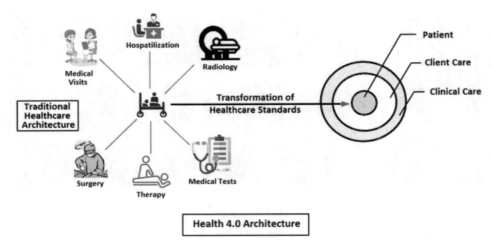

Why Health 4.0 Blockchain?

The necessity of data management is understood by Health 4.0 (Mukherjee & Singh, 2020). The movement knows that a patient-centered system and better user experience need consistent, safe, and effective storage and analysis techniques. The burden for preserving medical records and tracing planned inspections is lifted from the patient's shoulders by Health 4.0 standards and is instead digitized and safeguarded. In addition, if allowed by the patient, these data can be transmitted without hassles between providers.

It is no easy undertaking to perform this gigantic duty. Blockchain belongs to a class of databases by design and definition. The data saved in the decentralized blockchain ledger is called the transaction and takes 1 kB or less space. This material is restricted by a mechanism of access, which allows access to only the owner with private keys. The owner can move this data through the Inter-Planetary File System (IPFS) from one computer system to another. This transfer is rapid and secure and is preferable economically to a conventional centralized database.

Blockchain technology is utilized in medical record storage due to its range of capabilities, including file backup, error-free restoration, and data integrity. The data is disseminated around the network in a blockchain structure, significantly reducing the likelihood of failure, given that no single point of failure exists. In addition, each node copies one version of the data, which is most recently updated, which significantly reduces the volume of interactions across the information systems. These aspects collectively reduce the strain on the healthcare ecosystem, making it

Figure 3. Healthcare blockchain architecture
(Mukherjee & Singh, 2020)

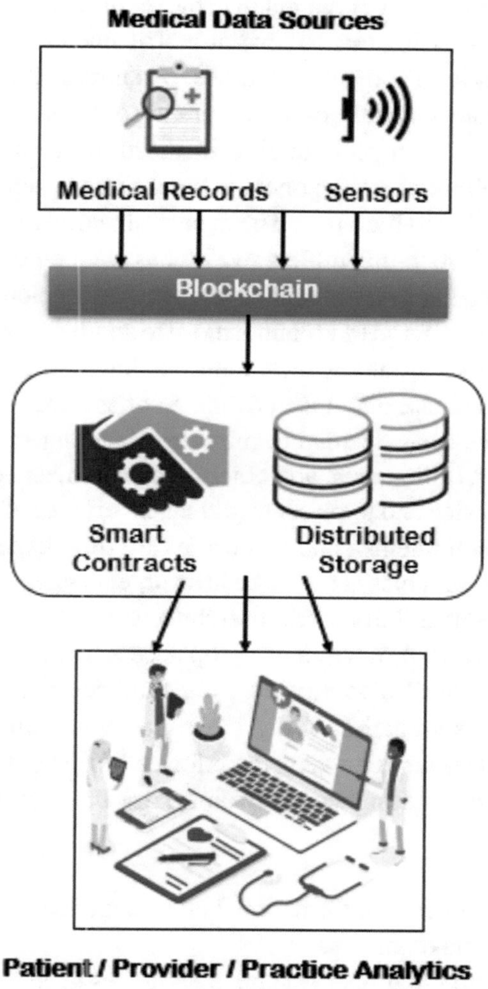

possible for service clientele to analyze data better and provide healthcare solutions. Fig. 3 shows how blockchain architecture can be used in the health sector.

This is a collection of principles of Industry 4.0 that comprise essential standards of health 4.0, which can be achieved using blockchain technology (Mukherjee & Singh, 2020).

1. *Data Management and Decentralization:* For Industry 4.0 applications, a distributed decentralized architecture is desirable when its calculation loads are middle- to high. Centralized servers are first and foremost costly, and the deployment

and correct maintenance of these structures continue to increase. Healthcare is a complicated system of interconnected businesses that operate within strict regulatory limits. Patients' data are widely fragmented in the traditional context, and healthcare provision costs are fast rising due to several inefficiencies within the system and reliance on third-party staff and intermediaries. If centralized solutions increase the already costly healthcare sector, the excessive pricing of medical services discourages prospective employees from participating in the movement. This decentralized design is the most spellbinding component of blockchain technology, typically cited to characterize the notion in literature. The decentralization of blockchain promises to reduce the supplier's lock-up problem, which has plagued the health business for millennia. When custodians rely on one cloud provider in cloud environments, the vendor lock-in problem emerges and cannot move to another provider simply without the high cost, legal issues, and/or technique incompatibility. A similar situation occurs when the patient can only take advantage of services in a particular health center. Once the patient has decided to migrate to another clinic, it is difficult to transmit prior records, billing data, and other information, and often legal concerns leading to delayed service and unpleasant patient experience. Crucial data are often inaccessible because middlemen and authorities are fragmented and authenticated on several levels, and valuables are secured in an urgent context. Health Information Exchange (HIE) introduces the blockchain architecture using a decentralized, trusted database. This framework provides a one-stop access method, via which all health care providers and medical practitioners are given access to a patient's complete medical history for examination. Only after the owner sanctioned an activity, participants and stakeholders can view the information. The blockchain concept of digital decentralization is designed to revolutionize the extension of Industry 4.0 in several ways.

- Real-time exchange of information between patients, healthcare workers, physicians, and stakeholders.
  - Collaboration and data exchange could result in steep learning curves and increased medical research by practitioners giving various drugs to individuals with comparable symptoms.
  - Decentralized apps (dApps) inter-link the shared network of hospital data systems, enabling information to be exchanged from one end to another. The patient data, which eliminates the vendor lock-in problem regarding medical treatment, is continuously updated and saved on the distributed ledger.
- Secured medical record storage.

In hospitals and clinics with discrete and independent core servers, cybercriminals and hackers are easy to achieve.

- Decentralized blockchain concepts offer a significantly more safe paradigm when compared to conventional recording systems for storing and distributing digital information. While a blockchain network is technologically advantageous, it introduces a whole new set of data protection challenges handled by carefully designing consensus mechanisms and cryptographic protocols in the nodes.
- In this regard, the main advantage of a decentralized design is exchanging information among various network nodes and the lack of a single failure point. The storage system is resilient and defect-tolerant, making the network challenging for hackers.
    ◦ Better management of the hospital.
- healthcareEasy access to patient data will keep everybody engaged in the medical practice well informed if permission is granted.
- Decentralized applications shall streamline communication amongst healthcare workers, professionals, and staff. This is a significant contributor to the consistency of day-to-day procedure and overall administration and improved insurance claims policies.
    ◦ Management of the Electronic Medical Record (EMR).

The modern Internet of Things (IoT) enabled wearable gadgets to gather relevant health information and update the database constantly while exchanging this data in real-time with doctors if allowed.

- Decentralized applications permit patients not to store the same data in a remote electronic health-medical record system held by doctors, clinicians, or non-partisan bodies but to gather, own, and manage their data. This technology supports patient-centered systems, giving the individual concerned ultimate ownership of sensitive medical information.
- The program could otherwise store access control specifiers determined by an individual instead of keeping patient data. The notion generates the same impact as the previous framework and saves the actual data in the remote EHR. The flexible design allows for a slow transition to health 4.0 standards to survive specific characteristics of traditional health care.

2. *Confidence and traceability*: The fundamental pillars of Industry 4.0 are precision analyzes of information and digital confidence. There may be considerable changes to corporate formats in the industrial revolution. The one area that firms

cannot afford to overlook is digital confidence with these tremendous changes in store. To work effectively, an integrated technology ecosystem requires that all parties trust data and communication security and have confidence in the digital framework and the intellectual property protection that safeguards the entire system. Protecting a business demands large investments and clear data integrity and security requirements while ensuring digital trust. Confidence and traceability are of prime importance in the healthcare industry. Data drive health institutions, and there is a considerable increase in the volume of data created during the age of wearable sensors and overall surveillance techniques. Ensuring the transmission and storage of sensitive information and worries about privacy discourages people from converting to health 4.0 medical standards. Violating the security of illegal users has damaged numerous institutions' reputations and has battered their assets considerably.

Various members play a variety of functions in the healthcare network. By these roles and significance, the health 4.0 system demands adequate access credentials. The blockchain principles might readily address these problems about trust and traceability. In reality, these are the network's two fundamental pledges, resolving generic trust problems at public, federal, and corporate levels. Extensive research has been carried out in cryptographing protocols and consensus mechanisms to construct a solid fail-safe system. Several assaults have been studied in the literature on blockchain networks. Attack strategies have various variations, ranging from using a hybrid machine learning algorithmic game theory approach to protecting against a Majority Attack with a Distributed Denial of Service Attack (DDoS). These measures have been mitigated by the use of a proven activity protocol. An eclipse attack occurs when most people are malicious at a node and do not connect to the main network. This exploit is aimed at obtaining sensitive information about interest transactions. The assault usually targets a particular user, and additional procedures to save confidential I.P. addresses in the network and utilize the specific intrusion detection techniques on the nodes are taken to counteract these malicious nodes.

The attacks of Sybil damage the network as a whole. The phenomenon is called Sybil Attack when one opponent controls several network nodes. In obtaining control over these nodes, the Internet stays unconscious about the operations of the opponent. Without attacking Sybil, thresholds are set to the block production capabilities within the Bitcoin network. Bitcoin's monetary supply is tied to the computation effort required to generate new blocks, thus constraining the total number of blocks that an adversary could produce. Several other systems, such as zero-knowledge evidence, may be used as well. The compatibility and privacy-resistant architecture of the supply chain systems, including healthcare and suppliers, ensure that distributed ledger technology is supported by sophisticated safety protocols that constitute a core component of key Industry 4.0 applications.

3. *Supply Chain Solutions*: Supply Chain Management (SCM) is designed to encompass the industry's best practices, from ordering products to supplying the items to simplify the entire delivery process. SCM is a tough and significant potential in the healthcare sector to ensure that the manufacture and tracking of medical distribution products are transparent. In traditional medical markets, the problem is that the scattered ordering methodology provides fragmented information on mass orders of surgical equipment, medications, and vital supplies. The compromise in the supply chain process could directly affect the health and safety of patients. The adequate framework design must be taken extremely carefully. The illegal sale of counterfeit pharmaceuticals lies in this area recently. Accordingly, over 100,000 deaths in Africa have to do with unsuitable doses of fake medicines obtained from unknown vendors, according to the World Health Organization (WHO) survey.

The first adopted by Congress in 2013, the Drug Quality and Safety Act (DQSA), defines the measures to develop an interoperable electronic medicines system to identify and track certain prescription drugs sold in the U.S. The FDA's capabilities to safeguard consumers from exposure to falsified, stolen, tainted, or otherwise dangerous medicines are projected to be improved by this approach. This method also provides rapid detection and removal from the supply chain networks in the States of potentially harmful pharmaceuticals. The blockchain ensures the authenticity of the drug supply chain security law prescriptions through its trustworthy and traceable architecture and transparency of its transactions. As well as counterfeiting of product and drug products, the absence of a trustworthy database and packing errors could disrupt the entire supply chain network and cost the treatment center heavy-duty. Blockchain can monitor the whole process, tap into any transaction and transport the goods throughout the chain.

Whenever the item changes hands, the transaction is recorded and replicated to each node on the public ledger. Without a single fault, the systemic approach simplifies the drug origin, seller credentials, and distributor identification to be verified. With an increase in knowledge of supply chain activity and essential authentication measures, pharmaceuticals and healthcare providers may ensure that authentic medicines flow without fail from source to destination. In addition, blockchain technology promises considerable improvements in other SCM areas, such as demand forecasting, data sources, protection of fraud and transactions.

NEAR-FUTURE HEALTHCARE BLOCKCHAIN PREDICTIONS

Blockchain in Healthcare Today (BHTY) has reached out to health professionals to show how the blockchain can benefit the healthcare industry. Based on their answers, presented in detail below, ten important topics (Table1) will emerge in the following years for the future of blockchain in health care (Halamka et al., 2020).

ISSUES AND CHALLENGES / LIMITATIONS

According to a new research company report (https://www.technologynetworks.com), ten main challenges blockchain must overcome to be implemented in health care, medical technology, and biopharmaceutical industries (IEEE, 2021).

1. Data standardization
2. Management of change and innovation implementation
3. Blockchain interoperability
4. I.P. & Blockchain patents
5. Protected health information (PHI) data security
6. permissive/non-permissive blockchains scalability
7. Regulatory bodies on-boarding
8. Smart Contracts deployment
9. Operating costs
10. Service providers of Blockchain

EXAMPLES OF USES OF BLOCKCHAIN IN HEALTHCARE

Blockchain has a wide variety of healthcare applications and uses. The ledger technology promotes the safe transmission and management of the supply chain for medical records and supports unlocking genetic codes for medical researchers. The following examples of Blockchain are thought-provoking (Daley, 2021).

PATIENT DATA SECURING

The most popular blockchain healthcare use at present is maintaining our essential medical information safe and secure. This is no surprise. In the healthcare sector, security is a huge problem. Over 176 million records of patients were present in data violations between 2009 and 2017. Credit card and bank information can be stolen by perpetrators, including health and genetic details.

The potential of Blockchain to maintain an immutable, decentralized, and transparent ledger of patient data makes it a security application rife with technology. In addition to being public, Blockchain conceals everyone's identity with private

Table 1. Ten key topics for Blockchain's near-term healthcare future

S. No.	Theme	Description
1	About healthcare consent management, the distributed ledger (i.e., blockchain) will play an important role.	Firstly, consent is now stored in electronic medical records for individual providers, hospital medical departments, and fax machines in heaps of paper. For each surgery or visit, consent shall be obtained. Consent for each provider is local and not at the patient level for all care sites throughout their lives. Many startups undertake a fundamental reform of the consent process — patient permission to trade data/privacy preferences and blockchain treatment for all parties involved to access consents from one location and respect patient requests. This technique reduces the administrative burden and improves the experience of patient care.
2	Non-cash assets will be tokenized, including health outcomes.	In addition, while the cryptocurrency component of blockchain has been there from the beginning, a token can represent anything—a building, an object, or a product. Tokens help to manage health outcomes or consequences. A new startup, Proof of Impact, has begun to measure results for patients and offers NGOs the chance to 'complete' results. For example, patients treated effectively for a condition could be marketed. The foundation might pay for outcomes documented in the Blockchain instead of only offering grants.
3	Micropayments transfer to blockchain more and more.	Thirdly, medical practitioners are rewarded for wellness, not the amount of treatment they provide, in a world of value-added purchases. Many startups concentrate on wellness applications that encourage 'doing the right thing.' A universal payment interface is easy to use to provide patients with micropayments when meeting goals/outcomes. Similarly, a blockchain universal pay interface might facilitate tracking payrolls and the litany of staff share of the medical expense.
4	Providers are listed on the chain.	Fourthly, up-to-date maintenance of healthcare provider directories in health plans is essential and challenging for healthcare organizations. The Synaptic Health Alliance's initial project attempts to streamline this procedure by providing demographic information on a blockchain that is permitted access and maintenance for Alliance members.
5	Improving the blockchain infrastructure reduces power needs and enhances speed and scalability.	Proof-of-work approaches use fifth, Ireland's annual power output. Building confidence via alternative ways will retain trust but lower the computing footprint dramatically. Transactional speeds rise as a service increases the simplicity of use and Blockchain (Using a platform that hides the complexity of Blockchain behind a set of cloud-hosted functions with simple APIs, all users need to know is how to use the buttons on the screen.).
6	The integrity of the supply chain is tracked.	Sixthly, when you purchase medicine in a local pharmacy, the legitimacy of the lot numbers and the compound pureness could not be monitored. The integrity of products would be ensured by a blockchain approach to the supply chain.
7	Stakeholder education will refine the use cases and speed up adoption.	Seventh, we don't know who posts blockchain transactions. The Blockchain is used for numerous purposes, such as consent, credentials, data integrity guarantees, supply chain management, and micropayments. There are additional reasons as well. Blockchain is gaining popularity among staking parties as they learn about its advantages and disadvantages. As a result, high-value instances are becoming more widely adopted.
8	Chances to monetize the data, including the genome using Blockchain, will be boosted.	Eight, many entrepreneurs realize the new "oil" is the data. The retailing of data without complete disclosure and approval has proven difficult – look only at the issues faced by Facebook. What if a marketplace for data enables data collectors to get compensated for their data every time they make use – for some public good such as clinical trials, clinical research, and people's health? Patients can engage with wide-open eyes in this marketplace and share any gains achieved from their anonymized data. For example, Nebula Genomics is researching this idea of collecting genomic data more swiftly to develop tools for precision medicine. Or, Dustin Hoffman might be told to monetize information rather than plastics for those who recall viewing The Graduate in 1967.
9	Blockchain will play a critical role in maintaining the integrity of medical records.	Ninth, the claims of malpractice occur. Good health outcomes are not always present, and someone is always held responsible. Lawyers who demand documents from previous generations frequently claim the records are falsified or doctored to omit evidence of medical malpractice. The lawyers contend that the tracks of the audit have been changed (which is impossible). To confirm that records have not been modified, we provide audit trails. To secure the integrity of the medical record, the burden for physicians, I.T. departments, and attorneys would be minimized if distributed ledger technology with an unbreakable trust were utilized. The records are not saved in the chain themselves, simply a hash (every document contains a one-way mathematical transformation that is unique.). If a record is established today and its hash matches the blockchain, every stakeholder may be assured of never changing the record.
10	An increasing number of healthcare startup organizations already utilizing the blockchain will be acquired. Blockchain in healthcare solutions will be substantially consolidated.	Finally, the marketplace of blockchain enterprises is larger, and more PowerPoint presentations than products are available. Because of the lack of a business model, many of these starters are gone. If not, promising firms like Change Healthcare with Pokitdok (and its Dokchain) will be bought and consolidated;

and secure codes that preserve sensitive medical data. Because of the decentralized nature of the system, doctors, patients, and medical professionals can share their personal and confidential medical information quickly and securely.

See how Blockchain is being applied to health security in the four companies listed in Table 2.

Medical Recourse May Be Used for Blockchain and Costly Mistakes

The health care sector costs $11 billion every year for the miscommunication of medical experts. It takes a lot of time and effort to gain access to a patient's medical record, which means that healthcare professionals waste time and delay the patient's treatment. Medical records based on Blockchain provide a remedy for certain diseases.

The decentralized structure of this technology produces one ecosystem of patient data that doctors, hospitals, pharmacists, and anybody else involved in care can rapidly and efficiently reference. This can lead to quicker diagnoses and customized care schedules.

The four companies listed in Table 3 embrace the concept of blockchain health records to produce shared databases and individual health plans.

Medical Aid for Managing and Drug Traceability/Sophistication

How much are we truly aware of our medicine? Can we be sure that it wasn't manipulated? Is it from a lawful supplier? The main problems of the medical supply chain or the link between laboratories and the market are these questions.

Blockchain has severe consequences for managing the pharmaceutical supply chain, and its decentralization ensures practically complete transparency in the shipping process. Once a medication leaflet is made, it marks the source (i.e., a laboratory). Each step along the route, including who handled it and where it has been before reaching the consumer, will be recorded by the ledger. The procedure can also monitor labor costs and emissions of garbage.

The companies listed in Table 4 are rethinking the medical supply chain using Blockchain.

Genomic breakthroughs

Genomics, long a dream, is a scientific and financial reality to help improve the future of human health. The processing of a human genome cost $1 billion in 2001. The cost is now about $1.000, and companies like 23andMe and Ancestry.com provide DNA tests to millions of households that unveil insights into our health and past.

Table 2. List of companies that apply blockchain for health security

S. No	Company Name	What they do	Blockchain application
1	BURSTIQ	BurstIQ's Platform supports the safe management of huge amounts of patient information by healthcare firms. Its blockchain technology allows for data protection, sale, share, or licensing while maintaining rigorous compliance with HIPAA requirements.	The company employs Blockchain to facilitate the sharing and utilization of medical data.
2	FACTOM	Factom provides tools that securely let the healthcare sector keep digital records n the enterprise Blockchain network, accessible solely to healthcare administrators and hospitals. Special data protection chips can be fitted with physical papers containing patient information and preserved as private data only to authorized individuals.	Factom uses blockchain technology to store digital health records securely.
3	MEDICALCHAIN	Medicalchain's Blockchain keeps health records integrity and establishes a single truth point. Doctors, hospitals, and labs may all seek information from patients recorded initially, protecting the patient's identity from outside sources.	Medicalchain's blockchain keeps a record of the patient's origin and safeguards their identity.
4	GUARDTIME	Guardtime helps healthcare companies, governments, and their cybersecurity systems implement blockchains. In assisting to integrate Blockchain in Estonia's healthcare systems, the company recently struck an agreement to bring Blockchain to its data protection systems with a private healthcare provider in the United Arab Emirates.	Guardtime uses Blockchain, including for healthcare applications.

Blockchain is an ideal fit for this booming business because it can safely contain billions of genetic information. An open marketplace where coded data can be bought and sold so that scientists can obtain more essential data than ever before.

The three companies listed in Table 5 use blockchain to comprehend the most basic building blocks better.

Table 3. List of companies that embrace the concept of blockchain health records for the productions of shared databases and individual health plans

S. No	Company Name	What they do	Blockchain application
1	SIMPLYVITAL HEALTH	SimplyVital Health provides the healthcare industry with its decentralized technology. The Health Platform in Nexus is an open-source database that includes healthcare providers with access to relevant information on the Blockchain of a patient. Since open access to critical medical information enables health care professionals to coordinate their efforts better, it benefits health care organizations more than traditional techniques to do so.	To provide an open-source database, SimplyVital employs Blockchain to allow healthcare practitioners to access and coordinate patient information.
2	CORAL HEALTH RESEARCH & DISCOVERY	Blockchain is used in Coral Health to improve the quality of care, make it faster, and cut administrative costs. Information stored in a distributed ledger connects scientists, doctors, lab technicians, and public health authorities faster than before. To maintain accurate and up-to-date records, SCoral Health uses smart contracts between patients and healthcare providers.	Coral's blockchain technology speeds up care, automates management processes, and uses intelligent patient-doctor contracts.
3	ROBOMED	Robomed blends A.I. and Blockchain to provide patients with a single treatment point. To collect patient information, the startup uses wearable diagnostic technologies, chatbots, and telemedicine. Patients can participate in smart contracts on the Panacea platform, Robomeds, which gives them motivation and advice to strive for better health care.	Robomed leverages Blockchain to securely collect and distribute patient information with healthcare professionals of a patient.
4	PATIENTORY	End-to-end encryption of Patientory ensures the safe and efficient sharing of patient information. The Company Platform allows access, store, and transfer all relevant information using Blockchain by patients, health care providers, and professionals. The patient care business is assisted by patient information being housed more swiftly under a single roof.	The blockchain architecture of the Patientory offers secure medical storage and transmission.

Table 4. List of companies that are rethinking the medical supply chain using Blockchain

S. No	Company Name	What they do	Blockchain application
1	CHRONICLED	Chronicled constructs blockchain networks that show the chain of guardianship. The networks are designed to help pharmaceutical businesses efficiently arrive and enable law enforcement to check suspect activities, such as drug trafficking. In 2017, Chronicled established the Mediledger Project, a leading medical supply chain security, privacy, and efficiency technology.	The Chronicle'd blockchain Network is deployed to guarantee the safe arrival and thorough evaluation of pharmaceutical shipments.
2	BLOCKPHARMA	Blockpharma offers a traceability and counterfeiting solution to medicines. The company's application scans the supply chain and checks all transport items so that patients can know if they are using counterfeit drugs. Blockpharma is weeding 15 percent of all fraudulent pharmaceuticals worldwide using a blockchain-based SCM system.	The blockchain system of the company can assist prevent the use of falsified drugs in patients via its app.
3	TIERION	To maintain a clean record of possessions, the Blockchain Tierion audits documents, records, and medicines. The medical supply chain stores evidence of ownership with timestamps and credentials.	It retains a documented history of possession inside medical supply networks via Blockchain.
4	CENTERS FOR DISEASE CONTROL AND PREVENTION (CDC)	To monitor diseases in a supply chain way, the Disease Control and Preventing Centers look at blockchain. Blockchain's timestamps, health reporting by individuals, and data processing skills may help report disease outbreaks in real-time. By investigating the trail of reported outbreaks, scientists can determine the genesis of a condition develop models to prevent disease. The CDC may potentially track the drug problem via blockchain.	The CDC monitors and reports epidemics via blockchains in real-time.

THE CURRENT AND FUTURE RESEARCH DIRECTIONS OF BLOCKCHAIN TECHNOLOGY IN HEALTH CARE

In recent years, the literature on blockchain-controlled applications has increased tremendously. The authors (Rejeb et al., 2021) of a series of bibliometric analyzes on

Table 5. List of companies that are using blockchain to comprehend the most basic building blocks better

S. No	Company Name	What they do	Blockchain application
1	NEBULA GENOMICS	Nebula Genomics uses distributed ledger technology to remove wasteful expenditure and intermediaries for genetic research. Biotech and pharmaceutical businesses spend billions of dollars every year purchasing third-party genetic data. Nebula Genomics cuts out the middlemen and encourages individuals to safely sell their coded genetic data, creating a massive genetic database.	They are using blockchain to make genetic studies simpler and to lower their costs.
2	ENCRYPGEN	The EncrypGen Gene-Chain blockchain-supported network for genetic information searches, shares, stores, and buys and sells. The company safeguards the privacy of its customers by making it possible for them to buy genetic information using traceable DNA tokens that are only offered to members. To expand on genetic knowledge and advance the industry, Member companies can use genetic information.	The company's blockchain platform facilitates the search, sharing, store, and acquisition of genetic information.
3	DOC.AI	Doc.ai employs intelligence machinery such as A.I. to decentralize blockchain medicine. To make their medical and genomic data accessible to a scientific community, users can provide this information on its platform for predictive modeling. No patient data is saved by doc.ai. After uploading, encrypting, and testing data on a blockchain, the data is wiped entirely to protect safety and privacy.	This company relies on machine learning to decentralize medical data on the blockchain. (as does A.I.).

the literature, which includes scholarly production, developmental patterns of total annual authors, and the identifying of productive academic institutions, countries, and leading authors, were carried out in (Rejeb et al., 2021). In addition, a keyword analysis was carried out, and essential research hotspots and trends indicated for the future were found. The research findings are helpful for researchers seeking to understand better developmental status, dynamics, and trends in health care related to BCTs.

Current Research in Blockchain Healthcare

A bibliometric analysis of current blockchain healthcare studies was carried out in (Rejeb et al., 2021). The primary purpose of this study was for the bibliometric analysis of 626 studies to review blockchain healthcare research.

The study results show that research in the field of blockchain healthcare in recent years has significantly risen. There is a quick increase in the number of researchers working in health research in the blockchain. It was also found that the prominent blockchain health research journals, including IEEE Access, Sensors, Electronics, and several medical publications, such as the Medical Internet Research Journal and the Medical Systems Journal, have been published from 2016 through 2020. The University of Electronic Science and Technology in China is the most prolific university in this field for leading institutions. There are also extensive research cooperation networks across several institutions.

International collaboration in research is valuable to generate new ideas for new projects, Leino-Kilpi et al. (Leino-kilpi et al., 2003) have pointed out. We urge collaboration between writers from various academic institutions to be encouraged by introducing joint research projects and integrating academics from underdeveloped nations to improve this relevant topic further. Collaboration contributes to varied abilities and scientific thinking, giving developed and newly developed countries access to scientific information and technology (Kim, 2006). We also encourage institutional collaborative efforts to support the overall strength of research and make more effective use of resources.

China and the USA provided the most significant contribution in academic blockchain healthcare from the standpoint of national contributions. This, of course, concerns solely English-language publications. It was also found a large number of Indian and English publications. The leading articles draw significant attention to scientific research and contribute to developing the blockchain paradigm in the healthcare sector. Collaborative research arrangements and links have generally been created throughout nations over a period of time to illustrate the quick expansion of blockchain health research into many related disciplines.

With regard to the knowledge base, the study (Rejeb et al., 2021) has identified the excellence of blockchain health research, researchers, and core content in recent years. These researchers contributed substantially to the conceptual development of blockchain medical care, touched upon numerous medical difficulties, and demonstrated the efficiency and effectiveness of blockchain's activities.

GOALS FOR FUTURE RESEARCH

Blockchain technology has emerged as a primary invention, with significant economic and social ramifications, notably in healthcare. It represents a whole new method to safe, efficient, and scalable management of healthcare information. Blockchain's ability will optimize medical processes, strengthen the control of the patients with medical data and finally improve the total health services outcome. The technology is promisingly available from efficient handling of health care data to prevent data protection breaches, increase interoperability, improve medical treatment delivery and traceability, and enhance the control of the pharmaceutical supply chain and any IoT device used. The technology offers a wide range of possibilities. However, the benefits of blockchain technology also present many challenges and barriers to be addressed before the technology is implemented on a large scale. For example, blockchain's technical problems are limited scalability, security threats, high energy consumption and non-authorized networks in public (Ismail et al., 2019; Monrat et al., 2019), increasing complexity (Kumar et al., 2020; Li et al., 2018), and data redundancy (Ismail et al., 2019), safety threats, and the need for a more flexible system. Due to an increase in the number of transactions and message transfers, there is an increase in the amount of scalability as the number of nodes and miners on the network increases. (Ismail et al., 2019). Thus, it is necessary to introduce more scalable blockchains and investigate them. In the future, the scalability parameters of blockchain medical systems, such as the pace of block propagation, consensus process, the throughput of transactions, and dimensions of blocks employed, may be examined.

While blockchain technology assists in ensuring the safety of the patient's medical data, blockchain systems are not immune from cyber threats. For example, public blockchain networks make patient information open to confidentiality incursion since linked data can reveal owners and their data (Radanović & Likić, 2018). It is possible to lose control of all of your saved data if you lose your private key. This means efforts are necessary to protect data storage, decrease privacy breaches and avoid assaults. Blockchain-based health systems need better security and usability.

Similarly, it should not be overlooked to adopt more energized and scalable blockchain systems. Hitherto has been substantial criticism about public and unauthorized blockchain networks about their demanding energy nature, excessive electricity usage, and computer resources (Hasselgren et al., 2020). Research should be aimed at boosting blockchain's efficiency in handling large-scale latency health data sets. Blockchain-based health systems should be built to simplify medical information retrieval and record maintenance. Many parties in the health industry are unwilling to host blockchain (Stafford & Treiblmaier, 2020). Physicians are reluctant to adopt technology, and health services providers are not prepared to share data because health regulations ban such sharing even anonymously (Zhang et al., 2018). In addition, blockchain adoption also means substantial investment in additional skills and resources, such as training, development of human resources and I.T. infrastructure, and adaptability in a new modus operandi. The absence of a legal framework for electronic health data interoperability and unclear legal responsibility for medical mistakes and privacy violations; Regulators should extensively explore this problem to use blockchain implementations to improve patient services and sustainable health systems for mobile pharmaceuticals. Research into how regulators and legislators can translate existing legal duties into the blockchain system is vital if legal language consistency is guaranteed and ambiguity is removed when law rules and codes are rewritten. Patients may also be discouraged and take advantage of the perks of participating in a blockchain healthcare system. Future research should concentrate in this respect on examining blockchain's patient acceptability, the expectations of users, and their satisfaction drivers. Faced with these issues, the design of blockchain patient-centered systems will also aid practitioners.

CONCLUSION

Providers, patients, and research organizations. Both in the field of computing and healthcare, blockchain technology is relatively new. In the healthcare subsectors, this technology has significant potentials to solve key problems with its properties and characteristics. The whole ecology can be revolutionized by technology. Full attention on its initial trip requires additional research, but intensive research must be done on health and pharmaceutical supply chains. Blockchain technology is also seen with a few issues while future research requires a solution. In our opinion, the content discussed in this chapter could lead to improved work in this field.

REFERENCES

Alla, S., Soltanisehat, L., Tatar, U., & Keskin, O. (2018). Blockchain technology in electronic healthcare systems. *IISE Annual Conference and Expo 2018, May*, 901–906.

Daley, S. (2021). *How using blockchain in healthcare is reviving the industry's capabilities*. Builtin. https://builtin.com/blockchain/blockchain-healthcare-applications-companies

Halamka, J. D., Alterovitz, G., Buchanan, W. J., Cenaj, T., Clauson, K. A., Dhillon, V., Hudson, F. D., Mokhtari, M., Porto, D. A., Rutschman, A., & Ngo, A. L. (2020). *Top 10 Blockchain Predictions for the (Near) Future of Healthcare*. Blockchain in Healthcare Today. doi:10.30953/bhty.v2.106

Hasselgren, A., Kralevska, K., Gligoroski, D., Pedersen, S. A., & Faxvaag, A. (2020). Blockchain in healthcare and health sciences—A scoping review. International Journal of Medical Informatics, 134. doi:10.1016/j.ijmedinf.2019.104040

Iansiti, M., & Lakhani, K. R. (2017). The Truth About Blockchain. *Harvard Business Review*. https://hbr.org/2017/01/the-truth-about-blockchain

IEEE. (2021). *How Blockchain Can Transform Healthcare*. IEEE. https://innovationatwork.ieee.org/how-blockchain-can-transform-healthcare/

Ismail, L., Materwala, H., & Zeadally, S. (2019). Lightweight Blockchain for Healthcare. *IEEE Access: Practical Innovations, Open Solutions, 7*, 149935–149951. doi:10.1109/ACCESS.2019.2947613

Kim, K.-W. (2006). Measuring international research collaborationof peripheral countries: Taking the contextinto consideration. *Scientometrics, 66*(2), 231–240. doi:10.100711192-006-0017-0

Kumar, A., Liu, R., & Shan, Z. (2020). Is Blockchain a Silver Bullet for Supply Chain Management? Technical Challenges and Research Opportunities. *Decision Sciences, 51*(1), 8–37. doi:10.1111/deci.12396

Leino-kilpi, H., Välimäki, M., Dassen, T., Gasull, M., Lemonidou, C., Schopp, A., Scott, P. A., Arndt, M., & Kaljonen, A. (2003). *Perceptions of Autonomy, Privacy and Informed Consent in The Care of Elderly People in Five European Countries: Comparison and Implications for The Future*. Academic Press.

Li, H., Zhu, L., Shen, M., Gao, F., Tao, X., & Liu, S. (2018). Blockchain-Based Data Preservation System for Medical Data. Journal of Medical Systems, 42(8). doi:10.100710916-018-0997-3

Monrat, A. A., Schelén, O., & Andersson, K. (2019). A survey of blockchain from the perspectives of applications, challenges, and opportunities. *IEEE Access: Practical Innovations, Open Solutions, 7*, 117134–117151. doi:10.1109/ACCESS.2019.2936094

Mukherjee, P., & Singh, D. (2020). The Opportunities of Blockchain in Health 4.0. In Blockchain Technology for Industry 4.0 (pp. 149–164). Springer. doi:10.1007/978-981-15-1137-0_8

Nakamoto, S. (2008). Bitcoin: A Peer-to-Peer Electronic Cash System. *SSRN Electronic Journal*. doi:10.2139/ssrn.3440802

New Age TechSci Research Pvt Ltd. (2020). *Blockchain in Healthcare Market to Grow at Staggering 70% CAGR until 2027*. New Age TechSci Research Pvt Ltd. https://www.einnews.com/pr_news/510619051/blockchain-in-healthcare-market-to-grow-at-staggering-70-cagr-until-2027-techsci-research

Nguyen, J. (2021). *Blockchains are the building blocks of better healthcare*. MedCity News. https://medcitynews.com/2021/03/blockchains-are-the-building-blocks-of-better-healthcare/?rf=1

Radanović, I., & Likić, R. (2018). Opportunities for Use of Blockchain Technology in Medicine. Applied Health Economics and Health Policy, 16(5), 583–590. doi:10.100740258-018-0412-8

Ray, P. P., Dash, D., Salah, K., & Kumar, N. (2020). Blockchain for IoT-Based Healthcare: Background, Consensus, Platforms, and Use Cases. *IEEE Systems Journal*, 15(1), 85–94. doi:10.1109/JSYST.2020.2963840

Rejeb, A., Treiblmaier, H., Rejeb, K., & Zailani, S. (2021). Blockchain research in healthcare: A bibliometric review and current research trends. *Journal of Data. Information & Management*, 3(2), 109–124. doi:10.100742488-021-00046-2

Stafford, T. F., & Treiblmaier, H. (2020). Characteristics of a Blockchain Ecosystem for Secure and Sharable Electronic Medical Records. *IEEE Transactions on Engineering Management*, 67(4), 1340–1362. doi:10.1109/TEM.2020.2973095

Thomas, L., & Coveney, S. (2012). *Blockchain Applications in Healthcare*. News Medical. https://www.news-medical.net/health/Blockchain-Applications-in-Healthcare.aspx

Wood, G. (2014). Ethereum: A Secure Decentralised Generalised Transaction Ledger. *Ethereum Project Yellow Paper*, 1–32.

Zhang, P., Schmidt, D. C., White, J., & Lenz, G. (2018). Blockchain Technology Use Cases in Healthcare. In *Advances in Computers* (1st ed., Vol. 111, pp. 1–41). Elsevier Inc. doi:10.1016/bs.adcom.2018.03.006

Chapter 3

Innovations in the Healthcare Industry Using Blockchain Technology:
Concept, Application Areas, and Research Agendas

P. S. Aithal

iD https://orcid.org/0000-0002-4691-8736
Srinivas University, Mangalore, India

Edwin Dias
Srinivas Institute of Medical Sciences and Research Centre, India

ABSTRACT

With blockchain technology, the healthcare sector can have data efficiency, data access flexibility, interconnection, transparency, and security. This chapter reviews the development of blockchain technology usage, current implementation challenges of blockchain technology, and includes references for the applications of blockchain technology in healthcare. A systematic review of current status, desired status called ideal status, and the research gap of use of blockchain technology in application areas of the healthcare industry are included along with identification of possible research agendas for future research.

DOI: 10.4018/978-1-7998-9606-7.ch003

1. INTRODUCTION

The twelve underlying emerging technologies of Information Communication and Computation Technology (ICCT) including blockchain technology are considered as general-purpose technologies of the 21st century (Aithal & Aithal, 2019b). A general-purpose technology or GPT is a technology that has potential applications in multiple industries with the new methods of producing, serving, and inventing opportunities with a protracted aggregate impact. Electricity and information technology (IT) probably are the two most important GPTs until the 20th century. A GPT can be a product, a process, technology or an organisational system. Whole eras of technical progress and growth appear to be driven by a few 'General Purpose Technologies' (GPT's), such as the steam engine, the electric motor, and semiconductors. GPT's are characterized by pervasiveness to many industry sectors, inherent potential for technical improvements, and innovation complementarities to many applications, giving rise to increasing scale of operation. Economist Richard Lipsey and Kenneth Carlaw (Lipsey et al., 2005) suggested that there have only been 24 technologies in history that have been identified as true GPTs. They define a transforming GPT follows four criteria which are listed below (Aithal & Aithal, 2018): (1) GPT is a single, recognizable generic technology. (2) Initially, GPT has much scope for improvement but comes to be widely used across the economy. (3) GPT has many different uses in many areas to solve problems or to provide comfortability. (4) GPT creates many spill-over effects to spread its base to many sectors. General purpose technologies have the potential to reshape the economy of the world and boost productivity across all sectors and industries. Such transformations are far more than simple technical innovation, or a new discovery. However, such technologies often require a wholesale remaking of infrastructure environments, of business models, and of cultural norms. There are three fundamental features of GPTs that differentiate them from other technologies which are (1) Pervasiveness – The GPT should spread to most sectors. (2) Improvement – The GPT should get better over time and, hence, should keep lowering the costs of its users. (3) Innovation spawning – The GPT should support to invent and produce new products or processes. Blockchain technology possess each of these characteristics to some degree, and considered as a potential tool for innovations in multiple industry sectors including primary industry sector, secondary industry sector, tertiary industry sector, and quaternary industry sector (Aithal & Madhushree, 2019b) (Aithal & Madhushree, 2019a).

Blockchain is one of the undeniably clever innovations under general purpose universal technology called Information Communication and Computation Technology (ICCT) (Aithal & Aithal, 2019b). Blockchain has been implemented over a decade. Like any blockchain digital technology, recognition experiments were carried out in various industries before successful use. Each block stores the transaction information, each block is saved with a single code called "hash". A blockchain-based system is a publicly shared digital block system (i.e., a decentralized one) in which all participant blocks are distributed geographically and linked across different network types. Blockchain networks can be segregated and permitted into two key styles as permissioned & permissionless Open-ended systems like Bitcoin and Ethereum are permissionless. They are open to the public. Any node will carry out transactions and also engage in a phase of consensus to advance the blockchain. Permissioned registered Networks, such as Hyperledger Fabric and Multichain, are aimed at consortia where limited options exist. Even though customers are permitted to request transactions, the blockchain's development is restricted to a defined community of peering nodes run by consortium members. Indian healthcare system has been one of the rapidly growing sectors with the goal of reaching more people every year.

It is a technology for record creation across many computers or digital devices of a process or an activity which cannot be altered retroactively, without altering its subsequent processes or activities. Blockchain technology allows a system to own digital goods, assets, and data and capable to trace the history of everything which is created as a footprint in the past transactions. Thus, an ideal blockchain technology is expected to have the capability to trace the history of everything which created a footprint in the past. In simple words, blockchain technology can be used in each financial transaction and is digitally signed to ensure its authenticity and not allowed to tamper it, so that a ledger created with the existing transactions within it are assumed to be of high integrity. It is expected that blockchain technology is expected to help total stoppage of financial frauds and hence contributing to eradicate corruptions in this world. Blockchain technology has applications in financial transactions, healthcare systems, education, supply chain systems, etc.

Block chain-based framework lets users to script transactions & contracts to enable transactions that go beyond money. Here the required verification resource would be ledger depending on the script size specified by the user (Luu et al., 2015). Chaum's work on the decentralized essence of the payment system enables the blockchain to inaugurate a new age beyond global payments (Wright & De Filippi, 2015). Blockchain can indeed be called a public ledger, as well as all agreed transactions is stored in a blocklist. The chains grow as it continually adds new links. Asymmetric encryption and distributed consensus algorithms were implemented for the user security and accuracy of a ledger. Usually, the blockchain has core characteristics of decentralization, longevity, accountability, and auditability. With these devices, Blockchain can significantly save on costs and increase efficiency (Yaga et al., 2019). Since it enables payment to be done without any bank or intermediary, blockchain can be used in various financial services, such as digital assets, transactions, and electronic payments (Peters et al., 2015), (Foroglou & Tsilidou, 2015). Blockchain is the decentralized transaction mechanism for Bitcoin, built to distribute and pass money for holders of the Bitcoin currency. This technique would support the public ledger for all ever-executed Bitcoin transactions, with no third-party entity control, the advantage of Blockchain is that after all nodes have approved the data, the public database cannot be modified or withdrawn. Blockchain is now well known for its data privacy and security features. Blockchain technology can also be applied to other applications. It has built an ecosystem within a cloud service for digital contracts and peer-to-peer data sharing (Gordon & Catalini, 2018). BCT acts as a digital exchange for healthcare while allowing patents to retain excessive control over their information, exposure to medical data and promote the transition to patients. (Reyes, 2016). In some medical systems, smart contracts could be used, like payment & insurance, that allows automate the process and reduce costs.

Blockchain technology offers several direct and indirect benefits of using in healthcare ecosystem which include (Tripathi et al., 2020):

(1) Distributed and Secured Storage of patient's medical and clinical Data.
(2) Enable Patient Centric System.
(3) Transparency in Audit Trials.
(4) Holistic Quality Management and tracking of facilities and services.
(5) Secured and Transparent Supply Chain Management.
(6) Trusted and Immutable Control and Management System.
(7) Promotes patient mediated communication, information sharing and exchange.
(8) Data is encrypted using immutable blocks forming a chain like structure.
(9) Remove central node dependency (everyone shares equal rights and privileges).
(10) Better engagement of patients in every aspect from diagnosis to treatment and cure.

In this paper, based on a systematic review, we have identified current status, desired status called ideal status and the research gap of use of blockchain technology in various application areas of healthcare industry including Healthcare Security & Authentication aspects, Clinical Trials & Precision Medicine, Personalizing the Healthcare Services, Healthcare Data Management, Strengthening Public Health Surveillance, e-Healthcare to Customers, Healthcare Administration & Medicine Management, Telehealth & Telemedicine, Managing Medical Imaging, Developing Smart Healthcare System, and Healthcare Information System along with identification of various possible research agendas for future research.

2. OBJECTIVES

This study is limited to the discussion on possible innovations in healthcare sector services using blockchain technology. The main objectives are:

(1) To learn blockchain technology as distributed ledger tool and its potential capabilities across industries,
(2) To find out the current status and potential usage of blockchain technology in the healthcareindustry sector through a systematic review,
(3) To predict the possible innovations in the healthcare sector using blockchain technology,
(4) To identify the opportunities and challenges of blockchain technology in various areas of healthcare service and stages of its implementation.
(5) To develop and analyse various research agendas by identifying the research gap on the use of blockchain technology in the healthcare industry.

3. METHODOLOGY

The study is descriptive and exploratory in nature. The related information is collected from various secondary sources for review. The secondary sources include published literature from various scholarly journals searched through Google scholar by means of identified keywords. The related research works published in these journal articles are summarised to know the current status of using blockchain technology.

4. BLOCKCHAIN AS DISRUPTION TECHNOLOGY IN HEALTHCARE

Blockchain, though introduced in 2008, a revolutionizing technology is widely known after the introduction of a Bitcoin network in 2009. With such an, incredibly transparent ledger system developed for Bitcoin and operating on the blockchain is therefore no longer just associated with cryptocurrencies, but the technology that is permanent, open, and stable makes it more relevant to various industries. Satoshi Nakamoto released the Bitcoin White Paper in 2008; 2009 saw the first Bitcoin block created. Because the Bitcoin protocol is open source, anybody can take the protocol, fork it (modify the code), and create their own P2P money version. BC is a shared ledger or system of records. This can also be referred to as blocks in a chain where, prior to them, the respective blocks apply to the blocks. If the specifics of the transactions or events are fed into the Blockchain, it is impossible to modify the data being exchanged with the network members. Blockchain network users are fully aware of the occurring transactions. For example, consider, book-based data structure where every page of the book corresponds to a paragraph of the previous edition. Here, the ledger refers to the Database, page refers to the ledger and the database transaction refers to an entry in either document. Whether a page or block has been tampered with or not is easy to detect. Pages can be organized in any way so pages in a distributed ledger aren't relevant. Currently, each block is constructed on top of the preceding block in Blockchain and it uses the nonce and signature of the latter as a key to go into the next block. Network miners do the job of constructing a block and connecting the block to the chain. A random string or nonce is easy for the miners to guess to tamper with the block just by knowing the signature in a Public Blockchain. Adding blocks in the Blockchain isn't easy and there is a 12.5 bitcoins incentive for that. The miners are granted a contract in a private blockchain, and as a result, they can connect to the chain on blocks. It can therefore also be described as a consensus-oriented public / private distributed ledger that stored data across a peer-to-peer network (Chatterjee & Chatterjee, 2017).

Blockchain is temper-clear and temper-protecting ledgers implemented in a distributed mode that involves how well it operates through ledgers for full transactional background with a protected feature and distributed between numerous parties with various categories of blockchain i.e., permissionless and permissions that seem complicated but when examined it seems easy to use hash functions (Yaga et al., 2019). The framework with traditional consensus algorithms used in various private public and consortium blockchains continues to pose some technological challenges such as scalability, privacy leakage and selfish mining (Gordon & Catalini, 2018). Main concept of blockchain is a distributed database with transactions and records most work is based on network efficiency protection and creative applications basic problems in blockchain techniques are generally not appropriate for the Internet of Things (IoT) due to limited computing capacity are very limited powered (Reyes, 2016). Blockchain is a platform for decentralized network storage applications. Blockchain, however, not only is used for financial applications. But you could also build a transaction to fit in with our application. Blockchain. Yes. Trust and traceability are the two basic blockchain promises obtained from the box that solves the problem of generic trust at all levels of the public, federated, and organization. These features, however, aren't always enough to have a complete solution, and that is why we always see blockchain combined with strong cryptographic protocols such as zero-knowledge proofs (Bhuvana & Aithal, 2020a; Bhuvana & Aithal, 2020b; Bhuvana et al., 2020a; Bhuvana et al., 2020b; Gade & Aithal, 2020; Katuwal et al., 2018; Rangi & Aithal, 2020; Sai Manoj & Aithal, 2020).

Blockchain technology uses various techniques which are listed below (Bhuvana et al., 2020a):

Table 1. Typical consensus algorithm comparison (Bhuvana et al., 2020a)

Property	PoW	PoS	PBFT	DPoS	PoET	Ripple
Blockchain type	permissionlees	open	permissioned	open	open	open
Transaction finality	probabilistic	probabilistic	probabilistic	probabilistic	probabilistic	probabilistic
Transaction rate	Low	High	High	High	Medium	High
Token needed	Yes	Yes	No	Yes	No	Yes
Cost of participation	Yes	Yes	No	Yes	No	Yes
Scalability of peer network	Yes	Yes	Low / High	Yes	Yes	Yes
Trust model	Untrusted	Untrusted	Semi- trusted	Untrusted	Untrusted	Untrusted
Adversary	< = 25%	< 51%	< 33.3%	<51%	Unknown	<20%
Example	Bitcoin	Peercoin	Hyperledger fabric	Bitshares	Hyperledger fabric	Ripple

4.1 Consensus Mechanism

Consensus is a method for validation in time for the completion, modification, or development of requests, transactions (deployment and invoking) and details. Proper ordering is important because ownership and additional rights and obligations can be established. On the blockchain network, there really is no centralized hub or authority that determines the transaction order, recognizes transactions, and defines rules about how nodes communicate. Alternatively, a network consensus protocol is implemented with multiple validating 'parent' nodes, and all nodes have the knowledge available – restricted to their authorization. The documents are also transparent and trackable. In addition to the various forms and approval protocols proposed so far, the agreement guarantees that the node quorum agrees on the exact order of new records to the shared ledger (Aste et al., 2017).

4.2 Decentralized Ledger System

Referring explicitly to a distributed network technology that allows users to upload programs and abandon programs to self-execute, maintains a persistent and transparent record with current and past system states, uses public key cryptography, and uses economic incentives to ensure that the network retains technology. Therefore, the Decentralised ledger system is broad enough to cover the blockchain underpinning the application for bitcoin payments, which is currently receiving incredible attention, but is not so narrow as to exclude other forms of the technology or other practical applications other than payments (Reyes, 2016).

4.3 Decentralized Data Mining

Data mining helps to automatically discover new information that is useful in describing or predicting unknown phenomenon from vast quantities of data. Decentralized data mining is especially suitable for applications which usually handle very large quantities of data (e.g. transaction data, science simulation and telecom data) that cannot be analysed in a reasonable period using a conventional paradigm. (Wu et al., 2013).

4.4 Decentralized Data Storage

Security breaches have occurred since the internet was introduced and organizations have managed to cope with them, but it is worth noting that new technology may help repair parts like decentralized storage system that can store files without having to react to massive centralized data collections and do not compromise important values such as privacy and freedom of information (Do & Ng, 2017).

4.5 Encryption Algorithm

An algorithm is a collection of instructions which produce a result or an output. It can be a simple script, or it can be a complex program. The algorithm in the blockchain verifies signatures, confirms balances, decides if a block is legitimate, specifies how a block is validated by miners, defines the protocol for telling a block to pass. Establishes the process for generating new coins, and informs the system how consensus algorithms can be decided to tell the miners how to validate a block. They set conditions, as do protocols, but the instructions are central, and there is a desired outcome: processing transactions, deciding the blocks join the chain and reaching consensus on which chain is correct.

4.6 Smart Contracts

Smart contracts are a form of digital electronic contract wherein the terms of the transaction are encoded into computer code to be performed automatically by the software upon receipt of a specific input. Smart contracts are, in their simplest form, a set of digital commitments, including protocols in which the parties fulfil certain promises (Deshpande et al., 2017). Smart contracts are programs which execute on blockchains autonomously. The primary intended uses (e.g. financial instruments) allow data from outside the blockchain (e.g. stock quotes) to be accessed. This will make trustworthy data feeds that serve a wide range of data requests important for smart contract ecosystems (Zhang et al., 2016).

Table 2. Blockchain and Distributed technology terms (Bhuvana et al., 2020a)

S. No	Term	Description
1	**DApp (decentralized applications)**	System device that stores network-wide data (Swan, 2015)
2	**Blockchain**	A form of DLT where blocks of data are added sequentially & linked together with respective hash values (Francisco & Swanson, 2018)
3	**Transparent**	The ledger share of the decentralized network can be seen by everyone in the node (Wang et al., 2019)
4	**Miner**	Transaction verifier (MacKenzie, 2019)
5	**Nonce**	A random value used once to ensure the correct hash value is set during blockchain mining (Wang, Hoang, Xiong et al, 2018)
6	**Consensus**	A system used for the transaction verification (Luu et al., 2016)
7	**Smart contracts**	Programme or scripts are written on Ethereum blockchain that execute if a given set of specific requirements are met & that require no governing body to ensure their 'payouts' are met properly (Biais et al., 2019)
8	**Forks**	The issue ascends when a node is used for different blockchain versions (Wang, Duan, & Zhu, 2018)
9	**Hash**	One-way hash function to test transaction/message integrity (Lin & Liao, 2017)
10	**Node**	The blockchain ledger (Di Pierro, 2017)
11	**Timestamp**	Date and time of the transaction in the computer system used as electronic timestamp (Maull et al., 2017)

4.7 Blockchain as Distributed Ledger Technology

A technology that can be easily understood to be a database that exists through several locations or amongst several participants is achieved by (remunerated) consensus by the network of users rather than having to rely on confidence in a third party intermediary users may 'deposit' digital assets (e.g. documents, actions, and statements) on the ledger (Johnston et al., 2014).

5. RELATED WORKS ON CURRENT USAGE IN VARIOUS RELATED AREAS

Blockchain has the potential to preserve an incorruptible, open, immutable database of all data that includes an individual's private and concealing identity with complex and protected codes that can protect the security of medical data. The collaborative design of the system also helps patients, physicians, and healthcare professionals to easily and safely share the same information (Pajooh et al., 2021). The following section reviews some of the specific applications of blockchain technology in healthcare sector.

5.1 Blockchain in Security & Authentication Aspects

Blockchain can be used for securing the health documents of all stages for a long period and any kind of intrusion or modification without the consent of people or departments involved are not possible. In blockchain based ledger storage models used in the healthcare sectors, a decentralized network of nodes is usually created using cryptographic processes computed by all members involved in various sections based on consensus mechanisms, digital signatures, and hash chains and hence it has highly reliable storage capabilities and provides numerous service qualities including traceability, integrity, security, and non-repudiation. These documents are usually stored in a public decentralized but in a privacy-preserving manner. A medical record can be both patient files and medical data related to the collection and usage of various resources during and after treatment in hospitals that are retrieved from various departments, patient body sensors and other automated applications. As medical records are now stored in digital formats, it requires additional security and role-based privileges to protect health information in the form of healthcare records security that includes access controls, authentication, nonreproduction of records by ensuring information and document integrity, confidentiality, and availability in the right time for authenticated users. Table 3 lists some of published research work on use of blockchain in security and authentication.

5.2 Blockchain in Clinical Trials & Precision Medicine

In healthcare industry, clinical trials are essential requirements to test the suitability of the medicine to a specific disease and the associated side effects. For clinical trials patient recruitment is known to be challenging aspect and failure to meet patient recruitment goals in time results in a waste of funds and time, incomprehensible statistical results, and unexpected delay in study period that could increase the planned recruitment timeline of patients. It is observed that 86% of clinical trials

Table 3. Published research work on Blockchain in Security & Authentication

S. No.	Area	Issues and Outcome	Reference
1	Blockchain based security	Securing and authenticating healthcare records	Pandey, P., et al. (2020). (Pandey & Litoriya, 2020)
2	Blockchain based security	Healthcare security based on internet of things	Srivastava, G., et al. (2020). (Srivastava et al., 2020)
3	Survey on blockchain based security	Privacy threats and potential applications	Soni, S., et al. (2019). (Soni & Bhushan, 2019)
4	Blockchain based security	Security challenges using IoT	Kumar, N. M., et al. (2018). (Kumar & Mallick, 2018)
5	Blockchain based health Applications	IoT based e-health solutions	Neto, M. M., et al. (2019). (Neto et al., 2019)
6	Blockchain based framework	For securing electronic health records	Vora, J., et al. (2018). (Vora et al., 2018)

don't achieve their recruitment goals on time3 and 19% of registered clinical trials were either closed or terminated due to failure to reach expected enrolment (Carlisle et al., 2015).

Systematic and valid patient enrolment is essential in clinical trials to get conclusive results failure which may cause premature trail termination. Blockchain technology features a peer-to-peer system with external audited transaction capabilities, data security supports, and privacy for patients are suitable for an innovative model to be used in clinical trial recruitment of stakeholders. Blockchain model also supports essential features like data decentralization, immutability, ensuring data provenance, and public auditability. In blockchain based model, all the transactions are distributively stored into each node in any active electronic device without hardware requirements. All transactions need to be validated by the user in the blockchain before it is written into the system. Since the system is fully decentralized, all the transactions can be audited publicly by all the users and hence it constitutes a fool proof system.

A blockchain based system called "Smart Contract" is developed which is a programmable self-executing protocol that regulates the blockchain transactions. Smart Contract system is a coded protocol agreed between senders and receivers initially proposed by Nick Szabo in 1996 to regulate all transactions on the distributed ledger system (Szabo, 1996). Most blockchain systems proposed in clinical trials have added a smart contract function to their protocols such as Ethereum and Hyperledger

Table 4. Published research work on Blockchain in Clinical Trials & Precision Medicine

S. No.	Area	Issues and Outcome	Reference
1	Clinical trials using Blockchain	Prototype of running clinical trials in an untrustworthy environment	Wong, D. R., et al. (2019). (Wong et al., 2019)
2	Clinical trials using blockchain	Improving data transparency smart contracts	Nugent, T., et al. (2016). (Nugent et al., 2016)
3	Using blockchain technology to manage clinical trials data	A proof-of-concept study	Maslove, D. M., et al. (2018). (Maslove et al., 2018)
4	Blockchain protocols in clinical trials	Transparency and traceability of consent	Benchoufi, M., et al (2017). (Benchoufi et al., 2017)
5	Clinical trials using Blockchain	For improving clinical research quality	Benchoufi, M., et al. (2017). (Benchoufi & Ravaud, 2017)
6	Role of blockchain and IoT in clinical trials	Recruiting participants for digital clinical trials	Angeletti, F., et al. (2017). (Angeletti et al., 2017)
7	Clinical trials using Blockchain	To improve the outcomes of clinical trials	Borioli, G. S., et al. (2018). (Borioli & Couturier, 2018)
8	Blockchain for clinical trials	A framework for managing and monitoring data in multi-site clinical trials	Choudhury, O., et al. (2019). (Choudhury et al., 2019)
9	Blockchain for clinical trials	Ensuring protocol compliance and data transparency using Blockchain smart contracts.	Omar, I. A., et al. (2020). (Omar et al., 2020)
10	Blockchain for clinical trials and precision medicine	Design of a blockchain platform for clinical trial and precision medicine	Shae, Z., et al. (2017). (Shae & Tsai, 2017)
11	Blockchain for clinical trials	A Hybrid Blockchain Design for Patient Recruitments and Persistent Monitoring for Clinical Trials	Zhuang, Y., et al. (2018). (Zhuang et al., 2018)
12	Blockchain for clinical trials	Blockchain-enabled clinical study consent management	Jung, H. H., et al. (2020). (Jung & Pfister, 2020)

(Christidis & Devetsikiotis, 2016). Since the Ethereum blockchain comes with a built-in Turing complete programming language used for the smart contract, any computational problem such as patient matching for recruitment, or checking the validity of a clinical trial can be coded as a smart contract (Buterin, 2014). Thus, blockchain based smart contract system can handle current recruitment challenges, patient engagement, automated subject matching, patient recruitment, and trial-based contracts management. Table 4 lists some of published research work on use of blockchain in Clinical Trials & Precision Medicine

5.3 Blockchain in Personalizing the Healthcare Services

The digital healthcare system has a biggest challenge of secured data sharing and interoperability between applications data sources and other external systems. Personal healthcare records created for digital healthcare system provides access to patients to some extent and allows them to control it by means of interoperability in order to deliver personalized care. But as per the government regulations, supports to protect personal and private data and there is a need of maintaining security and transparency in the areas of consent, anonymisation and data ownership (Leeming et al., 2019). Blockchain technology-based platform allows patients to provide permission to use the data by means of use of token-based permission. Patients can also provide permission to use the data for healthcare professionals and researchers to access their health history and wellbeing and to get medical services from global market to improve their health without any illegal modifications. Table 5 lists some of published research work on use of blockchain in Personalizing the Healthcare Services.

5.4 Blockchain in Healthcare Data Management

A blockchain is a particular type of database by its design and is a kind of read-only-once database. The blockchain databases are designed and created only once and not allowed to be edited or deleted by any one internal or external to it. The data stored is a blockchain decentralized ledger is a transaction type of database and others are not able to access it until the actual owner holds the private keys. These database file systems are more secure, faster, and economical compared to centralized databases. The potential for the use of blockchain technology in hospitals has developed a new field of healthcare data management and utilizes data encryption logics and supports to reduce data duplication via off-chain cloud components with cryptographic algorithms to create user sharing. Various types of possible healthcare data management systems include Blockchain for Electronic Medical Record (EMR) Data Management, Blockchain and Healthcare Data Protection, Blockchain for

Table 5. Related scholarly work in Blockchain in Personalizing the Healthcare Services

S. No.	Area	Issues and Outcome	Reference
1	Blockchain in Personalizing the Healthcare Services	A Novel Blockchain Based Smart Contract System for eReferral in Healthcare: HealthChain	Chenthara, S., et al. (2020). (Chenthara et al., 2020)
2	Blockchain in personalizing patient-centric health	A patient-centric health information exchange framework using blockchain technology	Zhuang, Y., et al. (2020). (Zhuang et al., 2020)
3	Blockchain-based personal health record exchange	An architecture and management platform for development and usability	Lee, H. A., et al. (2020). (Lee et al., 2020)
4	Blockchain for digital health	Prospects and challenges	Evangelatos, N., et al. (2020). (Evangelatos et al., 2020)
5	Blockchain in Personalizing Health Records	Blockchain-Based Personal Health Records for Patients' Empowerment.	El Rifai, O., et al. (2020). (El Rifai et al., 2020)
6	Blockchain, Interoperability, and Self-Sovereign Identity	Trust Me, It's My Data	StClair, J., et al. (2020). (St. Clair et al., 2020)
7	Blockchain for digital health	EDI with blockchain as an enabler for extreme automation in healthcare	Fiaidhi, J., et al. (2020). (Fiaidhi et al., 2018)

Table 6. Related scholarly work in Blockchain in Healthcare Data Management

S. No.	Area	Issues and Outcome	Reference
1	Blockchain for healthcare data management	Opportunities, challenges, and future recommendations	Yaqoob, I., et al. (2021). (Yaqoob et al., 2021)
2	IoT-healthcare using blockchain technology	A hybrid framework for multimedia data processing	Rathee, G., et al. (2020). (Rathee et al., 2020)
3	Blockchain for healthcare data management	Blockchain versus database: a critical analysis	Chowdhury, M. J. M., et al. (2018). (Chowdhury et al., 2018)
4	Healthcare Data Management Using Blockchain Technology	Challenges and Future Work Directions	Pustokhin, D. A., et al. (2021). (Pustokhin et al., 2021)
5	Blockchain for healthcare data management	Blockchain technology acceptance in electronic medical record system	Wanitcharakkhakul, L., et al. (2018). (Wanitcharakkhakul & Rotchanakitumnuai, 2017)

Personal Health Record (PHR) Data Management, Blockchain for Point-of-Care Genomics, and Blockchain for EHR Data Management (Dimitrov, 2019). Table 6 lists some of published research work on use of blockchain in Healthcare Data Management.

5.5 Blockchain in Strengthening Public Health Surveillance

Blockchain technology has an enormous scope to revamp the healthcare system in many ways as it improves the quality of healthcare by data sharing among all the participants, selective privacy and ensuring data safety. In many countries, blockchain is being used to promote patient-centered care by sharing patient data for remote monitoring and management. Furthermore, blockchain technology has the potential to strengthen disease surveillance systems in cases of disease outbreaks resulting in local and global health emergencies. The other real-time surveillance systems lack scalability, security, interoperability, thus making blockchain as a choice for surveillance. Blockchain offers the capability of enhancing global health security and also can ensure the anonymity of patient data thereby aiding in healthcare research (Bhattacharya et al., 2019).

In decentralized health data records network, all the transactions or changes in the data are recorded with real-time updates across the network so that the same information gets stored in each node of the network. In such networks the stored information is permanent and cannot be deleted or modified. Thus, decentralization based blockchain technology provides transparency, autonomy and has the potential to improve the quality of healthcare as data is shared among all the participants. It is a system of creating an immutable, secure, distributed database of transactions where cryptographic algorithms are used to validate the transaction. This cryptographic proof is used instead of the "trustin-the-third-party" mechanism for two willing parties to approve an online transaction which is protected by a digital signature. Hence blockchain technology integration will improve interoperability, immutability, tighter security, transparency, reduced costs, and faster care delivery (Chattu et al., 2019).

Any surveillance system should have characteristics of systematic, ongoing collection, collation, and analysis of data and the timely dissemination of information to those who need to know so that the action can be taken. Public surveillance is important for both infectious diseases and chronic noncommunicable diseases by all the national health systems, and according to the national priorities, the diseases under surveillance may be different through the nations must comply with the reporting of infections listed under WHO's International Health Regulations. Effective disease surveillance and response systems are needed for infectious disease control and preventing the spread of epidemics (Chattu et al., 2019).

The blockchain technology helps the disease surveillance at district level, country level, and global level. The district-level surveillance becomes effective through prompt reporting by the district level health workers. The laboratories at district level, country level, or global level can be integrated as a participating node of the chain when the certain positive test for a priority disease is observed act as a trigger so that timely public health action can be taken. There is also scope for integration with other technologies like geographical information system to expedite the routine epidemic investigations, drug and vaccine supply chain systems can also be made efficient by supplying them on time. These blockchain applications can also evaluate the cost-effectiveness of various available treatment methodologies and share the information at a fast pace thereby saving time by reducing duplication in reporting. The other critical aspect is that by ensuring transparency and correct reporting, as in case of reporting deaths from the particular outbreak, the blockchain overcomes the limitations of already-present district health information systems ().

5.6 Blockchain in e-Healthcare to Customers

The current electronic medical record systems are customized to be used by a particular hospital only. In most cases, electronic medical records cannot be connected other hospitals and hence other hospitals cannot access patients' medical profile and hence patients receive minimum benefit when they try to receive medical facilities from other hospitals. Further, due to inferiority in the software used, the hospitals also cannot support more to provide e-healthcare facilities from other hospitals and the patients are not confident about the security and privacy of their data. Such problems are derived from three key issues that include completeness of data, sources and status of information, and data security in sharing (Wanitcharakkhakul & Rotchanakitumnuai, 2017). Hence the e-healthcare system need patients records with correctness and completeness of the data. Blockchain in e-healthcare systems do not require multiple levels of authentication and provide access to data to everyone who is part of the blockchain architecture. In this system, the data is made visible and transparent for all stakeholders including patients, so that these features can be used to solve the various challenges faced by the healthcare industry for interoperability in a networked environment (Alla et al., 2018; Gul et al., 2021; Jeet & Kang, 2020; Khubrani, 2021; Kohli et al., 2021; Maseleno et al., 2020; Neto et al., 2020; Sivan & Zukarnain, 2021).

5.7 Blockchain in Healthcare Administration & Medicine Management

Based on its characteristics, blockchain can allow stakeholders in the healthcare ecosystem to share patient, treatment, and clinical information without compromising on security by ensuring information origin as well as change tracking. The blockchain based healthcare administration system gives patients a comprehensive, immutable log and easy access to their medical information across providers and treatment sites. Unique features of blockchain allows the administrators of healthcare systems to manage authentication, confidentiality, accountability and data sharing—crucial considerations when handling sensitive information. Integration of local data storage solutions to provide a modular design-based healthcare system. facilitates interoperability, system conveniency, and adaptability. Blockchain based Medicine Management system allows medical stakeholders such as researchers, public health authorities, etc. to participate in the network as administrators and researchers. This provides them with access to aggregate, anonymized data as mining rewards, in return for sustaining and securing the network via Proof of Work. Medical records enable the emergence of data economics, supplying big data to empower researchers while engaging patients and providers in the choice to release metadata. Blockchain based integration of medical records provides ability to analyse information from various reliable sources to identify public health risks, develop new treatments and cures, and enable precision medicine (AlShamsi et al., 2021; Chen et al., 2019; Ploder et al., 2021; Premkumar & Srimathi, 2020).

5.8 Blockchain in Telehealth & Telemedicine

Blockchain technology can improve telehealth and telemedicine services by offering remote healthcare services in a manner that is decentralized, tamper-proof, transparent, traceable, reliable, trustful, and secure. Telehealth and telemedicine systems aim to deliver remote healthcare services to mitigate the spread of chronical and pandemic diseases and can help to manage scarce healthcare resources to control the massive burden on hospitals (Ahmad et al., 2021).

Telemedicine enables healthcare professionals to remotely monitor, diagnose, and treat patients by offering cost-efficient services, thereby minimizing patient access and workforce limitations, expanding technology capabilities, and mitigating the risk of exposure of physicians, staff, or patients to pandemic diseases. Similarly, telehealth employs digital information and communication technologies to help the patients to manage their illness through improved self-care and access to education and support systems. The existing telehealth and telemedicine systems reveal virtual healthcare and potential to successfully mitigate the spread of airborne infectious diseases.

The adoption of blockchain technology into existing telehealth and telemedicine systems can bring numerous opportunities for secure digitization of healthcare, such as successfully establish the provenance of clinical data, legitimacy of users seeking patient data, manage identities of devices used for remote patient monitoring, preserve patient anonymity, and automate the payments settlement (Ahmad et al., 2021).Despite the convenience of telemedicine, blockchain technology solves enormous potential security concerns. If the virtual connection between a doctor and the patient is secure through blockchain, it is possible that patients' location, data and other sensitive information could be protected without any leakage (Hathaliya et al., 2019; Le Nguyen, 2018).

5.9 Blockchain in Managing Medical Imaging

One of the blockchain's most unique strengths lies in its ability to establish an anonymous record while still enabling participants to authenticate themselves when required. Blockchain technology implementation is serves as a tool to enable the patient-controlled, cross-domain sharing of medical images without the need for a central authority. There are a number of unique advantages that the blockchain satisfies many of the requirements of an interoperable health system (Patel, 2019).

Before invention of blockchain based image storing and sharing, the digital imaging through high-speed network connectivity, the medical image sharing processes were using a copy in a physical storage medium such as CD or DVD and couriered between providers/users. There is clear inefficiency and waste inherent in transcribing a digital asset onto optical media which commonly is read only once during image import at the receiving site. Further, this method imposes an undue responsibility upon the patient to ensure that the images are not lost, damaged, or intercepted in transit (McBee & Wilcox, 2020).

The blockchain concept has been considered as a prominent decentralized process, and is applicabile to the task of medical image sharing. A blockchain is, quite simply, a data structure consisting of an ordered sequence of batched entries, termed blocks. The ordering of these blocks is established by storing a cryptographic hash of the immediate prior record within each block and by use of an irreversible hash function as the chaining mechanism, and serves to verify the integrity of the previous block. This characteristic if blockchain gives rise to the key emergent property to store data immutably. Any attempt to tamper with the data in an established image block is easily detected since it changes the hash of the altered image block and consequently, the hashes of all subsequent image blocks in the chain. Some of the challenges of implementation such as public versus private key access, distributed ledger size constraints, speed, complexity, and security pitfalls are yet to be resolved. Potential use cases for blockchain specifically relevant to medical imaging include image sharing including direct patient ownership of images, tracking of implanted medical devices, research, teleradiology, and artificial intelligence (Koptyra & Ogiela, 2021; Kumar & Tripathi, 2021; Kumar et al., 2021; Shubbar, 2017; Sultana et al., 2020; Witowski et al., 2021; Xu et al., 2019).

5.10 Blockchain in Developing Smart Healthcare System

The combination of blockchain and smarthealthcare can alleviate the pain points of traditional smart healthcare in information sharing, data security, and privacy maintenance, optimize the user-centered smart healthcare systems, and establish a multiparty medical alliance chain involving government, enterprises, and society. Such system demonstrates the usage of automated and intelligent blockchain for healthcare. Smart healthcare systems make use of Information Communication and Computation Technology (ICCT) underlying technologies such as Artificial Intelligence & Machine learning, big data and business Intelligence, Cloud computing, Internet of Things, Wireless sensor networks, Mobile and wearable devices, Robotic surgeries, Information storage technology, Virtual reality, etc. Smart healthcare systems along with blockchain technology enhances confidentiality, integrity, authorization, and availability of data to the stakeholders in centralized, decentralized, and distributed environment (Bhawiyuga et al., 2019; Demirkan, 2013; Farhin et al., 2021; Haque et al., 2021; Khubrani, 2021; Kumar et al., 2020; Qiu et al., 2018; Shukla et al., 2020). The importance of creating secured electronic health records for easy sharing and access through ICCT underlying technologies and blockchain provides a secured yet faster way of medical information exchange in current scenario.

5.11 Blockchain in Healthcare Information System

Blockchain information system integrates various subsystems in hospital industry both horizontally and vertically so that it brings a reliable, and effective information management in healthcare organizations and the healthcare systems of the country. Here the blockchain technology could be used as a bridge that can provide information systems interoperability within a hospital or between different hospitals.

Blockchain in healthcare information system allows to share records for information transactions. It enables all stakeholders in a team to securely share data with each other without a middleman and keep track of what was exchanged and when. Here the records are maintained across multiple computers, instead of being located on a single, hackable computer. This makes the information extremely difficult to tamper with or delete and hence provides the tamper-proof characteristic. Further, the process of information management ensures that any information added to the blockchain based healthcare system is valid, enables trust between the team members (Azogu et al., 2019; Marbouh et al., 2020).

5.12 Disadvantages of Blockchain Technology

Some of the disadvantages of blockchain technology are listed below: (Gatteschi et al., 2018; Soltanisehat et al., 2020)

(1) Complexity: Use of blockchain technology involves completely new environment of working with cryptography as mainstream.

(2) Network size: Blockchains requires large network of users, however if a blockchain is not a robust network with a widely distributed grid of nodes, it becomes more difficult to reap the full benefit of anti-fragility they respond to attacks and grow stronger.

(3) Transaction costs, network speed becomes issues as network size grows.

(4) Wasteful: Every Node runs the blockchain in order to maintain Consensus across the blockchain. This gives extreme levels of fault tolerance, ensures zero downtime, and makes data stored on the blockchain forever unchangeable and censorship-resistant. But all this is wasteful, as each Node repeats a task to reach Consensus burning electricity and time on the way. This makes computation far slower and more expensive than on a traditional single computer. There are many initiatives that seek to reduce this cost focusing on alternative means of maintaining Consensus, such as Proof-of-Stake.

(5) Human error: If a blockchain is used as a database, the information going into the database needs to be of high quality. The data stored on a blockchain is not inherently trustworthy, so events need to be recorded accurately in the first place. The phrase 'garbage in, garbage out' holds true in a blockchain system of record, just as with a centralized database.

(6) Unavoidable security flaw: if more than half of the computers working as nodes to service the network tell a lie, the lie will become the truth. This is called a '51% attack'. Hence continuous monitoring is required.

(7) Scalability Issues: Since each participating node has to verify a transaction in the network, the total number of transactions occurring per second is limited. It can take up to several hours for a transaction to commit. The scalability issues put the practical use of blockchain in a doubt. As the blockchain expands, data gets bigger and bigger, the loading of store and processing also gets harder and harder it takes a lot of time to synchronize data, but at the same time, the data continues to develop.

(8) Interoperability Issues: The lack of interoperability in healthcare systems and services, though, has long been identified as one of the major healthcare

challenges. Blockchain also suffers from the interoperability problem that means that blockchains from different providers of communication and services communicate seamlessly and properly with each other. This challenge creates obstacles to effective data sharing.

(9) The information is vulnerable to possible protection and privacy threats. Given that all nodes can access the transmitted data from one node, in blockchain the privacy of the data is not intact.

(10) The blockchain is susceptible to attacks by selfish miners involved in collusion. In general, it is convinced that the blockchain will reverse nodes with more than 51 percent computing power.

6. CURRENT IMPLEMENTATIONS OF BLOCKCHAIN IN HEALTHCARE

A blockchain is a chain of blocks apparently secured by cryptographic techniques (Bhuvana et al., 2020a). His immutability is among the most desirable aspects of this to other businesses. No alteration can be made to the data added to the blockchain therefore, a consensus-based, verifiable and reliable database can be created. This makes blockchain especially ideal for tasks where data integrity is of utmost importance a practical illustration of this immutability is ProvChain, an infrastructure developed on the blockchain to provide data artifacts on the cloud with a chain of custody (Kuo & Ohno-Machado, 2018; Lorenz et al., 2017; McConaghy et al., 2016). The advantages of blockchain are enormous in biomedical situations. Blockchain is suitable for implementations whereby biomedical / health care stakeholders independently regulated for example hospitals, manufacturers, patients, and contributors) choose to work together without giving power to a central management intermediary. Blockchain only allows functions that are very difficult to change data or registers to be developed and interpreted. As an unchangeable archive to store confidential information, blockchain is perfect for the example the history of insurance claims. Only under the cryptographic protocols can the owner change its ownership. The source of the assets can also be traced, which can be confirmed as sources or as data and documents, improving the reusability of the validated data, such as insurance transactions. Blockchain is, therefore, suitable for use in sensitive digital asset management for instance patient consent documents. The data redundancy can be accomplished by each node with a full copy of the historical data. Blockchain thus is perfect for maintaining and continued information availability for example EHR. The key advantage is to keep records secure with the use of cryptographic Algorithms (Liang et al., 2017). In order to exchange and collaborate on personal health care data, a mobile, blockchain-based mechanism will be placed in place, a Hyperledger Fabric system will be introduced, which is a licensed blockchain requiring verifications of network nodes, and a privacy-providing personal health infrastructure with broader coverage of the health environment from the end-computer to cloud (Angraal et al., 2017). Blockchain can fit into interoperability as the right player by hashing the existing MPIs in the form of blocks to help reduce clinical costs, maintaining access to large population data in a decentralized format through which the gap between interoperability and predictability can be filled, and multi-source data from smart wearable devices to mobile devices can be achieved with blockchain because they can co-operate with blockchain ().

7. IDEAL STATUS USING BLOCKCHAIN IN HEALTHCARE SECTOR

Blockchain consists of a growing list of records which are linked using cryptography and such chain has the property of transparency, decentralization, and immune to modifications. Ideal blockchain is capable to trace history of everything which created a footprint in the past. Blockchain consists of a growing list of records which are linked using cryptography and such chain has the property of transparency, decentralization, and immune to modifications.

Hence blockchain technology is optimum for medical record preservation for longer period especially for legal requirements in future days. Every aspect related to patient history, admission, treatment, discharge, and follow-up is recorded in non-destructive manner. Further any modification attempt is either not possible or will be known to everyone involved in the chain of activities. Though, achieving ideal status of non-destructiveness is impossible, the innovations and advents in blockchain technology has power to develop non-destructive chain of ledgers for secured documentation maintenance and cannot be modified individually at any point without the knowledge of others involved in it (Aithal, 2019; Aithal & Aithal, 2019a) (Chattu et al., 2019; Maseleno et al., 2020).

8. RESEARCH GAP & RESEARCH AGENDAS

Developing a method using Blockchain Technology to achieve 100% security, transparency, decentralization, and immune to modifications compared to present status security, transparency, decentralization, and immunity for modifications. Challenge is how to improve these characteristics of healthcare services.

Further various research agendas in innovations in the healthcare sector using blockchain technology include:

(1) Blockchain mediated Healthcare Security & Authentication aspects of networked hospitals and patients,

(2) Blockchain application in Clinical Trials & Precision Medicine to provide better information to stakeholders,

(3) Personalizing the Healthcare Services using Blockchain in terms of authenticity, completeness, and ubiquity,

(4) Healthcare Data Management assisted by Blockchain Technology as open access platform,

(5) Strengthening Public Health Surveillance using Blockchain Technology and provide current information to various monitoring bodies including government,

(6) Blockchain assisted e-Healthcare to Customers with comparative service accessibility and quality,

(7) Optimum Healthcare Administration & Medicine Management using Blockchain technology assisted security feature,

(8) Innovations and best practices in blockchain controlled Telehealth & Telemedicine and to make it customer friendly,

(9) Managing and protecting of Medical Images using blockchain Technology,

(10) Developing Smart Healthcare Systems assisted by blockchain with user friendly and advanced comfort features, and

(11) Use of Blockchain for developing Innovative Healthcare Information Systems with automated and secured decision making processes

9. FINDINGS BASED ON THE REVIEW

Blockchain technology has potential advantage in improving the healthcare services in the areas of Healthcare Security & Authentication aspects, Clinical Trials & Precision Medicine, Personalizing the Healthcare Services, Healthcare Data Management, Strengthening Public Health Surveillance, e-Healthcare to Customers, Healthcare Administration & Medicine Management, Telehealth & Telemedicine, Managing Medical Imaging, Developing Smart Healthcare System, and Healthcare Information System.

1. Adoption of blockchain in healthcare helps in establishing medical records which reduces the costs and also proper health data utilization.

2. Blockchain can help healthcare in maintaining health records, drug data, patient data and insurance information.

3. Transparency has the main function of blockchain helps to keep the information between medical facilities, insurance providers, and patients transparent.

4.   There are no universal health records for health data appropriate medical data management but blockchain has the potential to solve this problem.

5.   Understood about Blockchain technology and Distributed technology and how these technologies are changing the healthcare and financial services work.

6.   Interoperability being a major problem in healthcare blockchain can providing permission to digital access for clinical data, data availability, rapid access to clinical information, and patient identity and solve the problem.

7.   Blockchain improves contractual performance due to smart contracts

8.   Blockchain is mainly looked forward to the reason that it provides security

9.   When it comes to both healthcare and financial services blockchain promises security, transparency, trust, programmability, privacy, high performance, and scalability.

10.   Due to the programmable capabilities of blockchain, the code that addresses KYC can be built into assets themselves.

11.   Blockchain has become a disruptive technology with being used for different purposes from cost reduction to security in healthcare and financial services.

12.   The interest in testing and using the technology has drastically grown.

13.   Interoperability problem arises in blockchain because most of the blockchain work in silos and do not communicate with other peer networks as they are incapable of sending and receiving information from another blockchain based systems.

14.   The technology works on proof of work which needs a lot of computational power to solve complex mathematical puzzles, verify, and to secure the entire network.

15.   Identified various research agendas to carry out further research for patient satisfaction and comfortability.

10. CONCLUSION

This study analysed the emerging blockchain technology and its potential ramifications in healthcare and financial services. The blockchain technology provides a decentralized network and is considered to have tremendous potential for use in healthcare and financial services, due to the sensitive nature of the collection and management of data. The review aimed at defining the existing state of blockchain in healthcare and financial services and the current implementations in these industries. To achieve this aim, we have taken into account numerous scholarly publications concerning healthcare and financial services and challenges. Our findings indicate that blockchain technology has tremendously changed the healthcare sector and financial sector in the area of storage of data, processing of data, transaction, security, and so on based on its current implementation stage. Therefore, Blockchain technology help replaces paper-based and manual transaction processing in financial services and healthcare provides new models for electronic medical records and financial payments. It is found that blockchain technology facilitates for the improvement of quality services in the healthcare sector and various research agendas are proposed to carry out further research for patient satisfaction and comfortability.

REFERENCES

Aithal, P. S., & Aithal, S. (2019). Management of ICCT underlying Technologies used for Digital Service Innovation. [IJMTS]. *International Journal of Management, Technology, and Social Sciences*, *4*(2), 110–136.

Lipsey, R., Carlaw, K. I., & Bekhar, C. T. (2005). *Economic Transformations: General Purpose Technologies and Long-Term Economic Growth*. Oxford University Press.

Aithal, P. S., & Aithal, S. (2018). Study of various General-Purpose Technologies and Their Comparison towards developing Sustainable Society. [IJMTS]. *International Journal of Management, Technology, and Social Sciences*, *3*(2), 16–33.

Aithal, P. S., & Madhushree, L. M. (2019). Information Communication & Computation Technology (ICCT) as a Strategic Tool for Industry Sectors. [IJAEML]. *International Journal of Applied Engineering and Management Letters*, *3*(2), 65–80.

Aithal, P. S., & Madhushree, L. M. (2019). Emerging Trends in ICCT as Universal Technology for Strategic Development of Industry Sectors. Chapter in a Book - IT and Computing for all the Domains and Professionals: The Emergence of Computer and Information Sciences, Edited by P.K. Paul, A. Bhuimali, K.S. Tiwary, and P. S. Aithal published by New Delhi Publishers, New Delhi. pp 1-26, ISBN: 978-93-88879-66-8.

Aithal, P. S. &ShubhrajyotsnaAithal. (2019). Management of ICCT underlying Technologies used for Digital Service Innovation. [IJMTS]. *International Journal of Management, Technology, and Social Sciences*, *4*(2), 110–136.

Luu, L., & Teutsch, J., Kulkarni., & Saxena, P. (2015). Demystifying incentives in the consensus computer. *Proceedings of the 22nd ACM SIGSAC Conference on Computer and Communications Security, 1*(1), 706-719.

[] Wright, A., & De Filippi, P. (2015). Decentralized blockchain technology and the rise of lexcryptographia. Available at SSRN 2580664.

Yaga, D., Mell, P., Roby, N., & Scarfone, K. (2019). Blockchain technology overview. arXiv preprint arXiv:1906.11078.

Peters, G., Panayi, E., & Chapelle, A. (2015). Trends in cryptocurrencies and blockchain technologies: A monetary theory and regulation perspective. *Journal of Financial Perspectives*, *3*(3), 1–46.

Foroglou, G., & Tsilidou, A. L. (2015). Further applications of the blockchain. *Abgerufen Am.*, *3*(1), 1–9.

Gordon, W. J., & Catalini, C. (2018). Blockchain technology for healthcare: Facilitating the transition to patient-driven interoperability. *Computational and Structural Biotechnology Journal*, *16*(1), 224–230.

Reyes, C. L. (2016). Moving beyond Bitcoin to an endogenous theory of decentralized ledger technology regulation: An initial proposal. *Vill. L. Rev.*, *61*(1), 191–204.

Tripathi, G., Ahad, M. A., & Paiva, S. (2020, March). S2HS-A blockchain based approach for smart healthcare system. *Health Care*, *8*(100391), 1–13.

Chatterjee, R., & Chatterjee, R. (2017, October). An overview of the emerging technology: Blockchain. In 2017 3rd International Conference on Computational Intelligence and Networks (CINE) (pp. 126-127). IEEE.

Yaga, D., Mell, P., Roby, N., & Scarfone, K. (2019). Blockchain technology overview. arXivpreprint arXiv:1906.11078.

Katuwal, G. J., Pandey, S., Hennessey, M., & Lamichhane, B. (2018). Applications of blockchain in healthcare: current landscape & challenges. arXiv preprint arXiv:1812.02776.

Bhuvana, R., Madhushree, L. M., & Aithal, P. S. (2020). Blockchain as a Disruptive Technology in Healthcare and Financial Services-A Review based Analysis on Current Implementations. [IJAEML]. *International Journal of Applied Engineering and Management Letters*, *4*(1), 142–155.

Bhuvana, R., & Aithal, P. S. (2020). Blockchain based Service: A Case Study on IBM Blockchain Services & Hyperledger Fabric. [IJCSBE]. *International Journal of Case Studies in Business, IT, and Education*, *4*(1), 94–102.

Bhuvana, R., & Aithal, P. S. (2020). RBI Distributed Ledger Technology and Blockchain-A Future of Decentralized India. [IJMTS]. *International Journal of Management, Technology, and Social Sciences*, *5*(1), 227–237.

Gade, Dipak S.&Aithal, P. S. (2020). Blockchain Technology: A Driving Force in Smart Cities Development. [IJAEML]. *International Journal of Applied Engineering and Management Letters*, *4*(2), 237–252.

Rangi, P. K., & Aithal, P. S. (2020). A Study on Blockchain Technology as a Dominant Feature to Mitigate Reputational Risk for Indian Academic Institutions and Universities. [IJAEML]. *International Journal of Applied Engineering and Management Letters*, *4*(2), 275–284.

Bhuvana, R., Madhushree, L., & Aithal, P. S. (2020). Comparative Study on RFID based Tracking and Blockchain based Tracking of Material Transactions. [IJAEML]. *International Journal of Applied Engineering and Management Letters*, *4*(2), 22–30.

Sai Manoj, K., & Aithal, P. S. (2020). Blockchain Cyber Security Vulnerabilities and Potential Countermeasures. [IJITEE]. *International Journal of Innovative Technology and Exploring Engineering*, *9*(5), 1516–1522.

Aste, T., Tasca, P., & Di Matteo, T. (2017). Blockchain technologies: The foreseeable impact on society and industry. *Computer*, *50*(9), 18–28.

Wu, G., Zhang, H., Qiu, M., Ming, Z., Li, J., & Qin, X. (2013). A decentralized approach for mining event correlations in distributed system monitoring. *Journal of Parallel and Distributed Computing*, *73*(3), 330–340.

Do, H. G., & Ng, W. K. (2017, June). Blockchain-based system for secure data storage with private keyword search. *IEEE World Congress on Services (SERVICES)*, *1*(1), 90-93.

[] Deshpande, A., Stewart, K., Lepetit, L., &Gunashekar, S. (2017). Distributed Ledger Technologies/Blockchain: Challenges, opportunities and the prospects for standards. *Overview report The British Standards Institution (BSI)*, *1*(1), 1-34.

Zhang, F., Cecchetti, E., Croman, K., Juels, A., & Shi, E. (2016, October). Town crier: An authenticated data feed for smart contracts. *Proceedings of the 2016 ACM SIGSAC conference on computer and communications security*, *1*(1), 270-282.

[] Johnston, D., Yilmaz, S. O., Kandah, J., Bentenitis, N., Hashemi, F., Gross, R., Mason, S. (2014). The General Theory of Decen-tralized Applications, DApps.

Swan, M. (2015). *Blockchain: Blueprint for a new economy*. O'Reilly Media, Inc.

Francisco, K., & Swanson, D. (2018). The supply chain has no clothes: Technology adoption of blockchain for supply chain transparency. *Logistics*, *2*(1), 1–13.

Wang, W., Hoang, D. T., Hu, P., Xiong, Z., Niyato, D., Wang, P., & Kim, D. I. (2019). A survey on consensus mechanisms and mining strategy management in blockchain networks. *IEEE Access: Practical Innovations, Open Solutions, 7*(1), 22328–22370.

MacKenzie, D. (2019). Pick a nonce and try a hash. *London Review of Books, 41*(8), 35–38.

Wang, W., Hoang, D. T., Xiong, Z., Niyato, D., Wang, P., Hu, P., & Wen, Y. (2018). A survey on consensus mechanisms and mining management in blockchain networks. arXiv preprint arXiv:1805.02707, 1-33.

Luu, L., Chu, D. H., Olickel, H., Saxena, P., & Hobor, A. (2016). Making smart contracts smarter. In *Proceedings of the 2016 ACM SIGSAC conference on computer and communications security* (pp. 254- 269).

Biais, B., Bisiere, C., Bouvard, M., & Casamatta, C. (2019). The blockchain folk theorem. *Review of Financial Studies, 32*(5), 1662–1715.

Wang, M., Duan, M., & Zhu, J. (2018). Research on the security criteria of hash functions in the blockchain. *Proceedings of the 2nd ACM Workshop on Blockchains, Cryptocurrencies, and Contracts, 1*(1), 47-55.

Lin, I. C., & Liao, T. C. (2017). A survey of blockchain security issues and challenges. *International Journal of Network Security, 19*(5), 653–659.

Di Pierro, M. (2017). What is the blockchain? *Computing in Science & Engineering, 19*(5), 92–95.

Maull, R., Godsiff, P., Mulligan, C., Brown, A., & Kewell, B. (2017). Distributed ledger technology: Applications and implications. *Strategic Change, 26*(5), 481–489.

HonarPajooh, H., Rashid, M., Alam, F., & Demidenko, S. (2021). Multi-layer blockchain-based security architecture for internet of things. *Sensors (Basel), 21*(3), 1–26.

Pandey, P., & Litoriya, R. (2020). Securing and authenticating healthcare records through blockchain technology. *Cryptologia, 44*(4), 341–356.

[] Srivastava, G., Parizi, R. M., &Dehghantanha, A. (2020). The future of blockchain technology in healthcare internet of things security. *Blockchain Cybersecurity, Trust and Privacy*, 161-184.

Soni, S., & Bhushan, B. (2019, July). A comprehensive survey on blockchain: Working, security analysis, privacy threats and potential applications. In *2019 2nd International Conference on Intelligent Computing, Instrumentation and Control Technologies (ICICICT)* (Vol. 1, pp. 922-926). IEEE.

Kumar, N. M., & Mallick, P. K. (2018). Blockchain technology for security issues and challenges in IoT. *Procedia Computer Science*, *132*, 1815–1823.

Neto, M. M., Coutinho, E. F., Moreira, L. O., & de Souza, J. N. (2019, October). Toward blockchain technology in IoT applications: an analysis for e-health applications. In *IFIP International Internet of Things Conference* (pp. 36-50). Springer, Cham.

Vora, J., Nayyar, A., Tanwar, S., Tyagi, S., Kumar, N., Obaidat, M. S., & Rodrigues, J. J. (2018, December). BHEEM: A blockchain-based framework for securing electronic health records. In 2018 IEEE Globecom Workshops (GC Wkshps) (pp. 1-6). IEEE.

Carlisle, B., Kimmelman, J., Ramsay, T., & MacKinnon, N. J. C. T. (2015). Unsuccessful trial accrual and human subjects' protections: *An empirical analysis of recently closed trials. Clinical Trials*, *12*(1), 77–83.

Szabo, N. (1996). Smart Contracts: Building Blocks for Digital Markets. Extropy. *The Journal of Transhumanist Thought*, *16*(18), 2–20.

Christidis, K., & Devetsikiotis, M. (2016). Blockchains and smart contracts for the internet of things. *IEEE Access : Practical Innovations, Open Solutions*, *4*(1), 2292–2303.

Buterin, V. (2014). A next-generation smart contract and decentralized application platform. *white paper, 3*(1),1-36.

Wong, D. R., Bhattacharya, S., & Butte, A. J. (2019). Prototype of running clinical trials in an untrustworthy environment using blockchain. *Nature Communications*, *10*(1), 1–8.

Nugent, T., Upton, D., & Cimpoesu, M. (2016). Improving data transparency in clinical trials using blockchain smart contracts. *F1000 Research*, 5(2541), 1–7.

[] Maslove, D. M., Klein, J., Brohman, K., & Martin, P. (2018). Using blockchain technology to manage clinical trials data: a proof-of-concept study. *JMIR medical informatics, 6*(4), e11949, 1-7.

Benchoufi, M., Porcher, R., & Ravaud, P. (2017). Blockchain protocols in clinical trials: Transparency and traceability of consent. *F1000 Research*, *6*(1), 1–66.

Benchoufi, M., & Ravaud, P. (2017). Blockchain technology for improving clinical research quality. *Trials*, *18*(1), 1–5.

Angeletti, F., Chatzigiannakis, I., & Vitaletti, A. (2017, September). The role of blockchain and IoT in recruiting participants for digital clinical trials. In *2017 25th International Conference on Software, Telecommunications and Computer Networks (SoftCOM)* (pp. 1-5). IEEE.

Borioli, G. S., & Couturier, J. (2018). How blockchain technology can improve the outcomes of clinical trials. *British Journal of Healthcare Management*, *24*(3), 156–162.

Choudhury, O., Fairoza, N., Sylla, I., & Das, A. (2019). A blockchain framework for managing and monitoring data in multi-site clinical trials. *arXiv preprint arXiv:1902.03975.*, 1-13.

Omar, I. A., Jayaraman, R., Salah, K., Simsekler, M. C. E., Yaqoob, I., & Ellahham, S. (2020). Ensuring protocol compliance and data transparency in clinical trials using Blockchain smart contracts. *BMC Medical Research Methodology*, *20*(1), 1–17.

Shae, Z., & Tsai, J. J. (2017, June). On the design of a blockchain platform for clinical trial and precision medicine. In *2017 IEEE 37th international conference on distributed computing systems (ICDCS)* (pp. 1972-1980). IEEE.

[] Zhuang, Y., Atkins, A., Shyu, C. R., Shae, Z., Tsai, J. J., & Hsu, C. (2018). A Hybrid Blockchain Design for Patient Recruitments and Persistent Monitoring for Clinical Trials. *IEEE Standards Association: Blockchain for clinical trials*. 1-7.

Jung, H. H., & Pfister, F. M. (2020). Blockchain-enabled clinical study consent management. *Technology Innovation Management Review*, *10*(2), 14–24.

[] Leeming, G., Cunningham, J., & Ainsworth, J. (2019). A ledger of me: personalizing healthcare using blockchain technology. *Frontiers in medicine*, *6*(171), 1-10. *6*(171), 1-10.

Chenthara, S., Ahmed, K., Wang, H., & Whittaker, F. (2020, October). A Novel Blockchain Based Smart Contract System for eReferral in Healthcare: HealthChain. *International Conference on Health Information Science* (pp. 91-102). Springer, Cham.

Zhuang, Y., Sheets, L. R., Chen, Y. W., Shae, Z. Y., Tsai, J. J., & Shyu, C. R. (2020). A patient-centric health information exchange framework using blockchain technology. *IEEE Journal of Biomedical and Health Informatics*, *24*(8), 2169–2176.

Lee, H. A., Kung, H. H., Udayasankaran, J. G., Kijsanayotin, B., Marcelo, A. B., Chao, L. R., & Hsu, C. Y. (2020). An architecture and management platform for blockchain-based personal health record exchange: Development and usability study. *Journal of Medical Internet Research*, *22*(6), e16748.

Evangelatos, N., Özdemir, V., & Brand, A. (2020). Blockchain for digital health: Prospects and challenges. *OMICS: A Journal of Integrative Biology*, *24*(5), 237–240.

El Rifai, O., Biotteau, M., de Boissezon, X., Megdiche, I., Ravat, F., & Teste, O. (2020, September). Blockchain-Based Personal Health Records for Patients' Empowerment. In *International Conference on Research Challenges in Information Science* (pp. 455-471). Springer, Cham.

StClair, J., Ingraham, A., King, D., Marchant, M. B., McCraw, F. C., Metcalf, D., & Squeo, J. (2020). Blockchain, Interoperability, and Self-Sovereign Identity: Trust Me, It's My Data. *Blockchain in Healthcare Today*, *3*(1), 1–3.

Fiaidhi, J., Mohammed, S., & Mohammed, S. (2018). EDI with blockchain as an enabler for extreme automation. *IT Professional*, *20*(4), 66–72.

Dimitrov, D. V. (2019). Blockchain Applications for Healthcare Data Management. *Healthcare Informatics Research*, *25*(1), 51–56.

Yaqoob, I., Salah, K., Jayaraman, R., & Al-Hammadi, Y. (2021). Blockchain for healthcare data management: Opportunities, challenges, and future recommendations. *Neural Computing & Applications*, 1–16.

Rathee, G., Sharma, A., Saini, H., Kumar, R., & Iqbal, R. (2020). A hybrid framework for multimedia data processing in IoT-healthcare using blockchain technology. *Multimedia Tools and Applications*, *79*(15), 9711–9733.

Chowdhury, M. J. M., Colman, A., Kabir, M. A., Han, J., & Sarda, P. (2018, August). Blockchain versus database: a critical analysis. In *2018 17th IEEE International Conference on Trust, Security and Privacy in Computing and Communications/12th IEEE International Conference on Big Data Science and Engineering (TrustCom/ BigDataSE)* (pp. 1348-1353). IEEE.

Pustokhin, D. A., Pustokhina, I. V., & Shankar, K. (2021). Challenges and Future Work Directions in Healthcare Data Management Using Blockchain Technology. In *Applications of Blockchain in Healthcare* (pp. 253–267). Springer.

Wanitcharakkhakul, L., & Rotchanakitumnuai, S. (2017, December). Blockchain technology acceptance in electronic medical record system. In *The 17th International Conference on Electronic Business, Dubai, UAE*. 53-58.

Bhattacharya, S., Singh, A., & Hossain, M. M. (2019). Strengthening public health surveillance through blockchain technology. *AIMS Public Health*, 6(3), 326.

Chattu, V. K., Nanda, A., Chattu, S. K., Kadri, S. M., & Knight, A. W. (2019). The emerging role of blockchain technology applications in routine disease surveillance systems to strengthen global health security. *Big Data and Cognitive Computing*, 3(2), 25.

Sharma, S. (2019, December). pubHeal-A Decentralized Platform on Health Surveillance of People. In *2019 IEEE Pune Section International Conference (PuneCon)* (pp. 1-6). IEEE.

Coelho, F. C. (2018). Optimizing Disease Surveillance by Reporting on the Blockchain. *bioRxiv*, 278473.

Alla, S., Soltanisehat, L., Tatar, U., & Keskin, O. (2018, May). Blockchain technology in electronic healthcare systems. In *Proceedings of the 2018 IISE Annual Conference* (pp. 1-6).

Neto, M. M., Marinho, C. S. D. S., Coutinho, E. F., Moreira, L. O., Machado, J. D. C., & de Souza, J. N. (2020, March). Research Opportunities for E-health Applications with DNA Sequence Data using Blockchain Technology. In *2020 IEEE International Conference on Software Architecture Companion (ICSA-C)* (pp. 95-102). IEEE.

[] Jeet, R., & Kang, S. S. (2020). Investigating the progress of human e-healthcare systems with understanding the necessity of using emerging blockchain technology. *Materials Today: Proceedings*.

Gul, M. J., Subramanian, B., Paul, A., & Kim, J. (2021). Blockchain for public health care in smart society. *Microprocessors and Microsystems*, 80, 103524.

Maseleno, A., Hashim, W., Perumal, E., Ilayaraja, M., & Shankar, K. (2020). Access control and classifier-based blockchain technology in e-healthcare applications. In *Intelligent Data Security Solutions for e-Health Applications* (pp. 151–167). Academic Press.

Khubrani, M. M. (2021). A Framework for Blockchain-based Smart Health System. [TURCOMAT]. *Turkish Journal of Computer and Mathematics Education*, 12(9), 2609–2614.

Kohli, R., Garg, A., Phutela, S., Kumar, Y., & Jain, S. (2021). An Improvised Model for Securing Cloud-Based E-Healthcare Systems. In *IoT in Healthcare and Ambient Assisted Living* (pp. 293–310). Springer.

Sivan, R., & Zukarnain, Z. A. (2021). Security and Privacy in Cloud-Based E-Health System. *Symmetry*, *13*(5), 742.

AlShamsi, M., Salloum, S. A., Alshurideh, M., & Abdallah, S. (2021). Artificial intelligence and blockchain for transparency in governance. In *Artificial Intelligence for Sustainable Development: Theory, Practice and Future Applications* (pp. 219–230). Springer.

[] Ploder, C., Spiess, T., Bernsteiner, R., Dilger, T., &Weichelt, R. (2021). A Risk Analysis on Blockchain Technology Usage for Electronic Health Records. *Cloud Computing and Data Science*, 1-16.

Chen, Y., Ding, S., Xu, Z., Zheng, H., & Yang, S. (2019). Blockchain-based medical records secure storage and medical service framework. *Journal of Medical Systems*, *43*(1), 1–9.

Evangelatos, N., Özdemir, V., & Brand, A. (2020). Blockchain for digital health: Prospects and challenges. *OMICS: A Journal of Integrative Biology*, *24*(5), 237–240.

Premkumar, A., & Srimathi, C. (2020, March). Application of Blockchain and IoT towards Pharmaceutical Industry. In *2020 6th International Conference on Advanced Computing and Communication Systems (ICACCS)* (pp. 729-733). IEEE.

Ahmad, R. W., Salah, K., Jayaraman, R., Yaqoob, I., Ellahham, S., & Omar, M. (2021). The role of blockchain technology in telehealth and telemedicine. *International Journal of Medical Informatics*, ●●●, 104399.

Hathaliya, J., Sharma, P., Tanwar, S., & Gupta, R. (2019, December). Blockchain-based remote patient monitoring in healthcare 4.0. In *2019 IEEE 9th International Conference on Advanced Computing (IACC)* (pp. 87-91). IEEE.

Le Nguyen, T. (2018, August). Blockchain in healthcare: A new technology benefit for both patients and doctors. In *2018 Portland International Conference on Management of Engineering and Technology (PICMET)* (pp. 1-6). IEEE.

Patel, V. (2019). A framework for secure and decentralized sharing of medical imaging data via blockchain consensus. *Health Informatics Journal*, *25*(4), 1398–1411.

McBee, M. P., & Wilcox, C. (2020). Blockchain technology: Principles and applications in medical imaging. *Journal of Digital Imaging*, *33*(3), 726–734.

Xu, R., Chen, S., Yang, L., Chen, Y., & Chen, G. (2019, February). Decentralized autonomous imaging data processing using blockchain. In *Multimodal Biomedical Imaging XIV* (Vol. 10871, p. 108710U). International Society for Optics and Photonics.

Shubbar, S. (2017). *Ultrasound medical imaging systems using telemedicine and blockchain for remote monitoring of responses to neoadjuvant chemotherapy in women's breast cancer: concept and implementation* (Doctoral dissertation, Kent State University).

Kumar, R., & Tripathi, R. (2021). Building an IPFS and Blockchain-Based Decentralized Storage Model for Medical Imaging. In *Advancements in Security and Privacy Initiatives for Multimedia Images* (pp. 19–40). IGI Global.

Witowski, J., Choi, J., Jeon, S., Kim, D., Chung, J., Conklin, J., ... Do, S. (2021). MarkIt: A Collaborative Artificial Intelligence Annotation Platform Leveraging Blockchain for Medical Imaging Research. *Blockchain in Healthcare Today*, *4*(176), 1–9.

Koptyra, K., & Ogiela, M. R. (2021). Imagechain—Application of Blockchain Technology for Images. *Sensors (Basel)*, *21*(1), 82.

Kumar, R., Wang, W., Kumar, J., Yang, T., Khan, A., Ali, W., & Ali, I. (2021). An Integration of Blockchain and AI for Secure Data Sharing and Detection of CT images for the Hospitals. *Computerized Medical Imaging and Graphics*, *87*, 101812.

Sultana, M., Hossain, A., Laila, F., Taher, K. A., & Islam, M. N. (2020). Towards developing a secure medical image sharing system based on zero trust principles and blockchain technology. *BMC Medical Informatics and Decision Making*, *20*(1), 1–10.

Khubrani, M. M. (2021). A Framework for Blockchain-based Smart Health System. *Turkish Journal of Computer and Mathematics Education*, *12*(9), 2609–2614.

Demirkan, H. (2013). A Smart Healthcare Systems Framework. *IT Professional*, *15*(5), 38–45.

Shukla, R. G., Agarwal, A., & Shukla, S. (2020). Blockchain-powered smart healthcare system. In *Handbook of Research on Blockchain Technology* (pp. 245–270). Academic Press.

Qiu, J., Liang, X., Shetty, S., & Bowden, D. (2018, September). Towards secure and smart healthcare in smart cities using blockchain. In *2018 IEEE International Smart Cities Conference (ISC2)* (pp. 1-4). IEEE.

Haque, A. B., Muniat, A., Ullah, P. R., & Mushsharat, S. (2021, February). An Automated Approach towards Smart Healthcare with Blockchain and Smart Contracts. In *2021 International Conference on Computing, Communication, and Intelligent Systems (ICCCIS)* (pp. 250-255). IEEE.

Bhawiyuga, A., Wardhana, A., Amron, K., & Kirana, A. P. (2019, December). Platform for Integrating Internet of Things Based Smart Healthcare System and Blockchain Network. In *2019 6th NAFOSTED Conference on Information and Computer Science (NICS)* (pp. 55-60). IEEE.

Kumar, A., Krishnamurthi, R., Nayyar, A., Sharma, K., Grover, V., & Hossain, E. (2020). A Novel Smart Healthcare Design, Simulation, and Implementation Using Healthcare 4.0 Processes. *IEEE Access : Practical Innovations, Open Solutions*, 8(1), 118433–118471.

Farhin, F., Kaiser, M. S., & Mahmud, M. (2021). Secured Smart Healthcare System: Blockchain and Bayesian Inference Based Approach. In *Proceedings of International Conference on Trends in Computational and Cognitive Engineering* (pp. 455-465). Springer, Singapore.

Azogu, I., Norta, A., Papper, I., Longo, J., & Draheim, D. (2019, April). A Framework for the Adoption of Blockchain Technology in Healthcare Information Management Systems: A Case Study of Nigeria. In *Proceedings of the 12th International Conference on Theory and Practice of Electronic Governance* (pp. 310-316).

Chattu, V. K., Nanda, A., Chattu, S. K., Kadri, S. M., & Knight, A. W. (2019). The emerging role of blockchain technology applications in routine disease surveillance systems to strengthen global health security. *Big Data and Cognitive Computing*, 3(2), 25–38.

Marbouh, D., Abbasi, T., Maasmi, F., Omar, I. A., Debe, M. S., Salah, K., ... Ellahham, S. (2020). Blockchain for COVID-19: Review, Opportunities, and a Trusted Tracking System. *Arabian Journal for Science and Engineering*, 45(1), 9895–9911.

Gatteschi, V., Lamberti, F., Demartini, C., Pranteda, C., & Santamaria, V. (2018). To blockchain or not to blockchain: That is the question. *IT Professional*, 20(2), 62–74.

Soltanisehat, L., Alizadeh, R., Hao, H., & Choo, K. K. R. (2020). Technical, Temporal, and Spatial Research Challenges and Opportunities in Blockchain-Based Healthcare: A Systematic Literature Review. *IEEE Transactions on Engineering Management*, 1–16. doi:10.1109/TEM.2020.3013507

Kuo, T. T., & Ohno-Machado, L. (2018). Model Chain: Decentralized privacy-preserving healthcare predictive 154 modelling framework on private blockchain networks. arXiv preprint arXiv:1802.01746.

McConaghy, T., Marques, R., Müller, A., De Jonghe, D., McConaghy, T., & McMullen, G. ... &Granzotto, A. (2016). Bigchaindb: a scalable blockchain database. white paper, BigChainDB, 1-70.

Lorenz, J. T., Münstermann, B., Higginson, M., Olesen, P. B., Bohlken, N., & Ricciardi, V. (2017). Blockchain in Insurance–Opportunity or Threat? McKinsey & Company. http://www.mckinsey.com/~/media/McKinsey/Industries/Financial Services/Our Insights/Blockchain in insurance opportunity or threat/Blockchain-in-insurance-opportunity-or-threat.ashx. Accessed April 20, 2020.

Liang, X., Zhao, J., Shetty, S., Liu, J., & Li, D. (2017, October). Integrating blockchain for data sharing and collaboration in mobile healthcare applications. In *2017 IEEE 28th Annual International Symposium on Personal, Indoor, and Mobile Radio Communications (PIMRC)* (pp. 1-5).

Angraal, S., Krumholz, H. M., & Schulz, W. L. (2017). Blockchain technology: Applications in health care. *Circulation: Cardiovascular Quality and Outcomes*, *10*(9), e003800.

Rakic, D. (2018, March). Blockchain Technology in Healthcare. In *ICT4AWE* (pp. 13-20).

William, J. (2016). *Blockchain: The Simple Guide Everything You Need to Know*. CreateSpace. Independent Publishing Platform.

Aithal, P. S. (2019). Information Communication & Computation Technology (ICCT) as a Strategic Tool for Industry Sectors. [IJAEML]. *International Journal of Applied Engineering and Management Letters*, *3*(2), 65–80.

Aithal, P. S., & Aithal, S. (2019). Management of ICCT underlying Technologies used for Digital Service Innovation. [IJMTS]. *International Journal of Management, Technology, and Social Sciences*, *4*(2), 110–136.

Aithal, P. S., & Aithal, S. (2019, October). Digital Service Innovation Using ICCT Underlying Technologies. In *Proceedings of International Conference on Emerging Trends in Management, IT and Education* (Vol. 1, No. 1, pp. 33-63).

Chapter 4

Applications of Game Theory in a Blockchain–Based Healthcare Information System

Kamalendu Pal

ⓘD https://orcid.org/0000-0001-7158-6481
City, University of London, UK

ABSTRACT

Healthcare service providers are dependent on accurate information systems. Some crucial challenges are (1) improvement of patient caring services, (2) containing the deployment cost of information systems, and (3) avoiding any disturbances in its business processes at the time of data gathering and processing activities. Technological advancements are a significant driver of efficient healthcare information systems and services. By creating a rich healthcare-related data foundation and integrating technologies like the internet of things (IoT), blockchain technology, artificial intelligence (AI) techniques, and big data analytics, the digital transformation in healthcare is recognized as a pivotal component to tackle these challenges. For example, it can improve diagnostics, prevention, and patient therapy, ultimately empowering caregivers to use an evidence-based method to enhance clinical decision-making. Real-time interactions permit a physician to monitor a patient 'live' instead of interaction regularly (e.g., weekly, monthly). This way, healthcare operation can provide better services. However, the IoT system creates the risk of a sensitive data breach without a highly secure infrastructure. Blockchain technology improves the reliance on a centralized authority to certify information integrity and ownership and mediate transactions and exchange of digital assets. As a result, the mining process in the blockchain is very resource-intensive; hence, miners create coalition groups to cross-check each block of transactions in return for a reward. In addition, it creates enormous competition among miners, and consequently,

DOI: 10.4018/978-1-7998-9606-7.ch004

dishonest mining strategies (e.g., block withholding attack, selfish mining, eclipse attack) need to be controlled. Consequently, it is necessary to regulate the mining process to make miners accountable for any dishonest mining behaviours; game theory can help regulate it. Finally, this chapter presents a survey of game theory used to address the common issues in the blockchain network.

INTRODUCTION

The world has been going through a challenging time in recent years. On the one hand, the coronavirus pandemic (i.e., COVID-19) is placing enormous strain on the global healthcare sector's workforce, infrastructure, its supply chain and exposing social inequities in healthcare. In contrast, medical and technical advances are driving better healthcare for humanity across the globe. Several foundational shifts are arising from the COVID-19's spread. For example, patients are heavily involved in treatment decision-making processes, the rapid use of virtual consultation, the adoption of interoperable data and data analytics, and tremendous public-private collaborations in the healthcare industry and related service innovation.

The long-standing assumption that healthcare is '*sick care*' for the physical body, including patients' minds and spirits, has changed. Focus shifting from healthcare to health and well-being and providers should integrate this shift into the design of their service offering and delivery channels and locations. In addition, consumers (or patients) will expect care to be available when and how it is most convenient and safe for them. It includes virtual care, at-home prescription delivery, remote monitoring, digital diagnostic and decision support, self-service education applications, and social support.

Consequently, healthcare organizations invest in optimizing or replacing foundational structures, technologies, and business processes automation. Digital transformation helps individual healthcare organizations and the broader health ecosystem improve working methods, widen access to services, and provide a more effective patient and clinician experience. In addition, four critical aspects of computing are playing increasingly pivotal roles (i.e., IoT, blockchain, cloud computing, and artificial intelligence) in this transformation.

Along with technological advancement, healthcare service provision is changing rapidly. The IoT paradigm has revolutionized the healthcare industry. The IoT technology can help collect invaluable patient data, automate workflows, provide insights on disease symptoms and trends, and facilitate remote patient care. Over these years, several advanced IoT applications developed to support patients and medical officials. For example, IoT technology-based healthcare improves existing features by supporting patient management, medical records management, medical emergency management, patient treatment management, and other facilities, thus increasing the quality of healthcare information technology (IT) based applications.

However, many exiting IoT-based healthcare systems leveraged for managing data are centralized and pose potential risks of a single point of failure. Blockchain technology (Nakamoto, 2008) provides more intelligent and flexible handing of transactional data through appropriate convergence with IoT technology in supporting data integration and processing. This chapter describes a review of game theory models used to address common issues in the blockchain network. It includes different security issues (e.g., selfish mining, Denial of Service (DoS) attack, regarding mining management). Reward allocation, the verified transactional information is stored in a chain of blocks (a central data structure), and the chain grows in an append-only manner with all new verified blocks to it. This way, the whole process consists of many operations, for example, verifying transactions, disseminating blocks, and attaching blocks to the blockchain.

Blockchain-based information systems need several consensus nodes to participate in the information exchange network. The rational nodes perform actions or strategies to optimize their utility. In addition, the malicious nodes may launch attacks that damage the blockchain-enabled IoT information-sharing networks. Game theory-based techniques can mitigate consensus protocols such as Byzantine Fault Tolerance (BFT) protocol (Castro & Liskov, 2002). Nevertheless, the consensus protocols require a centralized permission controller and only achieve a tiny group of nodes. Such a consensus protocol is thus not useable to the blockchain network that is a decentralized and large-scale system. Different techniques and remedies (e.g., a Markov Decision Process (MDP) (Altman, 1999)) were deployed to optimize strategies of the blockchain nodes to stop their inappropriate behaviours. However, the minimization methods do not consider the interactions among the nodes.

In recent decades, game theory (Myerson, 2013) has been applied as an alternative solution in the blockchain network. Game theory uses mathematical modelling techniques for strategic interaction among rational decision-makers (Han et al., 2012). In this way, game theory can be used to analyze the strategies of the consensus node and the interactions among them. For example, in blockchain-based information systems that incentivize nodes to participate in the consensus process of the data stored with digital tokens, the consensus nodes are often called block miners, and their operations are referred to as *mining*. In the theory-based game analysis, the nodes can learn and predict mining behaviours of each other, then have optimal reaction strategies based on equilibrium analysis. Also, game theory can be used to develop incentive methods that discourage the nodes from executing inappropriate behaviours or launching attacks. This way, game theory-based mathematical models are natural in the decision making of all the consensus nodes in the blockchain networks.

There are reviews available regarding blockchain technology and its industrial applications. However, these research reviews do not provide the uses of the game theory in blockchain-based technology. For example, a group of researchers (Tschorsch & Scheuermann, 2016) provided a comprehensive introduction of the bitcoin network. Different groups of researchers (Pal & Yasar, 2020) (Conti et al., 2018) (Khalilov & Levi, 2018) describe security and privacy-related issues in blockchain technology (Pal, 2022).

This chapter provides a review with a reasonable literature survey on the game theory-based frameworks in the blockchain network. Simplistically, the related research works in this chapter review are grouped based on issues in the blockchain network. The significant technical issues consist of (i) security-related issues (e.g., Deniable of Service (DoS) attacks, selfish mining attacks), (ii) mining operational management related issues (e.g., pool selection, allocation of computational power, fork chain selection, and reward allocation); and (iii) energy trading in blockchain technology.

More specifically, this chapter first investigates the rational characteristics of smart contracts. For example, healthcare data privacy attackers may adopt rational, smart contracts and intelligent criminal contracts to maximize their incomes. Since the encouragement of the rational parties is economic incentives, they have enough motivation to sponsor rational attacks by leveraging incentive mechanisms in game theory. The primary function of the consensus layer is responsible for assigning rewards. This chapter outlines some rational consensus mechanisms. Finally, the chapter highlights the future directions concerning the combination of game theory and blockchain.

BACKGROUND PRELIMINARIES OF BLOCKCHAIN TECHNOLOGY

Blockchain technology was first proposed as a decentralized tamper-proof ledger that records transactions. Also, the individual transaction is verified by using a decentralized consensus mechanism between the trustless business partners (or agents) before including it in the chain. Some of the main benefits that blockchain networks can provide are discussed below.

Decentralized network: In simple, the distributed network permits each computing unit to use computing power in the blockchain. Besides, each transaction within the blockchain network must manage the agreement among all the nodes through the consensus protocol. The decentralized network management monopoly can be bypassed in blockchain technology.

Figure 1. The structure of a block

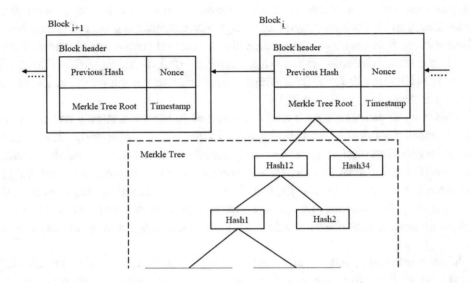

Tamper-proof ledger: The specialized encryption techniques (i.e., cryptographic) are used in blockchain to ensure that all the nodes in the network can observe any change in the transaction data in the blockchain. This way, the transaction recorded in the blockchain cannot be altered and tampered with unless blockchain nodes are compromised due to different vulnerabilities.

Transparent transaction: Transparency ensures that fund/information transfer agents can keep track of individual business transactional data/ information in real-time.

Trustless, secure trading: In blockchain technology, trustlessness means that one does not need to place sole trust in any stranger, institution, or third party for a network or payment system to work. Trustless systems work and achieve consensus mainly through code, asymmetric cryptography, and blockchain network protocols.

Data Organization and Workflow of Blockchain

Cryptographic data organization acts as an essential role in the blockchain structure. This section introduces some crucial components helping the data organization within blockchain-based P2P networks.

   Transaction: Transaction is the most common part of blockchain technology. The blockchain user describes a transaction, and it is composed of the transaction data, which specifies the value in concern.

Block: All blocks in a blockchain consists of the same components: (i) a block number, (ii) the hash of the previous block, (iii) Nonce, a random number, (iv) the transactions data, (v) timestamp with the time the block is found/ created, and (vi) the hash of the current block.

In other words, an individual block has a block number that, combined with the previous has and the present hash, determine the order in which the transaction took place. The accompanying timestamp determines when the transactions are recorded to have taken place. The data contains the transactions, consisting of nearly everything, not solely cryptocurrency value.

Hash Pointer: The hash is the complex mathematical problem (or the 'proof-of-work) the miner must solve to find a block. This goes as follows: (i) a random number is guessed (this is called the 'Nonce'), (ii) the 'Nonce' is included at the end of all the data in the block, (iii) this is all hashed according to SHA256 method, and (iv) if this hash begins with a calculated number of zeros, a new block is found. If this is not the case, the miner must start again at step 1 with guessing another Nonce.

The hash pointer of the current block must have the hash value connected to the previous block that also has a similar structure. Hence, the hash pointers can be used to build a link of records, i.e., blockchain.

Merkle Tree: Simply, a Merkle tree or hash tree with a leaf node contains the hash-value of the transaction data of a block. Also, non-leaf nodes are marked by the hash value of the concatenation of their child nodes. This structure makes it impossible to tamper with the data in blockchain privately. Figure 1 presents a blockchain data structure where the transactions are included in the block, and a Merkle root represents the block.

Blockchains are decentralized and distributed database systems that keep track of a continuously growing list of *blocks*. Every block has got a *timestamp* and a link to a previous block. By structural characteristics, blockchains are inherently resistant to modifying the data it holds. Functionally, a blockchain can serve as an open, distributed ledger that can record information exchanges (known as transactions) between a business partner in a healthcare business efficiently and in a verifiable and permanent way. To understand the basic concept of the verifiable and permanent way, let us present an example. For example, a health authority wants to provide the sales price of an item from a supplier, as shown in Figure 1.

The monetary value of transaction records on the blockchain does not need a third '*authority*' (e.g., a bank). The transaction does not need to be verified by a third authority (e.g., a bank); it is being 'checked' by everyone who participates in the system and everyone who will join the system in the future. Thus, releasing the need for a centralized third party has several benefits like fewer transfer costs (after all, there are no more person-hours needed to check everything). Moreover, it has the potential of being more anonymous while making it both simpler to pay globally and nearly impossible to 'reverse' transactions (which the third 'trusted' party could decide to do).

As shown in Figure 1, a simple blockchain is an appending only, ever-growing list of blocks connected sequentially using the hash pointers as a linear linked-list structure. Also, the block header includes a hash pointer that relates to the previous block, and transactional information (or data) is represented as Merkle tree structures.

The simple cryptographic data organization maintains the blockchain network's essential requirements for blockchain nodes to create the transaction, store the data into blocks, cross-check the transaction for verification purposes, and eventually reach a consensus.

The development of hardware technologies, typical standalone IoT-based applications may no longer satisfy the advanced need for efficiency and security in the high degree of heterogeneity of hardware devices and complex data formats. Firstly, centralized architecture's burdensome connectivity and maintenance costs result in low scalability. Secondly, the systems that are centralized become more vulnerable to outsider attacks (Pal & Yasar, 2020).

In this way, a decentralized approach based on blockchain technology may solve the above problems in a typical centralized IoT-based information system. Mainly, the above justification is for three reasons. Firstly, an autonomous decentralized information system is feasible for trusted business partners to join the network, independently improving the business task-processing ability. Secondly, multiparty coordination enhances nodes' state consistency that information system crashes are avoidable due to a single-point failure. Thirdly, nodes could synchronize the whole information system state only by coping with the blockchain ledger to minimize the computation related activities and improve storage load.

The success of information sharing using blockchain technology is based on its robust incentive mechanism. In this information-sharing framework, transactions are grouped in blocks to be verified by a subset of nodes in the network, known as *miners*. The mining activity, called *proof-of-work* (PoW), is computational resource intensive. Hence, nodes form *mining pools* under the supervision of *pool managers* to accomplish the mining task. The first mining pool that accomplishes the PoW is rewarded a certain amount of freshly mined information as an incentive for miners' works. This is the reason that why this process is also known as *mining*. Next, the verified block is attached to the list of existing verified blocks, known as the *blockchain*. Immediately after that, all miners stop the mining process of the already verified block and start working on the next block.

The first mining pool that accomplishes the proof-of-work is rewarded a certain amount of freshly mined healthcare data as an incentive for miners' works. That is why this process is also known as mining. Once a block is verified, it is attached to

Figure 2. Blockchain and mining

Block #	77		Block #	78		Block #	79
Nonce	272931		Nonce	171943		Nonce	**Try diff values**
Transactions	10B Alice → Bob ... 50B Alex → Mary		Transactions	10B Sara → Eli ... 50B Eve → Cory		Transactions	10B John → Ed ... 50B Dan → Geff
Previous	000937af19be17		Previous	007ae291da311		Previous	009da7537eb68
Current Hash	007ae291da311		Current Hash	009da7537eb68		Current Hash	**Find a valid Hash**

the blockchain's existing verified blocks. Immediately after that, all miners stop the mining process of the already verified block and start working on the next block.

The high-level idea of the proof-of-work/verification/mining is shown in Figure 2. Each block consists of a block number, a nonce value, a list of transactions, the hash value of the previous block (address of the previous block), and the hash value of the next block (address of the next block). During the mining process, the miners try to generate a valid hash value of a block that is less than a threshold (i.e., it starts with a certain number of zeros). The system will conduct this process by trying different nonce values.

The stochastic game theory-based model can be used efficiently to analyze the miners' selection of chains to mine regarding the data transactions of blockchain structure in healthcare information systems. The game begins at an initial state, and at a stage, each miner observes the blockchain structure and then chooses its strategy (i.e., select a chain to mine). Every miner receives an immediate payoff associated with the current state and the miners' strategies.

Excluding from the chain identification, the stochastic game can be used for mining management, for example, the selection between investing in computational power or leaving the mining (Dhamal et al., 2018) and the selection of chain to mine (Biais et al., 2019). Moreover, the stochastic game has also been widely applied to security issues and was utilized to analyze the identification between honest mining and selfish mining (Zhen et al., 2017), the decision of the appropriate time to release the mined block (Kroll et al., 2013), and the selection of adding a block to the chain (Kim, 2019).

AN INTRODUCTION TO GAME THEORY

Healthcare business decisions in a competitive situation do not depend on the organization's conclusion alone but the interaction between the decisions of the organization and those of competitors. For example, each business organization (e.g., hospital, ambulance service, pharmaceutical company) tries to select and execute its strategies and maximize its gains at the cost of its opponents (or competitors). Similarly, a competitor also selects the best strategies to counteract its opponent's gains. Finally, the game theory deals with such problems where actions and interactions of competing business organizations rise to conditions of business conflict (i.e., competitive situations).

John Von Neuman first introduced game Theory concepts in 1928 (Neuman, 1928), formalizing the idea of a game and providing proof for the famous Minimax theorem. His book titled "Theory and Practice of Games and Economic Behaviour", which he co-authored with Morgenstern, is considered a pioneer work by experts worldwide. These works significantly impacted the development of linear programming and Wald's statistical decision theory.

Terminology of Game Theory

Players: The participants who act as decision-makers are known as players. When two competitors oppose the other, the game is known as a *"two-person game"*.

Strategies: A finite number of possible *courses of actions* available to a player are called '*strategies*. For example, the mining process in blockchain technology is tremendously resources consuming. Hence, miners form groups (or *coalitions*) to cross-check each block of transactions in return for a reward where only the first coalition that achieves the proof-of-work will be rewarded. This rewarding mechanism creates intense competition among minors and, consequently, dishonest mining strategies, such as block withholding attacks, Denial of Service (DoS) attacks, and selfish mining-related attacks, are simple examples of theory-based game analysis.

Play: A play occurs when each player selects one of the available strategies. Two basic assumptions in a play are: (i) the choice of courses of action by players are made simultaneously, and (ii) no player knows the choice of the opponent(s).

Rational Player: A player is simply considered reasonable (e.g., self-interested) if the player tries to maximize personal payoff.

Outcome: Every combination of strategies of players determines an outcome called payoff.

Payoff Matrix: The gains resulting from a game are presented in a table called *"payoff matrix"*.

A payoff matrix comprises of "n" number of rows, n being a few strategies of the first player (e.g., Player A) and "m" number of column "m" being the number of strategies of the second player (e.g., Player B). The payoff for each combination of

Table 1. A payoff matrix

		Player B		
		I	**II**	**III**
	I	6	2	3
Player A	II	2	-1	-3
	III	5	4	5

strategies of the players is placed as elements within the matrix. A positive entry indicates gain to A (i.e., payment from B to A), whilst a negative entry denotes gain to B (i.e., payment from A to B).

A simple payoff matrix is shown in Table 5. The payoff matrix may be interpreted as under (i) there are two players, A and B in the game, (ii) player A has three strategies while player B has four strategies, (iii) elements such as 4, 2, 4, 3 against the first row; 2, - 4, 2 and 0 against the second row; and 3, -6, 4 and 2 against third row represent the payoff or gains of players. A positive entry represents a payment from B to A, whilst a negative entry denotes a payment from A to B. For example, if player A uses his second strategy and player B uses first, B pays A 2 units.

The strategies can be classified into two types: (i) pure strategy and (ii) mixed strategy. A *pure strategy* is the player's decision always to select the same strategy. A *mixed strategy* is the player's decision to select more than a strategy with fixed probabilities in advance of all plays. A mixed strategy is advantageous since the opponent is always kept guessing.

There are different types of games that are used for forming theory-based game strategies: (i) non-cooperative game, (ii) extensive-form game, (iii) Stackelberg game, and (iv) stochastic game are the only few considered in this chapter.

Non-Cooperative Game: These games are commonly analyzed through the scheme of non-cooperative game theory, which bids to anticipate players' sole plans (or strategies) and payoffs. A non-cooperative game needs action characterizing (i) the number of players, (ii) the conceivable deals applicable to an individual player, and any compulsions that may be required on them, (iii) the goal function of individual player which s/he pursuits to optimize, (iv) any time sequence of the execution of the actions of the players are permitted to take in consideration more than once, (v) any information gathering that takes place and how the information available to a player at an individual step in time depends on the previous actions of other players, and (vi) whether there a player whose action is the outcome of a possibilistic outcome with a known pattern of distribution.

Extensive-form Game: The extensive-form game is a characterizing of a game in game theory, permitting (as the name suggests) for categorical illustration of different crucial characteristics, like the step-by-step actions of players' good moves, their choices at every decision point, the (conceivable perfect) information individual player has about the other player's actions when they decide, and their payoffs for all permissible game outcomes.

Stackelberg Game: The Stackelberg stewardship game is a decision theory in economics in which the steward business moves first, and then the follower business move subsequently. The name of this game has been selected after the German economist Heinrich Freiherr von Stackelberg, who highlighted the 'Market Structure and Equilibrium' concept in a publication in 1943 and presented this model of game theory. In this game theory, the players belong to separate groups – leader and follower, and they contend.

Stochastic Game: A stochastic game, popularized by Lloyd Shapley in the early 1950s, is a duplicated game with probabilistic changeovers played by one or more players. This game is simple played in a step-by-step manner. At the start of each step, players select actions, and each player gets an estimated payoff for that situation. Next, the initial procedures repeat the initial step and play advances for successive stages.

Blockchain-based healthcare information system's collaborations are mainly designed and used to model different selfish mining techniques. In these models, two-player games (changeable to any number of players) are formed in which both players (e.g., attacker, defender) try to maximize the utility that each can achieve. For example, the defenders of information systems will be able to provide value to design and, as a result, achieve utility by enabling features, shifting the attack surface, and minimizing the attack surface measurement. Similarly, the attackers will execute utility if features are disabled, or the attack surface measurement is increased.

APPLICATIONS OF GAME THEORY FOR SELFISH MINING ATTACK

Selfish mining is a type of subversive strategy in PoW based blockchain system (Eyal & Sirer, 2014) that hackers (i.e., malicious miners or mining pool managers) may not broadcast the newly mined blocks but chooses to (i) keep the block isolated or (ii) hide and then release the block at a particular time. In this circumstance, honest miners waste their computational power finding the block discovered already, and malicious miners can enhance their possibility of finding the consequent block in the chain. The Pool Block WithHolding (PBWH) attack is one typical selfish mining attack (Courtois, 2014); in the PBWH attack, the attacking pool infiltrates the attacked pool, and the infiltrating miners perform the Block WithHolding (BWH) attack, i.e., withhold all the blocks newly discovered in the attacked pool.

To prevent a selfish attack, it is crucial to analyze the strategies of the miners and pools and the interaction among them. For example, a Markov Decision Process (MDP) (Sapirshtein et al., 2016) can analyze the strategy and utility of the individual player, i.e., the miner or the pool; however, the MDP does not consider the interaction among multiple players. Alternatively, game theory can be effectively applied.

In a research project, the researcher (Eyal, 2015) adopted a non-cooperative game to analyze the interaction among the pools. It used the well-known *'Prisoners' Dilemma'* of game theory (Han et al., 2012) to experiment. To circumvent the miners' dilemma, the miners can select one of the following options: (i) The miners can join private pools that will not involve the Block WithHolding (BWH) attack. As an outcome of this strategy, big mining pools may need to divide into many small pools, and consequently, it might lead to a favourable environment for blockchain-based information sharing. (ii) The other use of the game theory-based solution is that the miners perform so-called Zero Determinant (ZD) strategies (He at el., 2016). Another group of researchers (Zhen et al., 2017) presented a model consisting of a two-miner mining case as a stochastic iterative game. This is a bit different from a stereotype strategy that aims to enhance players' profits; the ZD strategy is used to manipulate an outcome of the opponents in a typical range to get rid of common social welfare (i.e., the complete pool's profit) (Zhang et al., 2016). This way, in the game, two players are philanthropic miners (i.e., in other words, a minor tries to maximize social welfare) and a selfish miner (i.e., the miner only tries to maximize the profit).

This includes the strategies of cooperation. The main characteristics are – mining honestly and purging the BWH attack on the other miners. This way, the altruistic miner and selfish miner choose their combatting plans using possibilistic reasoning based on each other's planning method iteratively. The research result presents that so long as the altruistic miner use strategies relating to the determinant function (i.e., a liner function which is related to players' profit factor), the profit of the selfish miner is in a range from cooperation to mutual attack irrespective of strategies used by the selfish miner. Therefore, the altruistic miner can inspire the selfish miner to cooperate by using ZD planning techniques to restrict the selfish miner's profit to gain the maximum social welfare. Experimental results demonstrate that the proposed game model can accomplish better social welfare than the proposed pool (Eyal, 2015).

Nonetheless, the described game does not consider the profit of the altruistic miner. In other words, it means that the altruistic miner may not have a payoff to use the ZD selfish planning method. Thus, the two-pool-attacker business use case in (Zhen et al., 2017) can also be found (Eyal, 2015). However, besides the PBWH attack, a researcher (Eyal, 2015) treated the miners' migration among the pools;

specifically, the pool miners can be migrated to another pool and launch the PBWH attack to increase the payoff value.

A group of researchers (Chatterjee et al., 2018) described the average payoff of the miner and miners' stochastic migration process (known as Concurrent Mean-payoff Game (CMPG)) is used. In this process, the players are pool one and pool two, and the state of the game includes the number of migrated miners of pool one and that of pool two. In doing so, a strategic technique is to evaluate: (i) the number of its miners to be relocated to the other pool and (ii) the miners who perform the PBWH attack. The number of relocated miners need to evaluate the dependency of the attractiveness levels of the other pool. By doing so, it evaluates the mining reward to the total computational power of its miners. This way, the pool's profit can formulate an appropriate strategy. Moreover, the research approaches (i.e., (Eyal, 2015) (Zhen et al., 2017) (Chatterjee et al., 2018)) are used only two pools for their experimentation and a multi-pool approach where the researchers consider more than two pools (Luu et al., 2015) (Laraki, 2002) to model the PBWH attack.

In recent years, researchers have been involved in researching strategy options to provide a maximum payoff for blockchain-based information systems modelling. Their projected payoffs, the players (i.e., the miners, the pools) are selecting affirmative computational power and selecting: (i) distributed computational ability to lunch the BWH attack, (ii) honestly follow or randomly deviate from the pool's protocol. In addition, it provides opportunities for broader game theory-based applications design and development.

CHALLENGES AND FUTURE RESEARCH DIRECTIONS

This chapter provides a brief review of applications of game theory to address a wide range of issues in blockchain networks and related systems. However, with the fast evolution of blockchain technologies and their applications, many emerging problems remain open for further studies, which can be solved using game theory.

In the context of healthcare data collaboration, this chapter presents a review of game theory-based approaches within a blockchain network. In future, this research will consider the following aspects of blockchain technology: (i) the smart contract automatically runs relating to the code agreed initially that are not affected by the outside world during the execution process, (ii) the incentive technique is one of the essential methods of blockchain technology, and to maximize their benefits, rational miners need to be investigated, and (iii) study the evolution effects of rational behaviours.

Moreover, the future intends to provide new solution concepts in which the extra utility incentivizes the attackers to act according to the defenders' strategies (i.e., deception).

CONCLUSION

The digital healthcare systems have produced efficiencies, new innovative customer-focused services, and patient relationships globally by using IoT technology, mobile services, social media, data analytics, and service-orient computing applications to generate models for better decisions. Blockchain technology is recently introduced and revolutionizing the digital healthcare world brings a new perspective to information systems' security, privacy, and efficiency.

This chapter introduced a game-theoretical solution concept that can be adopted to tackle collusion attacks in P2P based networks. It has presented a review of existing research literature of game theory in the blockchain. The chapter has given an overview of blockchain with its structure, workflow, and incentive compatibility. Then, it has introduced the basic knowledge of game theory and several game models to realize the prompt of using game theory to analyze interactions among different components in the blockchain. Afterwards, the chapter has provided surveys of some existing literature. Finally, it analyses the applications of game theory to deal with various problems regarding security, mining management in blockchain-based information systems. Finally, the chapter has described existing challenges and future research directions.

REFERENCES

Altman, E. (1999). Constrained Markov decision processes. CRC Press.

Biais, B., Bisiere, C., Bouvard, M., & Casamatta, C. (2019). The blockchain folk theorem. Review of Financial Studies, 32(5), 1662–1715.

Castro, M., & Liskov, B. (2002). B. (2002). "Practical byzantine fault tolerance and proactive recovery. ACM Transactions on Computer Systems, 20(4), 398–461.

Chatterjee, K., Goharshady, A. K., Ibsen-Jensen, R. & Velner, Y. (2018). Ergodic mean-payoff games for the analysis of attacks in cryptocurrencies. *CONCUR 2018*, 11:1 – 11:17.

Conti, M., Kumar, S., Lal, C., & Ruj, S. (2018). A survey on security and privacy issues of bitcoin. IEEE Communications Surveys and Tutorials.

Courtois, T. (2014). On The Longest Chain Rule and Programmed Self-Destruction of Crypto Currencies. *CoRR: Computing Research Repository*.

Dhamal, S., Chahed, T., Ben-Ameur, W., Altman, E., Sunny, A., & Poojary, S. (2018). *A stochastic game framework for analyzing computational investment strategies in distributed computing with application to blockchain mining*. Academic Press.

Eyal, I., & Sirer, E. G. (2014). Majority is not enough: Bitcoin mining is vulnerable. *Proc. of the International Financial Cryptography and Data Security Conference*.

Eyal, I. (2015). The miner's dilemma. In *Security and Privacy (SP), 2015 IEEE Symposium on*. IEEE.

Han, Z., Niyato, D., Saad, W., Basar, T., & Hjørungnes, A. (2012). Game theory in wireless and communication networks: theory, models, and applications. Cambridge University Press.

He, X., Dai, H., Ning, P., & Dutta, D. (2016). Zero-determinant strategies for multi-player multi-action iterated games. IEEE Signal Processing Letters, 23(3), 311–315.

Khalilov, M. C. K., & Levi, A. (2018). A survey on anonymity and privacy in bitcoin-like digital cash systems. IEEE Communications Surveys and Tutorials.

Kim, S. K. (2019). The Trailer of Blockchain Governance Game. Computers & Industrial Engineering, 136, 373–380.

Kroll, J. A., Davey, I. C., & Felten, E. W. (2013). The economics of bitcoin mining, or bitcoin in the presence of adversaries. *Proceedings of WEIS, 11*.

Kroll, J. A., Davey, I. C., & Felten, E. W. (2013). The economics of bitcoin mining, or bitcoin in the presence of adversaries. *Proceedings of WEIS, 11*.

Laraki, R. (2002). The splitting game and applications. International Journal of Game Theory, 30(3), 359–376.

Luu, L., Narayanan, V., Baweja, K., Zheng, C., Gilbert, S., & Saxena, P. (2015). *Scp: A computationally scalable byzantine consensus protocol for blockchains*. Cryptology ePrint Archive, Report 2015/1168, 2015. http://eprint.iacr.org/

Myerson, R. B. (2013). Game theory. Harvard University Press.

Nakamoto, S. (2008). *Bitcoin: A peer-to-peer electronic cash system*. Selfpublished Paper.

Neumann, J. V. (1928). Zur Theorie der Gesellschaftsspiele. *Mathematische Annalen, 100*, 295–300. doi:10.1007/bf01448847

Pal, K., & Yasar, A. (2020). Internet of Things and blockchain technology in apparel manufacturing supply chain data management. Procedia Computer Science, 170, 450–457.

Pal, K. (2020). Information sharing for manufacturing supply chain management based on blockchain technology. In I. Williams (Ed.), Cross-Industry Use of Blockchain Technology and Opportunities for the Future (pp. 1–17). IGI Global.

Pal, K. (2021). Applications of Secured Blockchain Technology in Manufacturing Industry. In Blockchain and AI Technology in the Industrial Internet of Things. IGI Global.

Pal, K. (2022). Blockchain Integrated Internet of Things Architecture in Privacy Preserving for Large Scale Healthcare Supply Chain Data. In Blockchain Technology and Computational Excellence for Society 5.0. IGI Global.

Sapirshtein, A., Sompolinsky, Y., & Zohar, A. (2016). Optimal selfish mining strategies in bitcoin. In *International Conference on Financial Cryptography and Data Security*. Springer.

Tschorsch, F., & Scheuermann, B. (2016). Bitcoin and beyond: A technical survey on decentralized digital currencies. IEEE Communications Surveys and Tutorials, 18(3), 2084–2123.

Zheng, Z., Xie, S., Dai, H., Chen, X., & Wang, H. (2017). An overview of blockchain technology: Architecture, consensus, and future trends. In *Big Data (BigData Congress), 2017 IEEE International Congress on*. IEEE.

Zheng, Z., Xie, S., Dai, H., Chen, X., & Wang, H. (2017). An overview of blockchain technology: Architecture, consensus, and future trends. In *Big Data (BigData Congress), 2017 IEEE International Congress on*. IEEE.

Zheng, Z., Xie, S., Dai, H. N., & Wang, H. (2016). Blockchain challenges and opportunities: A survey. Work Pap., 2016, 2016.

Chapter 5
Integration of Blockchain and Supply Chain Management

Manish Verma
DRDO, India

ABSTRACT

Supply chain has been the main process of sustainable products/services flow from supplier to customer in various industries. Blockchain has been a revolution in cryptocurrency, and it is the tamperproof, timestamp, consensus-based algorithm with the decentralized ledger. There are emerging applications of blockchain from financials to healthcare and creating various jobs in service industries. Big data and Industry 4.0 with the blockchain ecosystems can bring efficiencies and real-time transactions in the pharmaceutical industry from origin to distribution in the healthcare supply chain. This chapter shall explain the physical aspects of the integration of blockchain and supply chain management in pharmaceutical industries.

1. INTRODUCTION TO BLOCKCHAIN

Satoshi introduced the first digital money, the bitcoin cryptocurrency based on blockchain technology in 2009 (Bernard, 2018; Verma 2021) and its consensus's based decentralized organization engineering approves the honesty of information. A blockchain guarantees that any change in information is immediately identified. (Aich, 2019)

Since all information in a PC is just an assortment of pieces and bytes, they can be changed by any individual who can get to the computerized record. Indeed, even scrambled information can be changed if the private key is uncovered. Nonetheless,

DOI: 10.4018/978-1-7998-9606-7.ch005

all exchanges in a blockchain are "connected" together, and a change to any current exchange breaks a connection in the chain.

1.1 Brief Discussion About the Topic

Information put away in the blockchain is permanent and cannot be changed effectively. Hence, the information is added to the square after it is supported by everybody in the organization and accordingly permitting secure exchanges. The individuals who approve the exchanges and add them to the block are called miners.

Blockchain is Decentralized just as an open record. The transaction is the record of the exchanges done and because it is noticeable to everybody, along these lines is called an open record. No individual or any association oversees the exchanges.

Every single association in the blockchain network has been tamperproof and has been highly expensive in information credibility. Hence, the consensus-based algorithm in the distributed ledger is secure for every transaction in a blockchain.

1.2 Integration Issues of Blockchain and Supply Chain Management

The field of public authority has been effectively attempting to tap on the maximum capacity and force of blockchain innovation. The program of identity management for government schemes and security issues are of the utmost importance to the good governance of every nation with the emphasis on protection from ransomware and counterfeit hackers. (Ramadhani, 2018) Alleviating these dangers is urgent for any administration. With the blockchain information structures conveyed for the secure capacity of such information, governments can solidify the organization's security and forestall any break. It decreases the single-point-of-disappointment hazard and guarantees the least digital penetration in the information.

Through decentralization, blockchain can offer more straightforwardness in government activities. It can determine its kin that there are zero debasements and they can investigate and confirm the information whenever they need. Besides, it likewise not attainable for any administration to hold huge lumps of assets in this. They should be proficient and reduce the overhead of cyber events.

Blockchain can be executed to diminish the redundancies in tasks, smoothing out it, and diminishing any weight on reviews. It could likewise accelerate the way toward accommodating assets and numerous other government tasks. The legislatures of numerous nations are now executing blockchain innovations in large numbers of their activities.

Followmyvote is a drive that can even be utilized by the United Nations to guarantee more noteworthy straightforwardness in political decision casting a ballot and diminishing the number of citizen cheats such as proxy voting, double-counting, etc. This will illuminate the fairness of the constitution of the voting nation. Utilizing blockchain innovation, diminishes the expense of races, guarantees citizen protection, permits secure internet casting a ballot, along these lines expanding voter turnout.

The public authority of Estonia's Guardtime has held hands with Ericsson to make another middle for information base stockpiling and the board so open information can be safely moved to the next level of blockchain.

Numerous nations are now attempting to inject blockchain innovations into large numbers of their government activities. There have been high expectations that this would be extremely valuable in putting away a wide range of data and information like government licenses, brand names, Social Security numbers, visas, international IDs, and so forth.

1.3 Significance of Blockchain In the Computing Systems

The key advantages we can hope to accomplish while receiving Blockchain innovation into the business are given:

a.   It is a changeless public advanced record, which implies when an exchange is recorded, it cannot be altered.
b.   Because of the encryption highlight, Blockchain is consistently secure.
c.   The exchanges are done in a split second and straightforwardly, as the record is refreshed naturally.
d.   As it is a decentralized framework, no delegate expense is required.
e.   The realness of exchange is checked and affirmed by members.

1.4 Types of Blockchain

Blockchain is of four different types and these four types are as listed below and shown in figure 1. (Sabry, 2019)

●   Public Blockchain

A public blockchain network is a blockchain network where anybody can join at whatever point they need. Essentially, there are no limitations about interest. More along these lines, anybody can see the record and partake in the agreement interaction. For instance, Ethereum is one of the public blockchain stage models.

●   Private Blockchain

Figure 1. Overlapping diagram of four types of blockchains

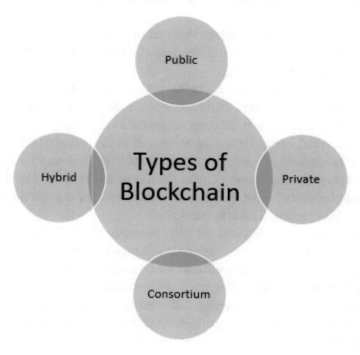

In a private blockchain, just a solitary association has authority over the organization. Thus, it implies that it is not open for the public to participate. All the private blockchain arrangements will have some type of approval plan for a personality who is entering the stage.

- Consortium Blockchain

A consortium blockchain is a blockchain innovation where rather than just a solitary association, different associations oversee the stage. It is anything but a public stage rather than a permission stage. More along these lines, it is very like private blockchains too.

- Hybrid Blockchain

Hybrid blockchain is a progressive kind of blockchain innovation. The blockchain is remarkably changing the world. It empowers ventures, governments, and different associations to more likely handle their work process and improve their frameworks with better arrangements.

1.5 Comparison Between the Blockchain Types with Examples

Blockchain has possible applications in numerous ventures, from bookkeeping to horticulture. It is anything but a disseminated record, which records exchanges between each client in the chain.

There are various kinds of blockchain: some are open and public and some are private and simply available to individuals who are allowed to utilize them. (Casino, 2019) A public blockchain is an open organization. Anybody can download the convention and read, compose or take an interest in the organization.

A public blockchain is conveyed and decentralized. Exchanges are recorded as squares and connected to frame a chain. Each new square should be timestamped and approved by every one of the PCs associated with the organization, known as hubs before it is composed into the blockchain.

All exchanges are public, and all hubs are equivalent. This implies a public blockchain is unchanging: once checked, information cannot be modified. The most popular public blockchains utilized for cryptographic money are Bitcoin and Ethereum: open-source, shrewd agreement blockchains.

A private blockchain is a greeting just organization administered by a solitary substance. Contestants to the organization expect consent to peruse, compose or review the blockchain. There can be various degrees of access and data can be scrambled to secure business secrecy. Private blockchains permit associations to utilize conveyed record innovation without disclosing information.

Be that as it may, this implies they come up short on a characterizing highlight of blockchains: decentralization. A few pundits guarantee private blockchains are not blockchains by any means, however, unified information bases that utilization dispersed record innovation. Private blockchains are quicker, more proficient and savvier than public blockchains, which require a ton of time and energy to approve exchanges.

1.6 Permissionless and Permissioned Blockchain

Permissionless blockchains will be blockchains that require no consent to join and collaborate with. They are otherwise called public blockchains. Often, permissionless blockchain is ideal for running and overseeing advanced monetary standards. (Verma, 2021)

In a permissionless blockchain, a client can make a street number and afterward collaborate with the organization by either assisting the organization with approving exchanges or send exchanges to another client on the organization.

The absolute first sort of permissionless blockchain is Bitcoin. It empowered clients to move computerized monetary forms among themselves. Likewise, clients can cooperate with the organization by taking an interest in the mining interaction. It is an interaction of tackling complex numerical conditions and afterward utilizing it to approve exchanges. The agreement calculation utilized by bitcoin is Proof-of-Work (PoW).

There are additionally other blockchains that are permissionless. Ethereum (ETH) is another well-known public permissionless sort that uses another agreement technique Proof-of-Stake (PoS). (Verma, 2021) It additionally presents different ideas like keen agreements.

Permissioned blockchains can be viewed as an extra blockchain security framework, as they keep an entrance control layer to permit certain activities to be performed simply by certain recognizable members. Consequently, these blockchains contrast from public and private blockchains.

Permissioned blockchains are additionally not quite the same as private blockchains, which permit just realized hubs to partake in the organization. For instance, a bank might be running a private blockchain worked through an assigned number of hubs inside the bank. Interestingly, permissioned blockchains may permit anybody to join an organization once their character and job are characterized.

2. SUPPLY CHAIN MANAGEMENT IN PHARMACEUTICAL INDUSTRIES

Supply Chain Management (SCM) is the way toward arranging, executing and controlling the tasks of the production network with the reason to fulfill client prerequisites as productively as could be expected. (Aich,2019; Azzi 2019) Production network the executives traverses all development and capacity of crude materials (Helo, 2020) work-in-measure stock and completed merchandise from point-of-origin (POO) to point-of-consumption (POC). (Ko, 2010)

SCM is a cognizant and purposeful control, coordination, and the executives of the business capacities. SCM contributes and influences that supply move through the business to improve execution, costs, adaptability and so forth, which bring a definitive advantage to the end clients or customers. The store network work incorporates many sub-regions, for example, estimating and arranging, buying and acquirement, coordination, tasks, stock administration, transportation, warehousing, dispersion, client care and so on Be that as it may, it is hard to track down a standard model of Supply Chain Management working in the business local area especially in the drug area.

Store network the executives (SCM) is the oversight of materials, data and funds as they move in interaction from provider to producer to distributor to retailer to purchaser. Production network management involves organizing and coordinating these streams both inside and among organizations. SCM is both an even business work (for example dealing with the production network in a business) and an upward industry area (for example organizations associated with overseeing supply chains in the interest of their customers). An organization may work as a store network administrations supplier inside the upward store network industry area. However, every one of the customers adjusted by an organization will utilize production network staff inside their business working on a level premise across their associations.

All business needs to conjecture and plan. To look advance and foresee what will be needed as far as assets and materials to convey their items or administrations to their clients in a convenient way. In this space, we discover SCM exercises, for example, request arranging, stock arranging, scope quantification and so on. The business portion of the production network is the place where a business recognizes providers to give the items and administrations that it needs to obtain to make and convey its assistance or item. Expenses and terms of business are arranged and concurred and contracts are framed. From there on the providers' exhibition and future legally binding plans will be overseen around here.

2.1 Introduction to Supply Chain Management

Supply chain management with information technology tools has led to process efficiencies in lean manufacturing to product distribution by drones in Supply chain industries. Supply chain management (SCM) in Pharmaceutical Industries is characterized as the mixture of key business measures across the store network for the reasoning of creating an incentive for clients and partners. (Bocek, 2017) Production network the executives incorporate organic markets inside and across organizations in a proficient plan of action.

The Council of Supply Chain Management Professionals characterizes the production network the executives as arranging and the board of all exercises associated with sourcing, obtainment, transformation and all coordination exercises. There is an assortment of parts of assessing in the inventory network; wiping out bottlenecks, adjusting between smallest material expense and transportation, advancing assembling stream, keeping up the correct blend and area of manufacturing plants and stockrooms, vehicle steering investigation, dynamic programming and productive utilization of limits, inventories, and works are of fundamental parts of inventory network streamlining.

2.2 Recent Development in Supply Chain Management

As sources and capacities with regards to assembling have expanded, more organizations have moved away from zeroing in endeavors on plant-level creation arranging and are receiving to a greater degree an interest-driven focal point of attempting to impact and oversee requests more effectively. Supporting what your organization is best at selling, making and conveying, and adjusting the business power with that outlook, is basic to receiving an interest-driven model. The interest-driven methodology can assist an organization with making a more client-centered mentality, without forfeiting operational effectiveness. At last, an interest-centered way to deal with arranging can essentially improve request arranging and the executive's endeavors and help in general expenses and client care endeavors.

Progressed request arranging frameworks and legitimate methodologies can likewise help reveal information and recognize patterns covered in an organization's data frameworks. Organizations should lead an undertaking wide inner Demand Review to assemble data from all parts of the association. Objectives are then set to acquire agreement on what will be sold every month for every product offering or class and the subsequent income. The driver of the Demand Review measure is consistent improvement of figure precision.

Basic to the achievement of any Demand Plan is having all partners, including deals, showcasing, account, item advancement and store network concur upon an agreement Demand Plan. It is significant for all members to examine factors influencing client request designs (like new or erased items, contenders, or economic situations), the total interest designs and related income plans. When all interest for items and administrations has been perceived, the data is merged into one Demand Plan.

Request arranging is a critical contribution to the bigger deals and tasks arranging measure and can decidedly affect new item presentations, stock arranging and the executives, client care, supply arranging effectiveness and sourcing methodologies. Request arranging achievement is frequently attached to authoritative construction. Organizations with committed assets centered around request arranging and anticipating yield more grounded results and drive more worth to their organization. Associations that emphasize low maintenance on request arranging and determining endeavors, notwithstanding, regularly yield unsatisfactory outcomes. With the essential significance of interest arranging, organizations should be focused on this from both an asset and innovation viewpoint.

2.3 Framework of Supply Chain Management

Supply chain management flexibility has drawn the consideration of organizations and strategy producers. Various investigations and examinations have shown up lately that underline the significance of this subject in a globalized world. (Shoaib, 2020) Yet, should not something be said about the execution of store network strength?

Figure 2. Five-column investigation

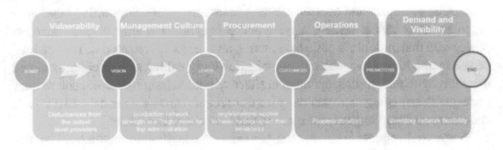

Can organizations address versatility? What is more, where do they have to improve to ensure that they are ready for the following calamity?

To resolve these inquiries, we led a study with nearly a hundred global organizations across ventures and directed a progression of tens plus organized meetings. Certain five-column investigations as shown in figure 2 gives definite experiences on the qualities and shortcomings of organizations concerning their danger to the board systems. The primary column (Vulnerability) evaluates the danger openness of an organization, trailed by the danger ID column (Management Culture) and the real relief columns (Procurement, Operations, and Demand and Visibility).

- Vulnerability

While investigating the weakness of an inventory network, a key test is to distinguish its bottleneck as some researchers at a significant pharma organization, calls attention to:

An interruption like a catastrophic event in specific areas where providers control the overall inventory of specific segments/items would influence all major parts of the business.

Taking a glimpse at interruptions along the worth chain as shown in figure 2, the researchers find that Request driven stockouts are exceptionally continuous, trailed by Disturbances from the outset level providers and disturbances in their tasks.

We distinguish product quality episodes, Request stuns and Fare/Import limitations as the top interruptions. Close to a Misfortune in income, organizations are punished with "Client objections" and "Loss of Productivity" among others.

- Management Culture

With regards to the consideration of top administration, one-third of our review members show that production network strength is a "High" need for top administration and a further one-third, it is even thought to be an "Exceptionally high" need. Figure 2 demonstrates that for more three a fourth of the organizations overviewed, the theme has an expanded significance either inside the whole association or in certain pieces of the association.

However, while organizations concur on the significance of the point, they come up short on a best-practice approach for estimating flexibility. Subjective, quantitative, or a combination of the two measures are near being similarly liked among overview members.

- Procurement

On the acquisition side, organizations appear to have distinguished their weakness brought about by interruptions from the start-level providers. They effectively double source their crude material by nearly ninety percentage, perform provider reviews or rate their providers as illustrated in figure 2. Nearly a hundred percent of the organizations follow long haul and shared associations with their key providers.

In any case, despite these endeavors, a solid weakness from the outset level providers stays. Proficient danger relief techniques require an expanded multi-partner discourse.

- Operations

Inside, organizations put resources into double/different sources inside the assembling interaction, hazard relief stock (on normal 21-40 days of stock for completed merchandise), or dexterity limit. These speculations mirror the significance of the point for top administration. Yet, with regards to execution, just one-fourth of the organizations figure out how to adjust the three alleviation systems comprehensively. Further operational alleviation systems are close to the exemplary "Process duration" and "Lead time decrease" additionally "Creation moving" or "Extra time and subcontracting."

- Demand and Visibility

On the interesting side, organizations center around perceivability related danger moderation procedures (for example EDI innovation or information sharing). Therefore, three-fourth of the organizations have "High" or "Medium" perceivability on their stockouts; and yet just a little extent of the organizations has "High" perceivability on wellbeing inventories conveyed by their dissemination accomplices or their clients. Furthermore, just one-fifth of the organizations have full perceivability on the expenses for their customers that are brought about by their stockouts.

While perceivability in their tasks is a decent route forward, further perceivability should be improved on the dispersion accomplice or client-side.

While the obligation to inventory network, flexibility is not the entire story, organizations battle with effective execution.

2.4 Applications of Supply Chain Management

In the present exceptionally aggressive commercial center, it is basic for organizations to advance better approaches to smooth out their store network and advance efficiency. With the guide of current store network innovation applications, you can make better perceivability inside your store network, which will empower you to have more power over your business and stay in front of the opposition. Innovation can assist with improving your store network, which will empower your business to work even more productively, give you greater perceivability and command over your stock, and help to diminish your operational expenses.

Furthermore, through a more steady and proficient production network, you can incredibly upgrade consumer loyalty and maintenance. Here are only a couple of approaches to incorporate present-day store network innovation applications into your plan of action and improve your inventory network with the executives.

Store network experts assume significant parts in the plan and the board of supply chains. In the plan of supply chains, they assist with deciding if an item or administration is given by the actual firm (adopting) or by another firm somewhere else (re-appropriating). (Dutta, 2020)

In the administration of supply chains, store network experts arrange creation among numerous suppliers, guaranteeing that creation and transport of merchandise occur with negligible quality control or stock issues. One objective of a very much planned and kept up with store network for an item is to effectively assemble the item at negligible expense. Such an inventory network could be viewed as the upper hand for a firm.

3. INTEGRATION OF BLOCKCHAIN AND SUPPLY CHAIN MANAGEMENT IN PHARMACEUTICAL INDUSTRIES

Integration of blockchain and SCM in pharmaceutical industries could ensure genuine and safer medicine supply to patients. (Radanović, 2018; Verma 2021) The incorporation would look to keep fake meds from entering the production network.

(Yaeger, 2019) The medication fabricates alongside wholesalers would likewise be included. (Roman-Belmonte, 2018)

3.1 Blockchain in Pharmaceutical Industries

Drug organizations need to manage the returned sedates intermittently. This happens considering overloading by the wholesalers. That is the reason they need to restore the unused stock to the makers.

At some random time, 2-3% of the medications are returned. Notwithstanding, when you match it with the volume of cash, it can reach a place between 7 to 10$ billion.

However, the greatest issue is that the profits contain fake medications. The pharma organizations' test is to recognize them and afterward separate them before they can offer the returned medications to the market. To guarantee that it occurs, each medication should be barcoded and serialized.

A unified authority does it in certain European countries. However, doing so can mean including another seller that controls the confirmation of the medications. In North American countries, there is an absence of an incorporated data set controller.

The arrangement is to use a decentralized blockchain. Thus, the drug makers can undoubtedly record the bundle chronic number on blockchain. This implies that the medication can be checked from any place. The blockchain drug store is the beginning of another time.

It enables the clients and wholesalers to check legitimacy without the need to rely upon a concentrated power.

3.2 Physical Aspects: Blockchain in Pharmaceutical Industries

Blockchain is the supporting innovation for digital forms of money, for example, bitcoin, and consequently numerous in the medical care area may have known about it regarding the different enormous scope ransomware assaults – which for the most part request installment as digital money – that have hit general wellbeing frameworks as of late.

Despite the conceivable regrettable underlying meanings encompassing blockchain and cryptographic forms of money, the potential for the blockchain to carry substantial advantages to the medical care area is extraordinarily high. At the MedCity Converge gathering in Philadelphia, the US in 2019, Merck partner chief for applied innovation, Nishan Kulatilaka, noticed that medical care could be the second-biggest area to embrace innovation, after monetary administrations.

For patients and general wellbeing frameworks, blockchain could, among different applications, be a characteristic facilitator for electronic wellbeing records that are shareable between various wellbeing associations without hindering the security of the information.

There is something truly cool about having their record follow certain any place they abandon requiring that information on their consistently, MedCity News cited Kulatilaka as saying. They are not, at this point, bound to their emergency clinic framework.

While there are various natural applications for blockchain in medical care, what might be said about the drug area that is liable for creating, producing and dispersing the prescriptions that are utilized in these settings consistently?

Various prospects are now being considered in the business, yet one aspect of the pharma scene is especially ready for development: the medication inventory network. (Agbo, 2019; Wang 2020) The issue of fake medications has gotten progressively squeezing, both as far as the monetary expense of this worldwide underground market and the danger to suffering patients that comes from ingesting fake medications that might not have similar dynamic drug fixings or measurement levels as the genuine medicine. (Pirtle, 2018)

A template of smart contract for pharma Supply Chain based on Blockchain in Healthcare has been provided below and its execution is shown in figure 3.

```solidity
pragma solidity ^0.7.0;
contract MedOwner {
    address private owner;
    string private medName="";
    event OwnerSet(address indexed oldOwner, address indexed newOwner);
    modifier isOwner() {
require(msg.sender == owner, "You are not owner");
        _;
    }
constructor() {
        owner = msg.sender;
        emit OwnerSet(address(0), owner);
    }
    function changeOwner(address _owner) public isOwner {
        emit OwnerSet(owner, _owner);
        owner = _owner;
    }
    function getOwner() external view returns (address) {
        return owner;
    }
```

Figure 3. Smart Contract "MedOwner" running in Remix IDE

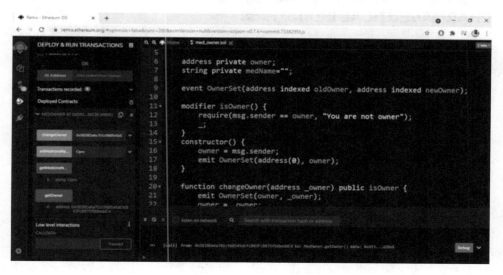

```
    function setMedicineName(string memory _medName) public
isOwner {
medName = _medName;
    }
    function getMedicineName() external view returns (string
memory) {
        return medName;
    }
}
```

Smart contracts are just projects put away on a blockchain that run when foreordained conditions are met. They regularly are utilized to mechanize the execution of an arrangement so all members can be quickly sure of the result, with no middle person's inclusion or time misfortune. The smart contract is executed through a blockchain network, and the code of the agreement is recreated on numerous PCs that contain the organization. This guarantees a more straightforward and got assistance and execution of the legally binding terms. Also, brilliant agreements do not need a mediator.

4. CASE STUDY OF BLOCKCHAIN IN PHARMACEUTICAL INDUSTRIES

CallHealth, the world's first and genuinely coordinated medical care stage, has cooperated with ThynkBlynk, the engineers of ChainTrail, to guarantee a medical care information mix on its foundation. This is India's first-ever blockchain administration organization with a medical care administration stage. It has the exceptional capacity to safely incorporate information from a wide range of medical care administrations and a great many medical services environment suppliers like Doctors, Nurses, Hospitals, Clinics and so forth in consistency with severe information protection guidelines.

EHR frameworks in India utilize distinctive data models. Because of this, hanging together information from different medical care sources is turning into a test. By normalizing Healthcare yields like solutions and reports, data is made irrefutable and interoperable, giving patients better power over their wellbeing data. Patients can take their unquestionable individual wellbeing information and execute with anybody they pick. Simultaneously, Healthcare suppliers can confirm and guarantee any information movement into their frameworks is exact. A mutually beneficial suggestion.

The reasonable utilization of CallHealth and ThynkBlynk'sChainTrail Blockchain Distributed Ledger approach in healthcare resolves main points of interest tormenting the Indian Healthcare framework, for example, Counterfeit or deceitfully changed documentation combined with an absence of advanced information check is prompting clinical errors and reliance on manual confirmations which thusly bring about high overhead expenses (Siyal, 2019). Interest for rehashed techniques and neurotic tests without believed information sources is causing high cash-based costs for patients and strains the all-around troubled medical services framework

By guaranteeing each information point is auditable, recognizable, controlled and is permanent, a believed data trade stage accommodates a better mix inside the health biological system. Printing and holding paper, giving duplicates to patients of their requested information, moving paper trail through the whole organization of specialists, emergency clinics indicative focuses and so on and physically confirming information at each stage is an awkward just as costly experience for suppliers and patients. Chaintrail makes the whole store network effective by giving a solitary direct interface toward more prominent operational effortlessness.

5. CONCLUSION

Blockchain is generally another next generation innovation that is in its early stage. It is an enormous achievement as Bitcoin has surely increased current standards of assumptions. In the coming years, we may see Blockchain disrupting the medical services industry and with that, there will be support in the medical care application improvement utilizing the blockchain innovation. Nonetheless, it is additionally evident that the execution of blockchain in medical care probably will not be a cakewalk as it would confront some genuine difficulties as examined in this chapter. This chapter has described the blockchain and its integration with SCM in the pharma industries. It will be interesting to see in the future, how actual implementation brought changes in the medicine supply chain.

REFERENCES

Agbo, C. C., Mahmoud, Q. H., & Eklund, J. M. (2019, June). Blockchain technology in healthcare: a systematic review. In Healthcare (Vol. 7, No. 2, p. 56). Multidisciplinary Digital Publishing Institute. doi:10.3390/healthcare7020056

Aich, S., Chakraborty, S., Sain, M., Lee, H. I., & Kim, H. C. (2019, February). A review on benefits of IoT integrated blockchain based supply chain management implementations across different sectors with case study. In *2019 21st international conference on advanced communication technology (ICACT)* (pp. 138-141). IEEE. 10.23919/ICACT.2019.8701910

Azzi, R., Chamoun, R. K., & Sokhn, M. (2019). The power of a blockchain-based supply chain. *Computers & Industrial Engineering, 135*, 582–592. doi:10.1016/j.cie.2019.06.042

Bernard, Z. (2018). *Everything you need to know about Bitcoin, its mysterious origins, and the many alleged identities of its creator.* Business Insider.

Bocek, T., Rodrigues, B. B., Strasser, T., & Stiller, B. (2017, May). Blockchains everywhere-a use-case of blockchains in the pharma supply-chain. In *2017 IFIP/ IEEE symposium on integrated network and service management (IM)* (pp. 772-777). IEEE.

Casino, F., Dasaklis, T. K., & Patsakis, C. (2019). A systematic literature review of blockchain-based applications: Current status, classification and open issues. *Telematics and Informatics, 36*, 55–81. doi:10.1016/j.tele.2018.11.006

Dutta, P., Choi, T. M., Somani, S., & Butala, R. (2020). Blockchain technology in supply chain operations: Applications, challenges and research opportunities. *Transportation Research Part E, Logistics and Transportation Review, 142*, 102067. doi:10.1016/j.tre.2020.102067 PMID:33013183

Helo, P., & Shamsuzzoha, A. H. M. (2020). Real-time supply chain—A blockchain architecture for project deliveries. *Robotics and Computer-integrated Manufacturing, 63*, 101909. doi:10.1016/j.rcim.2019.101909

Ko, M., Tiwari, A., & Mehnen, J. (2010). A review of soft computing applications in supply chain management. *Applied Soft Computing, 10*(3), 661–674. doi:10.1016/j.asoc.2009.09.004

Koens, T., & Poll, E. (2018). What blockchain alternative do you need? In *Data Privacy Management, Cryptocurrencies and Blockchain Technology* (pp. 113–129). Springer. doi:10.1007/978-3-030-00305-0_9

Leng, M., & Parlar, M. (2005). Game theoretic applications in supply chain management: A review. *INFOR, 43*(3), 187–220. doi:10.1080/03155986.2005.11 732725

Mettler, M. (2016, September). Blockchain technology in healthcare: The revolution starts here. In *2016 IEEE 18th international conference on e-health networking, applications and services (Healthcom)* (pp. 1-3). IEEE.

Niederman, F., Mathieu, R. G., Morley, R., & Kwon, I. W. (2007). Examining RFID applications in supply chain management. *Communications of the ACM, 50*(7), 92–101. doi:10.1145/1272516.1272520

Queiroz, M. M., Telles, R., & Bonilla, S. H. (2019). Blockchain and supply chain management integration: A systematic review of the literature. *Supply Chain Management, 25*(2), 241–254. doi:10.1108/SCM-03-2018-0143

Radanović, I., & Likić, R. (2018). Opportunities for use of blockchain technology in medicine. *Applied Health Economics and Health Policy, 16*(5), 583–590. doi:10.100740258-018-0412-8 PMID:30022440

Ramadhani, A. M., Choi, H. R., & Kim, N. R. (2018). Blockchain Implementation in Government: A Review. *Internet E-Commerce Research, 18*(2), 35-48.

Roman-Belmonte, J. M., De la Corte-Rodriguez, H., & Rodriguez-Merchan, E. C. (2018). How blockchain technology can change medicine. *Postgraduate Medicine, 130*(4), 420–427. doi:10.1080/00325481.2018.1472996 PMID:29727247

Sabry, S. S., Kaittan, N. M., & Majeed, I. (2019). The road to the blockchain technology: Concept and types. *Periodicals of Engineering and Natural Sciences, 7*(4), 1821–1832. doi:10.21533/pen.v7i4.935

Shoaib, M., Lim, M. K., & Wang, C. (2020). An integrated framework to prioritize blockchain-based supply chain success factors. *Industrial Management & Data Systems, 120*(11), 2103–2131. doi:10.1108/IMDS-04-2020-0194

Siyal, A. A., Junejo, A. Z., Zawish, M., Ahmed, K., Khalil, A., & Soursou, G. (2019). Applications of blockchain technology in medicine and healthcare: Challenges and future perspectives. *Cryptography, 3*(1), 3. doi:10.3390/cryptography3010003

Ullah, H. S., Aslam, S., & Anrjomand, N. (2020). *Blockchain in Healthcare and Medicine: A Contemporary Research of Applications, Challenges, and Future Perspectives.* arXiv preprint arXiv:2004.06795.

Manish, V. (2021, April). Building predictive model owned and operated by public infrastructure that uses blockchain technology. *International Journal for Science and Advance Research in Technology, 7*(4), 20.

Verma, M. (2021). Amalgamation of Blockchain Technology and Knowledge Management System to fetch an enhanced system in Library. IJIRT, 7(11), 474-477.

Verma, M. (2021). Emerging applications of blockchain technology. *International Research Journal of Modernization in Engineering Technology and Science, 3*(4), 1258-1260.

Verma, M. (2021). Modeling Identity Management System Based on Blockchain Technology. *International Journal of Research Publication and Reviews, 2*(4), 450-452.

Verma, M. (2021). Smart contract model for trust based agriculture using blockchain technology. International Journal of Research and Analytical Reviews, 8(2), 354-355.

Wang, M., Wu, Y., Chen, B., & Evans, M. (2020). Blockchain and supply chain management: A new paradigm for supply chain integration and collaboration. *Operations and Supply Chain Management: An International Journal, 14*(1), 111–122. doi:10.31387/oscm0440290

Weir, S. (2018). *Supply Chain Transparency.* Academic Press.

Yaeger, K., Martini, M., Rasouli, J., & Costa, A. (2019). Emerging blockchain technology solutions for modern healthcare infrastructure. *Journal of Scientific Innovation in Medicine, 2*(1), 1. doi:10.29024/jsim.7

ADDITIONAL READING

Ahmad, R. W., Salah, K., Jayaraman, R., Yaqoob, I., Ellahham, S., & Omar, M. (2021). The role of blockchain technology in telehealth and telemedicine. *International Journal of Medical Informatics*, *148*, 104399. doi:10.1016/j.ijmedinf.2021.104399 PMID:33540131

Alamri, M., Jhanjhi, N. Z., & Humayun, M. (2019). Blockchain for Internet of Things (IoT) research issues challenges & future directions: A review. *Int. J. Comput. Sci. Netw. Secur*, *19*, 244–258.

Anjana, P. S., Kumari, S., Peri, S., Rathor, S., & Somani, A. (2019, February). An efficient framework for optimistic concurrent execution of smart contracts. In *2019 27th Euromicro International Conference on Parallel, Distributed and Network-Based Processing (PDP)* (pp. 83-92). IEEE. 10.1109/EMPDP.2019.8671637

Anjana, P. S., Kumari, S., Peri, S., Rathor, S., & Somani, A. (2021). OptSmart: A Space Efficient Optimistic Concurrent Execution of Smart Contracts. arXiv preprint arXiv:2102.04875.

Kumar, A., Krishnamurthi, R., Nayyar, A., Sharma, K., Grover, V., & Hossain, E. (2020). A Novel Smart Healthcare Design, Simulation, and Implementation Using Healthcare 4.0 Processes. *IEEE Access: Practical Innovations, Open Solutions*, *8*, 118433–118471. doi:10.1109/ACCESS.2020.3004790

Sharma, V., & Lal, N. (2020). A novel comparison of consensus algorithms in blockchain. *Advances and Applications in Mathematical Sciences*, *20*(1), 1–13.

Stephen, R., & Alex, A. (2018, August). A review on blockchain security. *IOP Conference Series. Materials Science and Engineering*, *396*(1), 012030. doi:10.1088/1757-899X/396/1/012030

KEY TERMS AND DEFINITIONS

Ethereum: It is a public blockchain type that is also permissionless.
Smart Contract: It is a program that is used in Blockchain.

Chapter 6
Blockchain–Based Infrastructure for Product Traceability in the Medical Supply Chain

Tan Gürpinar
TU Dortmund University, Germany

Sk. Riad Bin Ashraf
TU Dortmund University, Germany

Natalia Broza-Abut
Fraunhofer IML, Germany

Dominik Sparer
Fraunhofer IML, Germany

ABSTRACT

This chapter introduces a blockchain-based infrastructure to support the traceability of medical products and implementation of unique device identification. Therefore, in the next pages, the characteristics of blockchain technology as well as benefits and challenges in supply chain management are described. After that, regulations for medical supply chains are gathered with a focus on American and European regulations and interlinked with the current concepts of the labling medical products. Finally, a technical blockchain-based solution is conceptualized with regard to full and light node system in medical supply chains before the chapter is concluded with an outlook and further scientific and technical research possibilities.

DOI: 10.4018/978-1-7998-9606-7.ch006

INTRODUCTION

Blockchain in Supply Chains

Over the last years, blockchain technology (BCT) evolved into a general-purpose IT infrastructure capable of dealing with a wide range of business challenges (Gurtu & Johny, 2019). Therefore, various branches recognize possible benefits and start proof-of-concepts in different application sectors – e.g., such as banking and energy, food, medical care, and many more (Treiblmaier, 2018). In most enterprise applications, a significant number of partners with various types of service contracts, such as manufacturers, dealers, suppliers, and logistics- and financial service providers are involved. All of them require a method for securely exchanging data (Wust & Gervais, 2018). As a result of this, as well as through increased globalization and the extension of business partnerships into new markets, enhancing the openness and visibility of supply chain processes is of considerable interest. In these situations, the benefits of blockchain technology can be critical. The ability to actualize opportunities without relying on a central authority, in particular, has the potential to disrupt numerous businesses. This potential is boosted by the fact that network partners can share specific data and transactions since data is kept tamper-proof throughout the network (Gao et al., 2018).

Tracking and tracing

The advantages of sharing information throughout supply chains are widely known for increasing productivity and lowering costs. However, as supply chains become more dynamic and adaptable, privacy concerns pose a severe threat to essential data retrieval. Because vital information for monitoring and tracing items is either inaccessible or only stored locally, advanced, multi-hop information flows are hampered by a lack of trust between various engaged parties (Bader et al., 2021). Blockchain-based tracking and tracing processes are critical can provide unified views on global supply chains consisting of several parties and help monitor supply chain key performance indicators (Helo & Shamsuzzoha, 2020). The advantages of sharing information throughout supply chains are widely known for increasing productivity and lowering costs. Tracking and tracing techniques have gotten a lot of attention in the previous two decades as future enablers for better supply chain connectivity, planning, and control, and hence greater overall supply chain surplus (Oluyisola et al., 2018). This has prompted studies to better understand the variables that have aided the digitization of supply chains and manufacturing systems in recent years.

Tracking and Tracing in Medical Supply Chains

Tracking and tracing have become increasingly important in medical supply chains to ensure the safety of patients and users, as well as the quality of medical products and equipment (Bayrak and Özdiler Çopur 2017). Medical supply chains are complex networks and are challenged by product impurities and erroneous information that emerge from a lack of transparency and restricted data provenance. As a result, previous research has underlined the importance of reliable, end-to-end track and trace systems for medical supply chains. Most contemporary track and trace systems are centralized in medical supply chains, resulting in data privacy and authenticity(Musamih et al., 2021). Because of that, new sophisticated and standardized approaches to track and manage medical products both within and between companies are required. Studies have shown that adequately implementing universal product identification can improve supply chain performance and reduce hazards, but solely they are not solving the stated problems (Sodero et al., 2013).

On the regulatory side, track and trace systems also have to consider country-specific requirements. In 2013 the US Food and Drug Administration (FDA) and the European Union (EU) released regulations about the Unique Device Identification (UDI) of medical products (Bayrak & Özdiler Çopur, 2017). The regulations were developed to ensure consistent traceability of individual products from the manufacturer to the end-user by utilizing a unique key, the UDI. Inventory transparency, consumer safety, product equivalence, and business intelligence are just a few of the advantages that the implementation of UDI provides to hospitals and patients (Abdulsalam et al., 2020). Nevertheless, legislative stakeholders have been working hard since then to harmonize the respective standards and regulations. Also, there are more challenges in implementing UDI: Both the American and European regulations don't provide sufficient details on how the UDI system should be implemented in enterprises and how the track and trace data should be securely stored and shared (Bayrak & Özdiler Çopur, 2017).

Motivation and Objectives of the Chapter

This chapter introduces a blockchain solution to support the traceability of medical products and implementation of UDI. Therefore, in the next chapters, background information about the characteristics of blockchain technology, as well as benefits and challenges are described. After that, a technical solution is explained in more detail before the chapter is concluded with an outlook and further research possibilities.

Figure 1. Blockchain Architecture
(Fill et al., 2020)

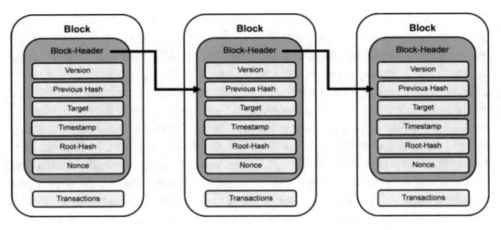

BACKGROUND

Characteristics of Blockchain Technology

Blockchain Technology can be seen as a distributed ledger technology (DLT) subclass that stores data in time-stamped consecutive blocks. By using hash functions, the single blocks are linked to their predecessors. A block is an ordered and grouped record containing at least two pieces of information presented in its header: the hash to the preceding block and its own block. The first genesis block, which has no antecedent, stores the initial state of the continuous transaction history. The blockchain is made up of a list of all headers and stored transaction information (Benčić & Zarko, 2018).

Different users, or so called "nodes," make up the blockchain and are brought to consensus on the current state by blockchain-inherent consensus mechanisms. While the proof-of-work algorithm is the most prominent one, it is primarily used in cryptocurrencies and is associated with high processing capabilities and electricity consumption. Blockchain frameworks are typically private in supply chain management and feature more efficient consensus mechanisms like proof-of-authority, round-robin, or practical byzantine fault tolerance (Hinckeldeyn, 2019). Due to the blockchain architecture, it is impossible to compromise the stored information, which means that, especially when interacting with external or previously unknown parties, a basis of trust is formed that is not based on intermediaries but is anchored in the data structure itself. This objective trust basis can span a complete value chain (Hildebrandt & Landhäußer, 2017).

Figure 2. Use Cases for Blockchain in Supply Chain Management
(Gürpinar et al., 2019)

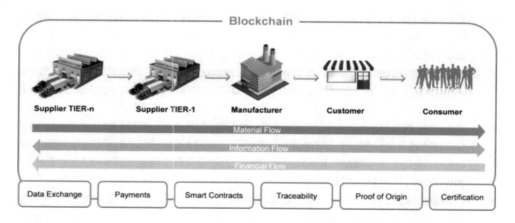

Benefits and Challenges of Blockchain in Supply Chain Management

Supply Chain Management (SCM) seeks to coordinate, optimize, and develop error-free value and supply chains, from raw material extraction to the finished product, while considering economic factors (Giese et al., 2016). The flows of goods, information, and finance are all interconnected in the supply chain (Beckmann, 2012). However, at this time, the monetary flow is only linked to a minor extent, and as a consequence, the service offering process is not synchronized (Jakob et al., 2018).

BCT is one of the technologies that has a noteworthy impact on supply chain management's continuous development and transformation in recent years (Terzi et al., 2019). It delivers advantageous qualities for an effective SCM because of inherent attributes such as data integrity and authenticity, pseudonymity, and irreversibility (Gürpinar et al., 2020; Treiblmaier, 2018).

In figure 2, use cases are listed that are accomplished by the stated blockchain functionalities and span the whole supply chain. Mostly these use cases are piloted in their interplay in current enterprise integration projects (Gürpinar et al., 2019).

Despite its use cases that benefit supply chain management processes, BCT brings several obstacles that prevent it from being fully adopted in most industries. These difficulties include the following:

- Scalability, which is primarily but not solely relevant for public blockchains. Long block intervals and small block sizes contribute to sluggish throughput. When it comes to having the best throughput, the block intervals and sizes must be well balanced. There is a compromise between blockchain's scalability, decentralization, and security (blockchain trilemma) (Sanka et al., 2021).

- Despite the reliability of BCT, several security threats and vulnerabilities have been discovered in blockchain applications, particularly in public blockchains. Due to their limited access, private and consortium blockchains are more secure. The most typically reported security flaws include scams, malware assaults, denial of service (DoS), Sybil attacks, application, and network vulnerabilities (Saad et al., 2019; Wang et al., 2019).
- Another key impediment to blockchain adoption is a lack of knowledge about the technology. Many individuals find blockchain technology challenging to comprehend or distrust it because they believe it is being utilized for criminal purposes (Huillet, 2019).
- Furthermore, from an organizational point of view, interdisciplinary challenges in cooperation and teamwork arise due to the high strategic impact of blockchain implementations and various involved enterprise departments and disciplines (Düdder et al., 2021)
- Also, another challenge for the technology integration is the difficulty in assessing its business value and developing a factual statement for potential cost savings (Gürpinar et al., 2020).
- Finally, compliance with governmental and legal regulations poses one of the most critical challenges in blockchain adoption and is focused on in this chapter (Reyna et al., 2018).

Integration of Blockchain in Supply Chains

When considering blockchain as a supplement for existing IT infrastructures of a supply chain, several integration levels have to be considered in all steps of the integration process (Große et al., 2020). On the shop floor, objects have to be made smart and interconnected to reach a fully flexible production environment, flexible structures, and decentralized, autonomous decision-making. On the system level, the formulation of rules and communication procedures that satisfy both technical and legal/business requirements needs to be taken care of. On the enterprise level, it is all about the integration and cooperation of different departments and disciplines to exploit all blockchain benefits. Finally, on the network layer, the integration of all blockchain stakeholders throughout the supply chain and beyond (external stakeholders, e.g. regulators, certifiers) are focused.

Figure 3. Vertical and Horizontal Integration of Blockchain
(Own Illustration)

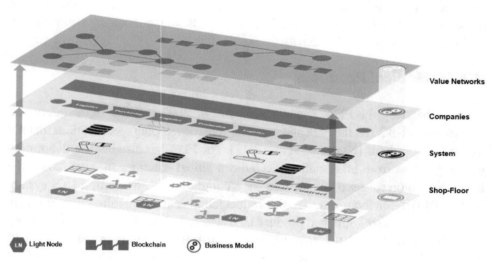

Challenges in Medical Supply Chains

Medical products comprise many different medical devices used for therapeutic or diagnostic purposes for humans and thereby contribute to healing and improving the quality of life or even saving it (Bundesministerium für Wirtschaft und Energie 2016). For the user at the point of treatment, specific product information on the condition and handling of the device must be provided in a simple, accessible and transparent manner to ensure the best possible treatment (Siyal et al. 2019). However, current initiatives by action alliances, associations, and legislative measures show that in advancing digitization, great potentials, especially concerning process automation and holistic, cross-facility data management, have so far remained untapped (Fedkenhauer et al., 2017). Complete traceability of the product is usually not possible at a later date. As a result, errors in product handling (e.g., during transport or reprocessing of sterile reusable products) are currently tolerated, as are products of poor quality (e.g., in the form of counterfeit products that enter the market due to inconsistencies in process documentation) (Kirmse, 2016).

A particular problem arises particularly for small and medium-sized enterprises (SMEs) involved in manufacturing medical products. A manageable software solution for tamper-proof traceability of medical products and methodological standards that enable the prescribed guidelines' implementation not yet exist (Miller, 2018; Walter, 2013). Both legislators and medical product manufacturers have recognized these shortcomings and have taken initial steps to advance connectivity and automation inpatient care (European Parliament, 2017). Safety concerns are to be countered by the significantly higher requirements for preparing clinical data, new regulations in market surveillance with shorter notification periods, and the staggered introduction of the UDI marking (Miller, 2018).

UDI for Medical Products

As authorized by the FDA Amendments Act of 2007 and the FDA Safety and Innovation Act of 2012, the FDA spent several years developing specifications for UDI for medical products (Normand et al., 2012). The FDA has also been collaborating with regulators from other nations to build a global solution. In April 2013, the European Union released suggestions for a common framework for a UDI system (FDA, 2013). Even though electronic product identification was already common in the financial industry, medical product UDI was only introduced in 2014 (Tcheng et al., 2014). In April 2017, two different regulations (Regulation (EU) 745/2017 on medical devices and Regulation (EU) 746/2017 on in vitro diagnostic medical devices were adopted and came into force on May 25, 2017. The two regulations' application periods are 26 May 2021 for medical devices and 26 May 2022 for In Vitro Diagnostic Medical Devices; however, certain sections have alternative schedules. These Regulations establish an EU-wide medical device-identifying system based on UDI (EU Health Programme, 2017).

The UDI system should apply to all medical devices under the new regulations. All economic operators must implement it to maintain the medical device's traceability throughout the supply chain. For example, the manufacturer must adhere to the UDI system's obligations (Clause 24) and the registration obligations (Clause 24a, 24b, and 25a). At the same time, the importer and distributor must issue and attach the UDI code. Furthermore, the company's Quality Management System must contain UDI attribution verification, and the labeling for the Technical File and conformity evaluation must be changed for UDI coding. A new UDI-DI should be introduced whenever a change potentially leads to uncertainty in device traceability and identification. Changes to the device's brand name or trade name, the device's version or model, the number of devices delivered in a package, the device being packaged as sterile / the requirement for sterilization before use, and so on, all necessitate a new UDI-DI. Furthermore, when a stakeholder repackages and relabels a device under their label, they must keep track of the original equipment manufacturers (OEM) UDI to ensure traceability. The European Databank on Medical Devices (EUDAMED) (referred to in Clause 27 of the new Regulation) is a secure, web-based portal whose purpose is to facilitate information exchange between competent national authorities and the European Commission, thereby ensuring market surveillance and transparency. The European Commission is convinced that the best method to

Figure 4. UDI System
(Bianchini et al., 2019)

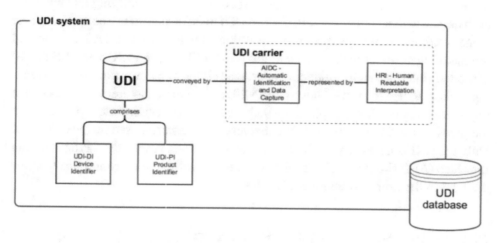

maintain effective medical device traceability in the EU is to employ a harmonized UDI system across Europe, thus the necessity for an electronic UDI system as part of EUDAMED (referred to in Clause 24a of the new Regulation). To help ensure patient safety, the device and its UDI must be registered in the EUDAMED database, and the UDI must be printed on the label, making vigilance and market surveillance easier (Bianchini et al., 2019)

Labeling of UDI

On the label or on the device itself, as well as on all higher levels of labeling, the UDI Carrier [Automated Identification for Data Capture (AIDC) and human-readable interpretation (HRI) representation of the UDI] must be present. If substantial constraints prevent both AIDC and HRI from being used on the label, only the AIDC format must be used (EU Health Programme, 2017). Furthermore, the device labeler should provide dates on device labels and packaging consistent manner that follows international standards and practice (YYYY-MM-DD) (FDA, 2019). The term "label" is defined under Section 201(k) of the Federal Food, Drug, and Cosmetic Act (FFDCA) as a "display of written, printed, or pictorial matter upon the immediate container of any object." The term "label" refers to a regulatory notion rather than a physical item in terms of UDI. When the manufacturer can't fit the UDI on the present label adding a separate UDI label to the device container is still FDA-compliant (Bianchini et al., 2019).

Device labelers are expected to provide information to the Global Unique Device Identification (GUDID) Database, which the FDA manages). GUDID comprises

ONLY the device identifier (DI), which serves as the key to retrieve device information in the database, and provides a standard set of essential identifying attributes for each device with a UDI (FDA, 2019). The UDI must be placed by the manufacturer alone. Authorized entities must provide coding standards. The FDA has approved three issuing agencies in the United States (GS1, HIBCC, and ICCBBA/ISBT-128) to produce internationally unique, standardized UDIs. The European Commission is quite likely to use the same ones to deal with device manufacturers. The European regulations require UDI to be placed on both the software user interface and, if relevant, the physical media used for software delivery for software-based medical devices. Only the HRI is necessary on the electronic display. An Application Programming Interface (API) should be offered for applications without a user interface to show the UDI to the user (Bianchini et al., 2019).

BLOCKCHAIN-BASED TRACKING AND TRACING OF UDI

BCT can be used to ensure the transparency of the value chains of medical products. Goods belonging to a damaged or contaminated batch must be immediately identifiable to protect end-users effectively. The secure and unchangeable storage of event data in the blockchain enables end-users and other stakeholders to keep track. It forms a link to central databases in the medical sector. In the case of the EU, Eudamed is a central database to store medical product event data and is used as an example in the following explanations.

The chapter's objective is to introduce a concept to make BCT usable to realize fully traceable and trustworthy value chains in the medical sector. For this purpose, a software solution for tamper-proof traceability of medical products is conceptualized. The solution supports enterprises in meeting the increasing challenges of the market for medical products, especially the fulfillment of the requirements explained above.

Solution approach

Figure 5 shows a concept of a permissioned blockchain network for the medical sector. A fundamental distinction is made between full and light nodes in permissioned blockchains, which have different read or write permissions to the blockchain. For example, the application partner's server would represent a full node and contains a copy of the entire blockchain history. Cyber-physical systems (CPS), such as scanning devices for reading UDI identifiers, on the other hand, represent light nodes and are implemented to track event data. The implementation based on permissioned blockchain solutions has the advantage that many benefits of public blockchain networks, such as decentralized data storage, manipulation security,

Figure 5. A concept of a permissioned blockchain network in the medical sector (Own Illustration)

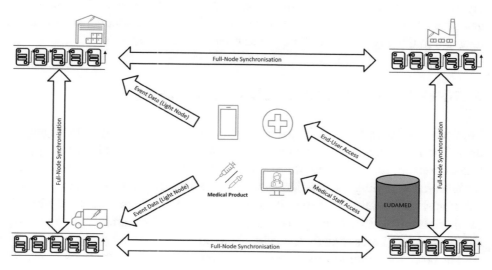

and participants' unique identification, are made possible. In addition, forming a consortium compensates for most of the disadvantages associated with public blockchain networks such as Bitcoin or Ethereum. In particular, the use of BCT in permissioned networks eliminates the problem of energy consumption due to mining, the possibility of majority attacks (51% attacks), and public access to data.

By recording the life cycle of a medical product from its pre-products to the end product and finally, to its consumption, complete traceability based on reliable data can be enabled. Transactions in the blockchain can also be easily enriched with information about the medical product's condition to determine the time and location of contamination.

In the solutions envisaged here, legal requirements must be observed, which stipulate a retention obligation of between 6 and 10 years, depending on the document type, which presents BCT with new challenges. For the data retention obligation, a participant must read its business data from the blockchain. A way to query the blockchain similar to a database is needed.For example, it could be essential to know which copies still belong to the batch in contaminated plaster. It may be necessary to trace back the defective product's value chain to check which other products had a point of contact with this specimen. In this way, the source of the contamination could be searched step by step to identify all products that came into contact with the source. Some blockchain framworks already implement solutions for data structuring "key value stores" (e.g. Tendermint, Multichain), "worldstates" (e.g. Tendermint, Hyperledger Fabric), or mechanisms for active/inactive data sets and also integrated databases. In general, it should be noted that blockchains are not intended to master data and in that regard do not function as effectively as databases.

FUTURE SCIENTIFIC AND TECHNICAL TASKS

To view data from a blockchain, a mechanism is needed that can specifically replay data. The BCT does not offer an efficient way to query captured data since only transactions and no resulting states are charged. Therefore, there is still a need for research regarding the efficient extraction of data from a blockchain. An ideal solution should combine the security aspects of the blockchain with the ability of a database to enable structured queries. This can be done, for example, by connecting centralized data bases directly to the blockchain.

The proposed solution already suggests a large volume of transactions. However, currently available BCT solutions do not all deliver possibilities to deal with such volumes and include a sufficient number of network participants. Therefore, a central task of future research should be to examine how blockchains can be parallelized so that they can be scaled for higher transaction volumes. Another technical task would be to investigate exit strategies for blockchain data that already reached the retention period of seven to ten years and could actually be deleted. In contrast to public blockchains like Bitcoin where only hashes are stored, in medical care enterprise solutions, more complex information is transacted and could therefore occupy more storage space. Finally, governance aspects need to be considered with respect to rules and obligations different stakeholder need to fulfill, as only by scaling the network to a critical number of stakeholders, blockchain benefits unfold entirely.

CONCLUSION

This chapter introduces a concept for a blockchain solution to support the traceability of medical products and the implementation of UDI. Therefore, background information is given about the characteristics of blockchain technology and its benefits and challenges in supply chain management. After that, the technical solution is explained based on a permissioned blockchain framework that connects the stakeholders of a medical supply chain and utilizes a light-node concept. With the solution, sources of contamination of medical products can be searched throughout the entire supply chain to identify all involved stakeholders or other products that originated from the same source.

The chapter shows that BCT can support in monitoring supply chain events starting from documenting the production history of a finished product that requires secured and trusted record keeping. A decentralized record that is not controlled by any company or other entity cannot be altered in a malicious way and ensures greater transparency. Moreover, medical product manufacturers and hospitals can use blockchain-based records to proof compliance with regulations. In this chapter, particulalrly American and European regulations for the deployment of UDI for medical products are described. Even though the targeted UDI systems are described with aids in increased traceability, target recall efficiency, and patient safety, enterprises lack in finding the right IT infrastrucutres to implement UDI in their processes. The developed blockchain concept should be a starting point to discuss a decentralized and scaleable implemenmtation of UDI for medical products. In future research, concrete business processes should be focused next to develop blockchain pilots and evaluate the meaningfulness as well as the profitability of such solutions. Finally, enterprise consortia should be targeted to test productive systems and integrate different kinds of stakeholders.

REFERENCES

Abdulsalam, Y., Alhuwail, D., & Schneller, E. S. (2020). Adopting identification standards in the medical device supply chain. *International Journal of Information Systems and Supply Chain Management*, *13*(1), 1–14. doi:10.4018/IJISSCM.2020010101

Bader, L., Pennekamp, J., Matzutt, R., Hedderich, D., Kowalski, M., Lücken, V., & Wehrle, K. (2021). Blockchain-based privacy preservation for supply chains supporting lightweight multi-hop information accountability. *Information Processing & Management*, *58*(3), 102529. doi:10.1016/j.ipm.2021.102529

Bayrak, T., & Özdiler Çopur, F. (2017). Evaluation of the unique device identification system and an approach for medical device tracking. *Health Policy and Technology*, *6*(2), 234–241. doi:10.1016/j.hlpt.2017.04.003

Beckmann, H. (2012). *Prozessorientiertes Supply Chain Engineering: Strategien, Konzepte und Methoden zur modellbasierten Gestaltung.* Springer Fachmedien Wiesbaden. https://site.ebrary.com/lib/alltitles/docDetail.action?docID=10627905 doi:10.1007/978-3-658-00269-5

Benčić, F. M., & Zarko, I. P. (2018). *Distributed ledger technology: Blockchain compared to directed acyclic graph.* https://www.researchgate.net/publication/326566509_Distributed_Ledger_Technology_Blockchain_Compared_to_Directed_Acyclic_Graph

Bianchini, E., Francesconi, M., Testa, M., Tanase, M., & Gemignani, V. (2019). Unique device identification and traceability for medical software: A major challenge for manufacturers in an ever-evolving marketplace. *Journal of Biomedical Informatics*, *93*, 103150. doi:10.1016/j.jbi.2019.103150 PMID:30878617

Düdder, B., Fomin, V., Gürpinar, T., Henke, M., Iqbal, M., Janavičienė, V., Matulevičius, R., Straub, N., & Wu, H. (2021). *Interdisciplinary blockchain education: Utilizing blockchain technology from various perspectives.*. doi:10.3389/fbloc.2020.578022

EU Health Programme. (2017). *Unique device identification (udi) system under the eu medical devices regulations 2017/745 and 2017/746*. https://ec.europa.eu/health/sites/default/files/md_topics-interest/docs/md_faq_udi_en.pdf

European Parliament. (2017, April 5). *Regulation (eu) 2017/745 of the European parliament and of the council of 5 April 2017 on medical devices, amending directive 2001/83 / ec, regulation (ec) no. 178/2002 and regulation (ec) no. 1223 / 2009 and repealing council directives 90/385 / eec and 93/42 / eec.*

FDA. (2013). *Unique device identification system*. https://www.federalregister.gov/documents/2013/09/24/2013-23059/unique-device-identification-system

FDA. (2019). *Udi basics*. https://www.fda.gov/medical-devices/unique-device-identification-system-udi-system/udi-basics#recognize

Fedkenhauer, T., Fritzsche-sterr, Y., Nagel. I., Pauer, A., & Resetko, A. (2017). *Datenaustausch als wesentlicher Bestandteil der Digitalisierung*. Academic Press.

Fill, H.-G., Haerer, F., & Meier, A. (2020). Wie funktioniert die blockchain? In Blockchain. Grundlagen, anwendungsszenarien und nutzungspotenziale. doi:10.1007/978-3-658-28006-2_1

Gao, Z., Xu, L., Chen, L., Zhao, X., Lu, Y., & Shi, W. (2018). Coc: A unified distributed ledger based supply chain management system. *Journal of Computer Science and Technology*, *33*(2), 237–248. doi:10.100711390-018-1816-5

Große, N., Leisen, D., Gürpinar, T., Forsthövel, R. S., Henke, M., & ten Hompel, M. (2020). *Evaluation of (De-)Centralized IT technologies in the fields of Cyber-Physical Production Systems*. Institutionelles Repositorium der Leibniz Universität Hannover. https://www.repo.uni-hannover.de/handle/123456789/9736 doi:10.15488/9680

Gürpinar, T., Harre, S., Henke, M., & Saleh, F. (2020). *Blockchain technology – integration in supply chain processes*. doi:10.15480/882.3117

Gürpinar, T., Straub, N., Kaczmarek, S., & Henke, M. (2019). *Blockchain-technologie im interdisziplinären umfeld*. Academic Press.

Gurtu, A., & Johny, J. (2019). Potential of blockchain technology in supply chain management: A literature review. *International Journal of Physical Distribution & Logistics Management, 49*(9), 881–900. doi:10.1108/IJPDLM-11-2018-0371

Helo, P., & Shamsuzzoha, A. (2020). Real-time supply chain—A blockchain architecture for project deliveries. *Robotics and Computer-integrated Manufacturing, 63*, 101909. doi:10.1016/j.rcim.2019.101909

Hinckeldeyn, J. (2019). *Blockchain-technologie in der supply chain: Einführung und anwendungsbeispiele.* Https://doi.Org/10.1007/978-3-658-26440-6

Huillet, M. (2019). *Blockchain not understood by almost 70% of firms in asiapacific.* Academic Press.

ildebrandt, A., & Landhäußer, W. (Eds.). (2017). *Management-Reihe Corporate Social Responsibility. CSR und Digitalisierung: Der digitale Wandel als Chance und Herausforderung für Wirtschaft und Gesellschaft.* Springer Berlin Heidelberg., doi:10.1007/978-3-662-53202-7

Jakob, S., Schulte, A. T., Sparer, D., Koller, R., & Henke, M. (2018). *Blockchain und smart contracts: Effiziente und sichere wertschöpfungsnetzwerke.* Academic Press.

Kirmse, G. (2016). Rückverfolgung der Aufbereitung. *OP, 6*(2), 75–80. doi:10.1055-0041-109841

Miller, D. (2018). Blockchain and the internet of things in the industrial sector. *IT Professional, 20*(3), 15–18. doi:10.1109/MITP.2018.032501742

Normand, S.-L. T., Hatfield, L., Drozda, J., & Resnic, F. S. (2012). Postmarket surveillance for medical devices: America's new strategy. *BMJ, 345*(2), e6848. doi:10.1136/bmj.e6848

Oluyisola, O. E., Strandhagen, J. W., & Buer, S.-V. (2018). Rfid technology in the manufacture of customized drainage and piping systems: A case study. *IFAC-PapersOnLine, 51*(11), 364–369. doi:10.1016/j.ifacol.2018.08.320

Reyna, A., Martin, C., Chen, J., Soler, E., & Díaz, M. (2018). On blockchain and its integration with iot. Challenges & opportunities. *Future Generation Computer Systems, 88*, 173–190. doi:10.1016/j.future.2018.05.046

Saad, M., Spaulding, J., Njilla, L., Kamhoua, C., Shetty, S., Nyang, D., & Mohaisen, A. (2019, April 6). *Exploring the Attack Surface of Blockchain: A Systematic Overview.* https://arxiv.org/pdf/1904.03487

Sanka, A. I., Irfan, M., Huang, I., & Cheung, R. C. (2021). A survey of breakthrough in blockchain technology: Adoptions, applications, challenges and future research. *Computer Communications, 169*, 179–201. doi:10.1016/j.comcom.2020.12.028

Sodero, A. C., Rabinovich, E., & Sinha, R. K. (2013). Drivers and outcomes of open-standard interorganizational information systems assimilation in high-technology supply chains: t. *Journal of Operations Management*, *31*(6), 330–344. doi:10.1016/j. jom.2013.07.008

Tcheng, J. E., Crowley, J., Tomes, M., Reed, T. L., Dudas, J. M., Thompson, K. P., Garratt, K. N., & Drozda, J. P. Jr. (2014). Unique device identifiers for coronary stent postmarket surveillance and research: A report from the food and drug administration medical device epidemiology network unique device identifier demonstration. *American Heart Journal*, *168*(4), 405–413.e2. doi:10.1016/j.ahj.2014.07.001 PMID:25262248

Terzi, S., Zacharaki, A., Nizamis, A., Votis, K., Ioannidis, D., Tzovaras, D., & Stamelos, I. (2019). Transforming the supply-chain management and industry logistics with blockchain smart contracts. In Y. Manolopoulos, G. A. Papadopoulos, A. Stassopoulou, I. Dionysiou, I. Kyriakides, & N. Tsapatsoulis (Eds.), *Proceedings of the 23rd pan-hellenic conference on informatics* (pp. 9–14). ACM. 10.1145/3368640.3368655

Treiblmaier, H. (2018). The impact of the blockchain on the supply chain: A theory-based research framework and a call for action. *Supply Chain Management*, *23*(6), 545–559. doi:10.1108/SCM-01-2018-0029

Walter, A. (2013). *Technologietransfer zwischen Wissenschaft und Wirtschaft: Voraussetzungen für den Erfolg*. Springer-Verlag.

Wang, X., Zha, X., Ni, W., Liu, R. P., Guo, Y. J., Niu, X., & Zheng, K. (2019). Survey on blockchain for internet of things. *Computer Communications*, *136*, 10–29. doi:10.1016/j.comcom.2019.01.006

Wust, K., & Gervais, A. (2018). *Do you need a blockchain? In 2018 crypto valley conference on blockchain technology (cvcbt)*. IEEE. doi:10.1109/CVCBT.2018.00011

Chapter 7
Securing Healthcare Data With Blockchain

Harsh Gupta
Indian Institute of Information Technology, Bhopal, India

Rahul Bharadwaaj
Indian Institute of Information Technology, Bhopal, India

ABSTRACT

This chapter shows that blockchain has a lot of potential for revolutionizing the traditional healthcare industry. When attempting to completely integrate blockchain technology with existing EHR systems, however, a number of research and operational hurdles remain. The authors evaluated and discussed some of these issues in this chapter. After that, they discovered a variety of possible research topics, such as IoT, big data, machine learning, and edge computing. They offer a methodology for implementing blockchain technology in the healthcare industry for electronic health records (EHR). The goal of the proposed structure is to first integrate blockchain technology for EHR and then to enable safe storage of electronic data for users of the framework by setting access controls. They hope that this review will help us gain a better understanding of the development and deployment of future generation EHR systems that will benefit humankind.

1. INTRODUCTION

The advancement of technology has resulted in numerous improvements in all aspects of our life. It's also looking of innovative methods to enhance the medical industry. EHR (Electronic Health Record) and EMR (Electronic Medical record)

DOI: 10.4018/978-1-7998-9606-7.ch007

systems are reaping the benefits of technological advancements such as reliability and user satisfaction. They do, though, have certain concerns about the privacy of health records, user data governance, data quality, and so on. Blockchain technology provides a bulwarked framework for holding health information, which addresses these concerns. Authorities and allied industrial sectors are becoming increasingly interested in digitalizing medical systems, as shown by a variety of projects currently happening in many nations and industries. [1] Electronic health records and the capacity to communicate patient data digitally will help you offer better and faster treatment for your patients even while improving your organization's overall performance. During the point of service, it offers reliable, up-to-date, and full data of patients. It also saves money by reducing documentation, improving safety, reducing laboratory redundancy, and improving health. The current 2019 new novel coronavirus crisis, in which remote medical surveillance and other healthcare delivery are being employed to manage the condition, demonstrates the potential of EHRs. There are indeed a variety of scientific and practical obstacles, like any growing commercial technology. Several existing Health systems, for example, employ a centralised server paradigm, and as a result, such implementations retain the centralised server model's confidentiality restrictions. Furthermore, as EHR services grow more prevalent and the significance of information (especially medical information) becomes more widely recognised, fair but inquisitive servers may secretly capture sensitive data from users while they go about their daily lives. The use of blockchain in a wide variety of uses, notably healthcare, has become increasingly popular in recent years. This is unsurprising, given that blockchain is a distributed system that is unchangeable, clear, and decentralised and can be used to create a safe and trustworthy supply chain (Akkaoui et al., 2020). Furthermore, because the information in the blockchain is duplicated across all devices in the system, an environment of transparency and availability is created, allowing healthcare users, particularly patients, to realize how their data is managed, by whom, when, and how. Moreover, because the data in the blockchain is duplicated across several nodes within the network, resolving any one node in the blockchain system has no effect on the ledger's state. As a result, by its very structure, blockchain can protect medical information against data loss, theft, and security concerns like ransomware. Furthermore, due to blockchain's absoluteness, it is difficult to edit or amend any information that has been uploaded to the blockchain. This is very much in line with the need to save healthcare records, which is to ensure the authenticity and validity of patients' medical data. ARRA 2009 mandates that all competent healthcare professionals implement or demonstrate "appropriate usage" of electronic health records. This act prompted a considerable growth in the use of electronic health records (EHRs). Unfortunately, one of the major problems of healthcare IT and EHR compatibility is that most technologies are incapable of

Table 1. Shows the difference between EHR and Blockchain-Based EHR

ELECTRONIC HEALTH RECORD	BLOCKCHAIN-BASED EHR
Every medical institute has their own EHR system	Can be viewable to any medical institute
Difficult to maintain confidential data	Confidentiality can be achievable easily
Data cannot be fully secured. Fraud may happen	Data is stored in a blockchain. It is highly secured

exchanging their health information. By serving as a single technological framework for effectively distributing digital health information, blockchain technology offers the ability to alleviate compatibility issues. The autonomous design of blockchain provides a greater monitoring choice and allows data to be refreshed immediately. Any attempt at data change should indeed be backed up by all the platform's blocks. Fresh information will become a fixed part of the public record after verification and cannot be altered or deleted. Blockchain has the potential to decrease financial failures while also significantly reducing fraud and illicit data transfer. According to a 2017 WHO study, 10% of pharmaceutical items in poor countries are either poor quality or faked. At least 1% of all medicines on the marketplace are fake, according to estimates. A blockchain-based solution can provide a highly efficient supply record that can be traced all the way back to the beginning of the medication supply chain. Additionally, add-on features enhance the drug supplier's reputation at every distribution stage and help to keep contracts between entities on track. The challenges of shuffling and data spying can be addressed using blockchain technology. The technology allows for the transmission of time-stamped documentary evidence of clinical studies and research results, reducing the risk of fraud and mistakes in relevant clinical reports. (Górski & Bednarski, 2020) It goes without saying that a health history is the most comprehensive record of a person's identity and must be maintained with care. Furthermore, blockchain has shown to be highly successful in ensuring the accuracy and confidentiality of medical records.

The one spot of breakdown can be mitigated with blockchain-based solutions. Furthermore, because information is stored in the shared ledger and all nodes inside the public blockchain have record duplicates and can retrieve this information at any place and any moment, such a method provides data integrity and aids in the development of decentralized node trustworthiness. It also makes data auditing and traceability easier by allowing users to track tamper-proof past records in the ledger. Content in the ledger can be maintained in encoded format using various cryptographic algorithms, maintaining data confidentiality, based on the exact implementation. People can also use sort of anti to conceal their true identity. To improve durability, smart contracts may be used to provide a variety of functionalities

Table 2. Shows the benefits and drawbacks of EHR systems

BENEFITS	DRAWBACKS
Decrease the number of medical mistakes	Starting fees, which might be too expensive
Improve the standard of treatment delivered to patients	There is a problem with protecting the privacy.
Reduce the expense of medical care	Hardware placement

for various business situations. User can specify the criteria of the smart contract, and the smart contract can only be performed if the conditions have been met.

We will concentrate on blockchain-based medical systems in this article. In the next part, we'll go through the EHR infrastructure and blockchain design. Later, we'll witness the effects of a blockchain-based EHR deployment.

2. BACKGROUND

2.1 Electronic Health Record (Ehr)

In general terms, an electronic health record (EHR) is a compilation of a patient's healthcare data. EMRs can be used as a data point for EHRs, primarily from clinical institutions' healthcare professionals. Patient data, such as that collected through portable tech maintained and managed by users, is stored in the personal health record (PHR). (Górski & Bednarski, 2020) Users and medical practitioners can access data gathered as part of PHRs. In general, EHR platforms must protect the data's security, accuracy, and reliability, and data may be safely exchanged between authorised users. Furthermore, if properly designed, such a system may decrease data duplication and the danger of lost records, among other things. Yet, the difficulty of protecting information in these kinds of platforms, whether it be in storage or transit, is exacerbated by their growing interconnectedness. Smart phones that may synchronize with the EHR platform, for example, are a possible threat vector.

The existence of huge amounts of data, which may be utilised to aid data analysis and pattern recognition, for example to influence other scientific research initiatives such as illness predictions, is one of the major advantages of electronic health records. Moreover, smart as well as other Internet of Things (IoT) gadgets can gather and transfer important data to electronic health records, including PHR data, facilitating medical surveillance and tailored quality healthcare.

Figure 1. Block of a blockchain

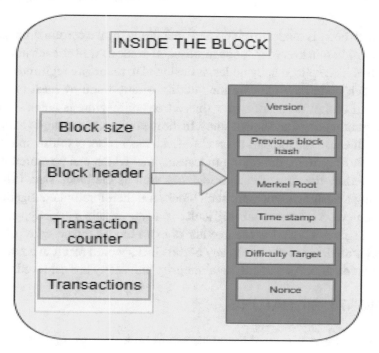

2.2 Blockchain

The development of Bitcoin helped popularise blockchain, which may be utilized to allow reliable and safe trades over an untrustworthy ecosystem without depending on a centralised 3rd person. A blockchain is a collection of full and legal transactional records in the form of a sequential succession of blocks. A link (hash value) connects each block to the one before it, establishing a chain. The parent block of a specific block is termed as genesis block. The block header as well as the block content make up a block.

The block header provides the following information:

- Block version: verification rules for blocks;
- Preceding block hash: the prior block's hash code;
- Timestamp: the present block's generation time;
- Nonce: a 4-byte unique parameter that miners change for each hash computation to tackle a PoW mining problem;
- Body root hash: hash of the Merkle tree root constructed by exchanges inside the block body;

- Target hash: it is being intended to define the PoW puzzle's complexity.

The block body is made up of verified operations from a certain time frame. The Merkle tree, wherein every leaf node represents a trade as well as each non-leaf node is the hash of its 2 spliced baby nodes, is designed to record all legitimate activities. Because each node may validate the validity of any trade by hash of associated forks instead of the full Merkle tree, thus a tree architecture is quick for verifying transaction authenticity and consistency. In the meantime, any changes to the transfer of funds will cause the top part to create a fresh hash code, resulting in a disproved root hash. Furthermore, the optimum transactions which can be stored in a block is determined by the size of each transfer as well as the block size. (Shala et al., 2020) Using a hashing algorithm, such blocks are therefore linked together like an exclave framework. Because it is difficult to change or delete already verified data, fresh data is always added in the manner of extra blocks linked with prior blocks. As already stated, every change to any of the blocks would result in a new hash and linkage relationship. As a result, data integrity and safety are achieved.

2.2.1 DIGITAL SIGNATURE

In an untrusted ecosystem, a digital signature built on asymmetric encryption is commonly employed for transaction verification. To execute transactions and validate transactional authenticity, blockchain employs an asymmetric encryption method. Before to being transferred via the Peer-to-peer network, the receipt is authenticated with the sender's secret key. In most extant blockchains, the elliptic curve digital signature method (ECDSA) is employed.

Once a payment is completed, it is published to all surrounding nodes via the peer-to-peer (P2P) protocol, in which neighbours have identical privileges. When additional nodes get the transactions, the sender's public key is employed to validate its validity using block verification criteria. If the trade is legitimate, it will be sent to additional nodes till they have all received and verified it. If not, it'll be rejected during the procedure. In the fresh block of the blockchain protocol, only legitimate activities could be recorded.

2.2.2. CONSENSUS ALGORITHMS

There really is no centralized entity in the blockchain ecosystem. As a result, obtaining a consensus for such transactions across untrusted nodes in a decentralized system, which is an adaptation of the Byzantine Generals (BG) Dilemma, is a critical challenge. The Byzantine legion is circling the city under the leadership of a collection of generals, and they also have little odds of succeeding the battle until they all strike at the same moment, according to the BG. They are unsure, though, if there will be cheaters in a dispersed setting. As a result, they must decide whether to assault or escape. The blockchain system is up against the exact problem.

Well, whenever fresh block is connected into blockchain, a variety of mechanisms have been devised to establish consensus between all dispersed peers, like the following:

- Bitcoin's consensus technique is known as PoW (Proof of Work). If the miners with a particular amount of computational (hashing) capacity wants to get any pay-outs, the miner first should show that he is not malevolent by mining. (Hafid et al., 2020) The miner must conduct hash calculations frequently in order to obtain an acceptable nonce number that meets the condition that a hash block head be below (or equal to) the desired hash. The nonce is complex to produce but simple to verify by other peers. Because of the large number of complex computations, the work is expensive. A 51 percent assault is a possible assault on the blockchain system in which a miner or a team of miners having greater than 51 percent of the computational capacity can prevent fresh blocks from being generated and produce false transaction logs that benefit the assailants.
- PoS (Proof of Stake) is a more energy-efficient version of PoW. Nodes having the most assets are thought to be least inclined to assault the system. The choosing depending on total balance, on the other hand, is unjust since the wealthiest node is much more prone to become predominant in the system, progressively becoming a centralised system.
- DPoS (Delegated Proof of Stake) is a kind of similar to PoS. The main distinction among DPoS and PoS is that PoS choosing is dependent on all nodes, whereas DPoS is democratically proportional. Users may choose who will produce and verify blocks by electing representatives. The faster the transactions are verified by neighbouring nodes, the fewer nodes that verify the block. Furthermore, fraudulent participants may be readily kicked out, making network monitoring easier.
- PBFT (Practical Byzantine Fault Tolerance) is a multiple amplification method that allows byzantine errors to be tolerated. Preparation, preparation, and commitment are the three steps. A fresh block might be created if it receives acceptable responses from more than two-thirds among all nodes in each step. In the event of fewer than 1/3 malevolent byzantine replication nodes, the network's accuracy may be assured. Permissioned Hyperledger Fabric validates transactions using the PBFT consensus technique.
- Raft is a consensus technique for managing emulated records across several computer nodes in a group. Only the chosen manager is accountable for

approving fresh transactions and duplicating them for other members throughout each term. The transactions will be executed once the manager obtains input from a specific number of members who have performed the transactions. Raft is suitable for private/consortium blockchains that can endure up to 50% crash hazard nodes.

- Proof of Authority (PoA) is a good consensus protocol. Those nodes with a permission to create fresh blocks are allowed to do so. Every node should first undergo an initial verification. This method, on the other hand, tends to create a concentrated design.
- Proof of Capacity (PoC) is an agreement technique that relies on accessible hard drive capacity rather than computer capabilities to achieve consensus. The more disk space you possess, the more answers you can record, and the more likely it is that a fresh block will be created.
- PoET (Proof of Elapsed Time) aims to select a block producer at irregular intervals and equitably depending on the amount of period each member has spent within a trustworthy runtime ecosystem.

2.2.3 BLOCKCHAIN NETWORKS CLASSIFICATION

Depending on the rights granted to network nodes, blockchain networks are classified into three categories:

Public Blockchain

The phrase "public blockchain" merely refers to blockchains that are available to the general public. The user and verifier are both unrestricted in these blockchain systems. The major benefit of this form of blockchain is its uncontrollability, which implies that no one has total command over the system ensuring that content is safe and documents are immutable. Each node linked to this public blockchain will always have equivalent power resulting in a completely distributed public blockchain.

Private Blockchain

As the title indicates, this blockchain needs participants to be authorized before they may join. Only people who are members of the blockchain network may see every transaction. These blockchain networks are significantly more controlled and regulated than public blockchains. In private blockchains, a system administrator is in charge of user permissions. These are commonly used in private companies to hold confidential information about the company.

Consortium or Hybrid blockchain

This is neither a public nor a private platform. This sort of blockchain is most useful when several companies engage in the same sector and need a common platform to conduct trades or transmit data. The main benefit of this blockchain is that it provides a collaborative atmosphere in which businesses may gain greater awareness and innovate.

2.3 Ethereum

Ethereum originally conceived in late 2013 and come to fruition in 2014 by Vitalik Buterin. Ethereum is a self-hosted environment for decentralised applications, or Dapps. What one needs to do is grasp the Ethereum coding language named Solidity and start writing to construct a decentralised software that no single individual owns, not even one who built it. The Ethereum network is totally decentralised since it is run by hundreds of separate computers. When a programme is uploaded to the Ethereum system, these machines, also called nodes, ensure that it runs correctly. Ethereum is the platform on which Dapps are built all around the world. It is a system, not a currency. Ether is the money that used to incentivise the platform. (Rathod et al., 2020) Hardly any online action takes place without the involvement of a third party or mediator. Most of the internet is controlled by Amazon, Google and other behemoths. However, as Bitcoin showed the notion of digital decentralisation, a whole new world of possibilities opened up. Now, we can begin to conceive and build an Internet that links people directly without the involvement of a centralised third party. Drivers may directly provide their services to customers, eliminating the need for "Uber." Ethereum enables people to communicate directly with one another without the need for a centralized entity to manage the process. It's a collection of devices that operate collectively to form a strong, distributed supercomputer. But this comes with a cost. Money to acquire the devices, charge those up, maintain them, if necessary, cool them. That's why Ether was invented. Whenever people speak about the value of Ethereum, they're talking about Ether, a cryptocurrency that encourages users to execute the Ethereum program on their computers. This is quite similar to how Bitcoin miner get compensated for keeping the Bitcoin network up to date.

2.3.1 ETHEREUM TRANSACTION

An activity begun by an externally-owned profile, that is, an account maintained by a person, rather than a protocol, is referred to as an Ethereum transaction. If Rahul gives Harsh 1 ETH, for instance, Rahul's account should be deducted and Harsh's account should be credited. Inside a process, this state-changing operation occurs. Operations that modify the EVM's status must be published to the entire system. A miner will perform the transaction and disseminate the resultant state update to the entire network whenever any node broadcasts a call for a transaction to be completed on the EVM. Transactions should be mined to remain legitimate and demand a charge. We'll discuss gas costs and mining somewhere to keep this summary short.

The following details is included in a reported transaction:

recipient – the sender's address

signature – the recipient's unique identification Whenever the sender's secret key confirms the transaction and verifies that the recipient has approved it, this is created.

value – the value of ETH to be sent from the sender to the receiver

data - a field that may be used to store any type of data.

gas Limit – the transaction's maximal gas consumption threshold. The computing stages are represented by gas units.

maxPriorityFeePerGas - the utmost quantity of gas that may be given to the miner as a gratuity.

maxFeePerGas - the utmost quantity of gas agreed to be given in exchange for a transaction.

There are some distinct sorts of exchanges on Ethereum:

A transaction between one account to another is known as a regular transaction.

Contract deployment transactions are those that don't have a 'to' location and instead utilise the data column to store the contract script.

2.3.2 Workflow of a Transaction

The following occurs after the transaction is published:

- Cryptography creates a transaction fingerprint after you submit a transaction.
- After then, the transaction is streamed live to the community and placed in a group with several other transactions.
- In order to validate your transaction and declare it "clean," a miner need to choose it and put it in a block.
  - "Approvals" will be sent to you for your transaction. The frequency of approvals refers to the frequency of blocks that have been generated since the block in which your transaction was contained. The larger the proportion, the more confident the network was in processing and recognising the transaction.
- Latest blocks could be re-ordered, creating the illusion that the transaction failed; nevertheless, the transaction could still be legitimate just in a distinct block.
- With each consecutive block mined, the likelihood of a re-organization decreases, i.e., the higher the number of approvals, the more unchangeable the transaction becomes.

2.4 Smart Contract

Nick Szabo coined the phrase "smart contract" in 1997, long prior Bitcoin. He is a coder, a computer programmer, and a law researcher. To record contracts, he intended to utilise a distributed ledger. Smart contracts now function in the same way that traditional contracts do. The only distinction is they're all computerized. Smart contracts are self-executing programmes that are implemented on the blockchain and are used in a variety of industries, including financial institutions, medical, and politics. By delivering a contract-invoking operation to the necessary contract location, such a system can accomplish sophisticated programmed tasks. The smart contract would then instantly implement the present conditions in the safe capsule. Smart contracts allow you to exchange cash, assets, stocks, or anything else of worth without the use of an intermediary in a clear, conflict-free manner. Smart contracts are based on if-then logic, making them very simple to understand. For instance, there are several internet-based e-commerce websites that we do not trust. Let's assume there's a site called abc.com where customers may purchase items online. Some consumers may well not purchase from them because of two reasons: firstly, they do not really trust them, and secondly, it isn't safe. Let's assume that consumers simply don't trust the website because they weren't able to provide the thing on time after collecting payment from costumer. What about if the e-commerce website is legitimate, but the delivery business, XYZ, is defrauding customers? As a result, we can create trust between them through using smart contracts. We may create smart contracts like this: a customer purchased something from ABC.com that was prepaid, and the customer began the payment, which will be collected by the website only when the customer receives the item. Similarly, ABC.com would pay the XYZ delivery firm, and they will only be paid whenever the item is delivered. That's how smart contracts establish network trustworthiness. Because smart contracts are placed on the blockchain, they are unchangeable. Ethereum is the very first accessible blockchain network to provide programmers with actually turning smart contract protocols, allowing them to build any decentralised application they want. (Dhiran et al., 2020) Such contracts can assist ease and accelerate different financial products in the finance industry. Insurance firms, for example, can utilise them to make legal commitments and pay disputes.

Depending on their uses, there are 3 kinds of smart contracts:

Smart Legal Contracts: These contracts are lawfully binding and compel the participants to carry out their commitments. If they do to comply, they may face severe legal consequences.

Decentralized Autonomous Organizations: These are blockchain societies governed by particular norms written into blockchain contracts and governed by

Figure 2. 3 kinds of smart contracts

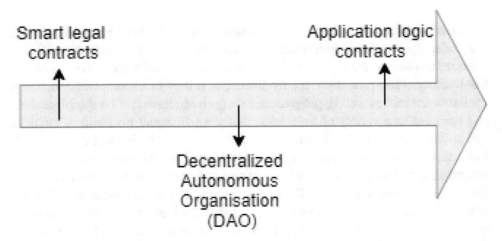

administration systems. As a result, each action made by individuals of the society is substituted by a self-enforcing algorithm.

Application Logic Contracts: These contracts include software code that keeps other blockchain contracts in sync. It allows interaction between disparate equipment, such as when the Internet of Things and blockchain technology are combined.

Table 3. Elements of smart contract

Technical Elements	Legal Elements	Economic Elements
self-validating	Legal responsibilities can be mapped into an automated procedure using smart contracts.	greater transparency
self-explanatory	They can give a higher level of legal protection if properly executed.	there are fewer middlemen
tamper-proof	Participants must follow the rules.	transaction costs are less

Every commitment, procedure, activity, and transaction may have a digital copy and sign that can be recognized, authenticated, saved, and distributed using smart contracts. Basic technical use cases include time-stamping systems like "Bernstein" (patent register) or governmental and semi-governmental databases (land titles, birth certificates, school and university degrees). The smart contract formalises the guidelines of an organisation, such as its laws, governing legislation, procedural rules, or articles of incorporation, and substitutes day-to-day functional administration with self-enforcing coding.

2.5 ETHEREUM VIRTUAL MACHINE

The Ethereum Virtual Machine (EVM) is a sophisticated, virtualized stack that executes contract bytecode and is contained into each complete Ethereum node. Contracts are usually created in high-level programming like Solidity and then compiled into EVM bytecode. This implies that the bytecode is entirely separated from the client computer's system, disc, and other activities. Each client in the Ethereum platform has an EVM replica, which enables them to rely on the same set of guidelines to be executed. EVM is Turing full, which means it can execute every logical phase of a process. Turing machine (for "automated system") is a fictional machine that represents the idea of non-human or machine intelligence. Algorithms are used to guide the cognitive approach. Such a computer, according to Turing's work, would have to handle a reel of tape containing a row of characters or operations that could be pushed back and forth. A read/write fork might also be used to switch among these operations. As a result, the machine will be proficient of digesting or changing a symbol. A system like this could only focus on one "state" at a moment. Using such a tape, no restriction has been specified. It is theoretically limitless and is only limited by practical constraints. The tape represents the memory of a device. As a result, the memory may be expanded indefinitely by increasing the capacity of the tape loop. When a computer is given a sequence of commands to execute, the data that may be used to carry out those commands is only restricted by physical restrictions. These concepts are essential to comprehending "What is Ethereum Virtual Machine?" since they form the foundation of its theory and structure. (Haveri et al., 2020) Others constructed a virtual equivalent from Turing's primarily "physical" notion of machine computation, with basically the same operational assumptions. EVM have indeed been effectively developed in a variety of coding languages such as C++, Java, JavaScript, Python, Ruby, etc. EVM designed to keep record of implementation costs provides a cost involved in Gas units to each and every operation implemented. Whenever a client wishes to start an action, they set aside enough Ether to cover the cost of the gas. Two significant difficulties are addressed by utilising the Gas method.

- Even if the transaction fails, a verifier is assured to get the original pre-paid payment.
- An implementation cannot go greater than the sum paid in advance. Rather of repeating endlessly, the execution will stop when it ran out of Gas.

Figure 3. Architecture of Ethereum Virtual Machine

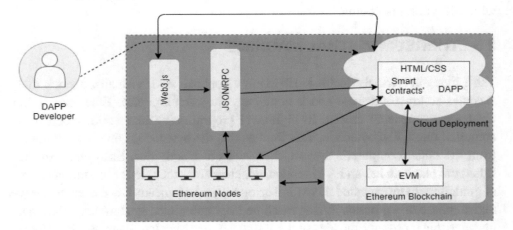

In recent times, Ethereum has attracted a lot of attention since it has shown to be a game-changing idea in blockchain and the construction of decentralised systems that do something other than handle simple financial operations.

The Ethereum Virtual Machine is Predictable. When a programme produces the same outcome for the identical collection of input data, it is said to be predictable. It doesn't make a difference how many instances the program is run. This is significant since Ethereum's decentralised programmes, or Dapps, can manage large-scale financial activities at any given moment. As a result, it's essential to understand how the program will behave at each level of operation. The EVM's underpinnings are built on determinism.

EVM has been isolated. Isolation is necessary because a smart contract may be protected against hackers or flaws. The functionality is in position to ensure that such faults or occurrences do not have an impact on the system as a whole.

The EVM is indeed Turing-complete, as discussed above, which implies that smart contracts can theoretically handle any issue. However, there is no method of knowing if any such smart contracts would be able to complete all of the tasks in a certain amount of time. As a result, a termination mechanism must be included in order to set precise boundaries. The idea of "gas" is utilised in Ethereum to enable mobility. Gas is also utilised as component of the network's reward system, with gas costs being used to decide which activities should be executed or prioritised. The gas limitations are established before the start. When certain limitations are reached, the system simply ceases to operate or process data. As a result, EVM can be terminated.

The EVM is responsible for the creation of an economy. It promotes peer-to-peer completely turning using gas rewards, allowing programmes to operate on the world 's assets. It achieves its goal of being a "global computer" by doing so. It enables anybody who enters the ecosystem to run their program in a trust - free way, with the result of every execution assured by completely predictable smart contracts.

2.6 Interplanetary File System (Ipfs)

Most of the data that makes up the web has shifted to "cloud services" during past decades. The majority of the apps people use on a regular basis save our confidential info in Aws, Google, or Microsoft storage facilities. Engineers are looking to decentralised network infrastructure as a method to enhance data robustness and establish new frameworks around data sovereignty in an attempt to build a stronger internet. (Naz et al., 2019) New innovations like the Interplanetary File System (IPFS) enable us to enhance the fundamental principles of Web 2.0, rendering the web safer and more efficient by spreading data throughout a wide, global network of individuals.

The goal of the interplanetary file system is to establish a decentralized web. IPFS is a peer-to-peer interactive media technology that aims to improve the internet more open, quicker, and healthier. Many problems arise as a result of centralization. Juan Binet, who is also the creator of Protocol Labs, developed IPFS. IPFS was designed to be a time-saving tool to transport scientific data. This implies datasets ranging in size from ten to one hundred terabytes. (Dai et al., 2018) It was created to resemble a mashup of GitHub plus BitTorrent. BitTorrent allows you to swiftly transport huge documents through a network, and GitHub provides integrated error handling for your information in a matter of seconds. IPFS is a platform where you may store information in several locations at the same moment. Data will not be kept in one location, but rather throughout the network. IPFS has evolved to serve a variety of use cases and is enhancing data handling for a variety of sectors, ranging from disintermediation in the entertainment industry to agricultural climate risk mitigation. IPFS is a decentralized storage and access platform for documents, webpages, apps, and data. It is transport level neutral, which means it can interact via a variety of ip layer, like TCP, uTP, UDT, QUIC, TOR, and also Bluetooth. IPFS contains protocols that govern the movement of data and online content throughout the network. (Nizamuddin et al., 2019) This storage system layer paves the way for a variety of intriguing distributed site use cases that may operate solely on client-side windows. Rather of addressing to data by its position or the servers on which they are kept, IPFS alludes to all by the hash of such a data, which is the information actually. IPFS would query the whole system, "Does anybody have the information that matches to this hash?" if you wish to view a certain article from your browser. The data will be returned via an IPFS nodes that includes the matching hash, enabling you to retrieve it from anyplace. HTTP is the present transmission protocol. Documents are saved on a central server via the HTTP protocol. The entire data will be destroyed if the server goes down. But IPFS won't work like that. Since it retrieves material from hundreds of peers rather than a single centralised server, IPFS is decentralised. (Hasan & Salah, 2018) Each bit of data is encrypted cryptographically, yielding a secure, one-of-a-kind content identifier: CID.

IPFS is a peer-to-peer mechanism for accessing and exchanging IPFS objects. An IPFS object is indeed a two-fielded data structure:

Data is a 256-kilobyte chunk of unorganized binary code.

Links is a collection of Link structures. These are connections to IPFS objects. There are 3 data columns in a Link structure:

Name — The Link's name.

Hash — the encryption of the IPFS item that is connected.

Size — the total size of the connected IPFS object, such as the connections that lead to it.

IPFS items are usually identified by the Base58 encryption.

IPFS is a simple way to describe a file system with files and folders. An IPFS object with information equal to the data files and no links, — in other words the links array is blank, represents a small file (256 kB). A huge file (> 256 kB) is expressed by a series of links to smaller file pieces and just minimum Data indicating that this object reflects a large file. The labels of the links to the file portions are empty characters. (Chen et al., 2017) IPFS is being used by businesses and institutions all around the world to create fantastic applications, platforms, and development tools.

Because the whole idea of putting up a DAPP is to seek to establish decentralisation, to get rid of a centralized power, to get rid of a single point of malfunction. IPFS accomplishes this. The platform we're utilising is Ethereum. It contains nodes that retain a record of all codes on the blockchain and disseminate the data files around the network. However, we cannot store big files on Ethereum blockchain because it will be incredibly expensive. IPFS helps here, as a result, every time we upload a content, it creates a hash, which we use to locate the file (Park et al., 2018).(Dhiran et al., 2020; Hafid et al., 2020; Rathod et al., 2020).

3. EHR PLATFORM BASED ON BLOCKCHAIN

We now will explain the major aims in the deployment of secured blockchain-based EHR platforms depending on the needs of protected EHR platforms and the features of blockchain:

- Confidentiality: personal details will be utilised in a private manner, and only authorised persons will have accessibility to the required information.
- Integrity: data in transit has to be correct and not be tampered with by an unauthorised party.
- Availability: accessibility to data and services is not prohibited to authorized individuals in an inappropriate manner.
- Traceability: is a crucial aspect of privacy. Audit reports, for example, primarily contain data on who has accessibility to which EHR (or specific PHR), for what purpose, and the timestamp of any activity throughout a whole supply chain.
- Responsibility: a person or an organisation will be audited and held accountable for their actions.
- Authenticity: the capacity to verify requestor credentials prior granting accessibility to critical information.
- Anonymity: for security, individuals have no apparent identification. Absolute anonymity is difficult to achieve, thus pseudo-anonymity is much more frequent.

Current blockchain-based work in the healthcare area comprises the following major components in order to meet the aforementioned objectives:

- Data storage: Blockchain may be used to record a wide range of confidential medical information in a secure ledger system. When secured storage is established, data confidentiality should be assured. In practise, though, the quantity of healthcare data is typically vast and complicated. As a result, a similar problem is figuring out how to cope with massive data storage without jeopardising the blockchain network's speed.
- Data sharing: Mostly in current medical systems, service firms are often the primary data custodians. With the concept of self-sovereignty in mind, it is becoming increasingly popular to restore copyright of medical information to the individual, who is free to share (or not share) his personal information as he sees fit. It's also important to establish safe data exchange between companies and domains.
- Data audit: When disagreements emerge, audit files may be used as evidence to make requestors responsible for their activities with EHRs. Some platforms use blockchain and smart contracts to keep track of transactions for auditability. Any action or demand will be documented on the blockchain database and accessible at any moment.
- Identity manager: The platform must ensure that each individual's account is legitimate. To guarantee system safety and prevent hacking attempts, only genuine individuals can perform the required tasks.

3.1 Proposed frame work

The blockchain is used to maintain patient information in this project (hybrid). Because data aren't kept on the blockchain, but access data is, it's a hybrid. There'll be 2 individuals: a doctor and a sufferer.

- By submitting your name, you may register as a doctor.
- By giving your name and age, you will be able to register as a patient.
- The patient submits files and gives a random nonce to encode them; the contents are then posted to IPFS, and the secret is kept in Ethereum.
- The patient grants authorization to a certain doctor.
- Once the patient has granted access, the doctor may be able to view the patient's location on his main page.
- The doctor may get all of the patient's files using the IPFS hash and make a request to the node app for file viewing.
- The Node app will download a file from IPFS, obtain a secret from the blockchain, decrypt the file, and transmit it to the doctor.

The projects require NodeJS and npm to work. Move to the project directory and open it in your terminal.

Run npm install to install project dependencies.

Ganache is a local blockchain and Meta mask is a browser extension available for Google Chrome, Mozilla Firefox and Brave Browser

Smart contract

- Install Truffle using npm install truffle -g
- Compile Contracts using truffle compile

The code has only been tested with ganache and not with any other TestNet.

Sign In

To login, the user must sign a challenge, following which a token will be provided.

Upload Files

We have two layers of security here.

1. IPFS provides a hash (i.e... files can be accessed only if file hash is known)
2. Private key encrypts the file sent to IPFS.

Access Files

Figure 4. High level use case

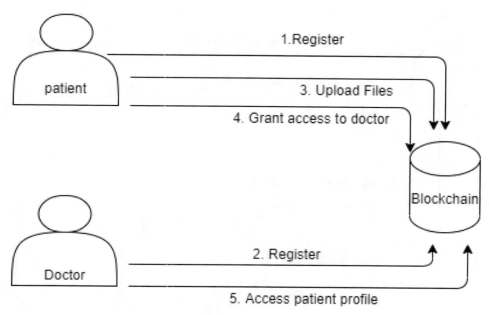

Figure 5. Sign in

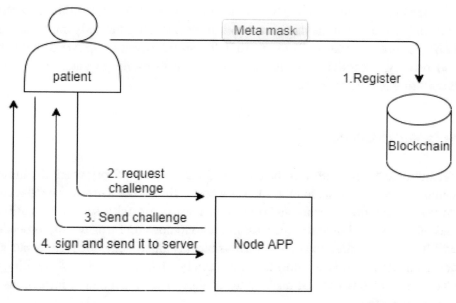

Figure 6. Upload file

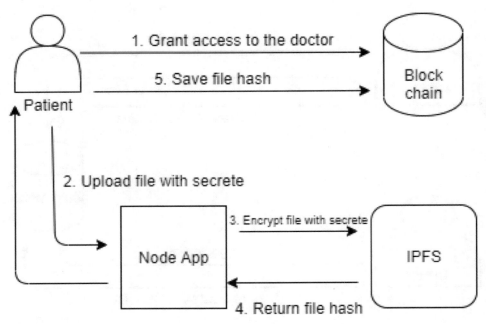

4. RESULTS

By using blockchain technology we can achieve data precision and truthfulness, Safety and confidentiality of the data as a result, if blockchain is properly implemented in EHR platforms, it may assist to secure EHR system privacy, improve data integrity and privacy, incentivize businesses and people to exchange data, and simplify monitoring and transparency.

5. CONCLUSION

Technological advances must be embraced with caution if they reach the industry without some sort of screening, such as a cost estimate. As a result, we must create universal guidelines, norms, and rules to increase conformity, safety, compatibility, and other issues. For instance, multiple autonomous and trustworthy procedures will likely be required to analyse various blockchain systems for various purposes and contexts in terms of confidentiality, safety, efficiency, delay, scalability, and so on. We'd also have to be enabled to regulate misconduct and/or infractions and impose penalties.

Figure 7. File access

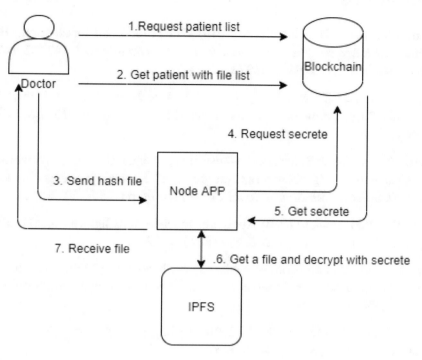

As this chapter shows, blockchain has a lot of potential for revolutionising the traditional healthcare industry. When attempting to completely integrate blockchain technology with existing EHR systems, however, a number of research and operational hurdles remain. We evaluated and discussed some of these issues in this chapter. After that, we discovered a variety of possible research topics, such as IoT, big data, machine learning, and edge computing. We offer a methodology for implementing blockchain technology in the healthcare industry for electronic health records (EHR). The goal of our proposed structure is to first integrate blockchain technology for EHR and then to enable safe storage of electronic data for users of the framework by setting access controls. We hope that this review will help us gain a better understanding of the development and deployment of future generation EHR systems that will benefit our humankind.

REFERENCES

Shahnaz, A., Qamar, U., & Khalid, A. (2019). Using Blockchain for Electronic Health Records. *IEEE Access : Practical Innovations, Open Solutions*, 7, 147782–147795. doi:10.1109/ACCESS.2019.2946373

Akkaoui, R., Hei, X., & Cheng, W. (2020). EdgeMediChain: A Hybrid Edge Blockchain-Based Framework for Health Data Exchange. *Access IEEE*, 8, 113467–113486.

Tomasz GÓrski. Jakub Bednarski, "Transformation of the UML Deployment Model into a Distributed Ledger Network Configuration", *System of Systems Engineering (SoSE) 2020 IEEE 15th International Conference of*, pp. 255-260, 2020.

Górski, T., & Bednarski, J. (2020). Applying Model-Driven Engineering to Distributed Ledger Deployment. *Access IEEE*, 8, 118245–118261.

Shala, B., Trick, U., Lehmann, A., Ghita, B., & Shiaeles, S. (2020). Blockchain and Trust for Secure End-User-Based and Decentralized IoT Service Provision. *Access IEEE*, 8, 119961–119979.

Hafid, A., Hafid, A. S., & Samih, M. (2020). Scaling Blockchains: A Comprehensive Survey. *Access IEEE*, 8, 125244–125262.

Rathod, J., Gupta, A., & Patel, D. "Using Blockchain Technology for Continuing Medical Education Credits System", *Software Defined Systems (SDS) 2020 Seventh International Conference on*, pp. 214-219, 2020.

Dhiran, A., Kumar, D., & Abhishek, A. A. "Video Fraud Detection using Blockchain", *Inventive Research in Computing Applications (ICIRCA) 2020 Second International Conference on*, pp. 102-107, 2020.

Pavitra Haveri, U. B. Rashmi, D.G. Narayan, K. Nagaratna, K. Shivaraj, "EduBlock: Securing Educational Documents using Blockchain Technology", *Computing Communication and Networking Technologies (ICCCNT) 2020 11th International Conference on*, pp. 1-7, 2020.

Čeke, D., & Kunosić, S. "Smart Contracts as a diploma anti-forgery system in higher education - a pilot project", *Information Communication and Electronic Technology (MIPRO) 2020 43rd International Convention on*, pp. 1662-1667, 2020.

Mukherji, A., & Ganguli, N. "Efficient and Scalable Electronic Health Record Management using Permissioned Blockchain Technology", *Electronics Materials Engineering & Nano-Technology (IEMENTech) 2020 4th International Conference on*, pp. 1-6, 2020.

Naz, M., Al-zahrani, F. A., Khalid, R., Javaid, N., Qamar, A. M., Afzal, M. K., & Shafiq, M. (2019). A Secure Data Sharing Platform Using Blockchain and Interplanetary File System. *Sustainability*, *11*, 7054. https://doi.org/10.3390/su11247054

Dai, M., Zhang, S., Wang, H., & Jin, S. (2018). A low storage room requirement framework for distributed ledger in blockchain. *IEEE Access : Practical Innovations, Open Solutions*, *6*, 22970–22975.Google ScholarCrossRef

Nizamuddin, N., Hasan, H., Salah, K., & Iqbal, R. (2019). Blockchain-Based Framework for Protecting Author Royalty of Digital Assets. *Arabian Journal for Science and Engineering*, *44*, 3849–3866.Google ScholarCrossRef

Hasan, H. R., & Salah, K. (2018). Proof of delivery of digital assets using blockchain and smart contracts. *IEEE Access : Practical Innovations, Open Solutions*, *6*, 65439–65448.Google ScholarCrossRef

Chen, Y., Li, H., Li, K., & Zhang, J. An improved P2P file system scheme based on IPFS and Blockchain. In Proceedings of the 2017 IEEE International Conference on Big Data (Big Data), Boston, MA, USA, 11–14 December 2017; pp. 2652–2657. [**Google Scholar**]

Park, J. S., Youn, T. Y., Kim, H. B., Rhee, K. H., & Shin, S. U. (2018). Smart contract-based review system for an IoT data marketplace. *Sensors (Basel)*, *18*, 3577.Google ScholarCrossRef

Suite, T. Available online: Https://truffleframework.com/tutorials/configuring-visual-studio-code (accessed on 23 April 2019).

Chapter 8

A Decentralized Privacy Preserving Healthcare Blockchain for IoT, Challenges, and Solutions

Kamalendu Pal

https://orcid.org/0000-0001-7158-6481
City, University of London, UK

ABSTRACT

Healthcare industry operation needs resources and information sharing between business partners. Internet of things (IoT) aims to simplify distributing data collection in the healthcare business, sharing and processing information across collaborative business partners using appropriate information system architecture. However, a large portion of existing IoT-based healthcare systems leveraged for managing data is centralized, posing potential risks of a single point of failure in natural disasters. The medical data privacy and security problems could result from a delay in treatment progress, even endangering the patient's life. This chapter describes the use of blockchain-enabled secure management of healthcare systems. Blockchain technology contributes to transactional data's intelligent and flexible handling through appropriate convergence with IoT technology in supporting data integration, processing, and providing data privacy and security-related issues. Finally, the chapter presents challenges and solutions on blockchain-based electronic healthcare record (EHR) systems.

DOI: 10.4018/978-1-7998-9606-7.ch008

INTRODUCTION

There are many potential benefits in the digitization of the healthcare administrative system. In this way, the digital healthcare system encompasses many items of interest – for example, prescription service, records of individual consultation with a medical practitioner, clinical examination reports (e.g., X-ray, blood test, and other pathological assessments), and patient's personal information (e.g., name, date of birth, age, height, weight, sexual orientation). All this information medical staff put in a digital database, commonly known as electronic healthcare record (EHR). It also stores patients' medical history; this way, the healthcare record keeps track of medications advice and appropriate preventative step by step guidance given. In addition, the advantage of digital healthcare systems providing benefits to the current coronavirus (i.e., COVID-19) pandemic, where remote patient monitoring and other healthcare deliveries are increasing used to contain the spreading of the virus in the community (Chamola et al., 2020).

The EHRs are a digital edition of a patient's paper-based medical records and charts that ensure that information is available instantly and securely to healthcare practitioners (e.g., doctors, nurses, pharmacists). They contain the medical and treatment histories of patients. They can also store information beyond standard clinical data collected in a healthcare provider's service.

The Internet of Things (IoT) technology has been adapted to collect and process the high volume of data generated in healthcare services. This way, IoT covers various healthcare applications for information gathering and processing purposes. For example, the IoT links individuals, objects, and goods to give the ability to collect data from sophisticated sensors and actuators, each transmitting data to centralized storage (e.g., cloud servers). In addition, the IoT analytics tools exploit IoT data to turn them into ideas and practices to influence healthcare business services.

Moreover, healthcare providers (e.g., doctor surgery, hospital, care home) commonly use EHR systems to monitor the individual patient medication data using a client-server architecture (Grant et al., 2006). Academics and practitioners have created different service-oriented computing (SOC) architectures (Bahga & Madisetti, 2013) to provide a system to monitor patient-specific medical data from different organizations for smooth healthcare regular operations. These SOC based EHR systems become complex, assessing the importance of data security and privacy-related issues (Azaria & Ekblaw, 2016).

Although, research initiatives of effective ways to share healthcare data among clinics and hospitals started in the early 1960s (Kim et al., 2019). Flowed by decades of research efforts and experimental results, research prototypes using different methods and technologies have been consolidated. World standardization organizations started to make interoperable services to exchange healthcare data; and healthcare data is isolated in silos (Reisman, 2017). In addition, the EHR systems have become complex, assessing the importance of data security and privacy-related issues (Azaria & Ekblaw, 2016).

The EHR system needs to ensure the confidentiality of the stored data and information. At the same time, the availability and integrity of stored data are also essential to regular healthcare operations. It must also have appropriate end-user authorization facilities for healthcare staff (e.g., nurses and doctors). Medical practitioners must access individual patients' data to provide correct diagnoses and pass medication prescriptions to the pharmacy.

This way, the EHR data often need to cross-organization boundary, and there is an initiative by healthcare practitioners and related industries to improve the automated systems in healthcare to share information by integrating the healthcare enterprise (IHE, 2019). It is worth noting that the research community has invested a substantial number of resources in finding a solution for the IHE initiative in recent years. Besides, academics and practitioners are promoting the advantages of establishing standards to address specific clinical requirements to support effective patient care.

Healthcare information system development practitioners initiated international standards for information encoding (e.g., Digital Imaging and Communications in Medicine (Pianykh, 2012), Health Level 7 (HL7, 2018)) were initiated to specify the standards of the electronic medical record and radiological images, respectively. Collaborative works between practitioners, academics and regulators produced a *governance* model for building the infrastructure to share medical records securely. This initiative identified different domains (e.g., eye care, cardiology, quality, and public health research) and clinical use cases focused on interoperability issues and the standards to overcome technical problems.

The profiles are categorized based on the domain into technical frameworks, and when published, are implemented by vendors. The IHE initiative experimentally validates the interoperability of the profile implementation between different commercial vendors' products. Also, the IHE methodology is endorsed by (i) the European Commission (Decision 2015/1302 and Recommendation 2019/800) as the European Electronic Health Record Exchange Format; (ii) the World Health Organization with the guideline: "Recommendation on Digital Interventions for Health System Strengthening" (World Health Organization, 2019); and (iii) the USA by the governmental Health and Human Services Interoperability Standards Advisory (National Coordinator for Health Information Technology, 2020).

The core of the IHT IT infrastructure is the cross-enterprise document sharing model. Logically, the cross-enterprise document sharing model defines: (i) a registry containing searchable meaningful (meta) data of documents, (ii) a repository of where the documents are physically stored, and (iii) consumers and sources of the (meta) data and documents. The interactions between this infrastructure and the users, known as transactions, define the messaging between architecture users. The cross-enterprise document sharing architecture with the IHE security models defines healthcare service's technical and integration requirements (e.g., hospital, pathological laboratory) for providing document exchange mechanism based on a standard set of policies and infrastructure.

The healthcare document exchange must comply with variegate legislation and policy requirements. The definition of data silos differs from hospital to region. The higher the mobility request is, the more the digital health infrastructures must evolve to support the demand. Worldwide (e.g., European Union, United Kingdom, United States of America, Australia), patients have the right to move to seek appropriate health services. Hence, the sharing of EHRs is a crucial requirement to mitigate patients' mobility while offering the expected level of health services. Besides, EHR systems should ensure the confidentiality, integrity and availability of the stored data, and data can be shared securely among authorized users.

In addition, hospitals in countries such as the United States of America (USA), the United Kingdom (UK), European Countries (EU), and Australia are subject to stringent regulatory control of healthcare data. There are also several challenges in deploying and implementing healthcare systems in practice. For example, centralized server models are vulnerable to single-point attack limitations and malicious insider attacks, as previously discussed. Users (e.g., patients) whose data is outsourced or stored in these EHR systems lose control of their data and have no way of knowing who is accessing their data and for what kind of purposes (i.e., violation of personal privacy). Such information can be at risk of being leaked by malicious insiders to another organization; for example, an insurance company may oppose insurance coverage to the patient based on leaked medical history.

Moreover, the security and privacy of the IoT ecosystem are significant concerns that have impeded its deployment on a broader scale. For example, an IoT network is often susceptible to security vulnerabilities, including Distributed Denial of Service (DDoS), Ransomware and malicious attacks. Further, as the number of devices joining an IoT network increases, a bottleneck problem can occur in the existing centralized systems while authenticating, approving, and connecting new nodes within the network.

Similarly, IoT-based technologies are used for different business process automation in healthcare systems. This way, IoT uses intelligent, interconnected cyber-physical systems to automate regular healthcare operations. The threat landscape concerning its deployment significantly impacts patients' safety, security, and privacy due to the IoT system's cyber-physical nature and inherent autonomy. As a result, IoT network is often susceptible to security problems that include Distributed Denial of Service (DDoS), ransomware and other malicious attacks. Besides, a system bottleneck

Figure 1. Blockchain-enabled healthcare application systems.

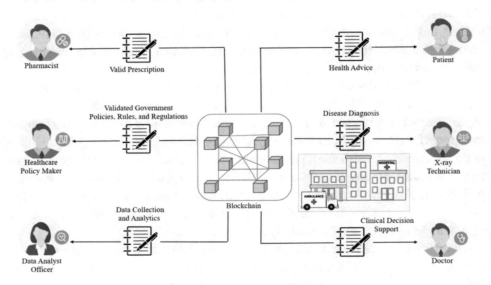

situation can occur as the number of devices increases in an IoT network due to authentication issues and connecting new nodes in the existing ecosystem.

Blockchain technology promotes the reliance on a centralized authority to certify data integrity and ownership and mediate transactions and digital asset exchange. Blockchain technology is an effective and efficient building block to deploy a healthcare system that needs interoperability and provide technology platforms to communicate securely and seamlessly. In addition, it provides technology and infrastructure to exchange healthcare data with trust. Practitioners and academics (Liu et al., 2018) (Kaur et al., 2018) (Al-Omar et al., 2019) designed blockchain with IoT digital healthcare systems to ensure patients and healthcare providers privacy. A group of researchers (Liu et al., 2018) advocated a privacy-preserving healthcare data exchange approach that integrated IoT networks and cloud storage. Their conceptual model comprises three layers: (in) data collection, (ii) data storage, and (iii) data exchange layer, and highlighted that how the architecture of EMR is securely stored in the cloud using smart contract technology. An architecture of blockchain-based healthcare systems is shown in Figure 1.

In the past few decades, there has been a marked tendency to deploy blockchain technology in a broad range of healthcare applications (e.g., public healthcare management, counterfeit drug prevention, and clinical trial) (Chamola, et al., 2020). This is not surprising since blockchain is an immutable, transparent, decentralized distributed database that can be leveraged to provide a secure and trusted value chain. Blockchain is a distributed ledger database on a peer-to-peer (P2P) network that chronologically comprises a list of ordered blocks.

It represents a decentralized and trustworthy distributed system (without relying on any third party). Mathematical methods establish trust relations among distributed nodes and cryptography technologies instead of semi-trusted central institutions. Blockchain-based systems can mitigate the limitation of the single point of failure. Since data is recorded in the public ledger, and all the nodes in the blockchain network have ledger backups and can access these data anytime and anywhere, such a system ensures data transparency and helps to build trust among distributed nodes. It also facilitates data audit and accountability by tracing tamper-resistant historical records in the ledger.

Depending on the actual deployment, data in the ledger can be stored in the encrypted form using different cryptographic techniques; hence, preserving data privacy. Users can also protect their real identities in the sense of pseudo-anonymity. To enhance robustness, the system can introduce smart contracts (i.e., a kind of self-executing program deployed on the distributed blockchain network) to support diverse functions for different application scenarios. Specifically, users' terms can be present, and the smart contract will only be executed if the terms are fulfilled. This hands over control to the owner of the data. Several real-world blockchain-based healthcare systems (e.g., Gem, Guardtime, healthbank) have been used (Mettler, 2016).

Blockchain, known as distributed transaction ledger (DTL), has emerged as a breakthrough technology to address some IoT security, privacy, and scalability problems with the solutions to many medical care business applications. Besides, blockchain technology has got many more advantages: (i) it is tamper-resistant that removes the need to trust the participating parties, (ii) blockchain could be a promising secured solution if IoT application requires to maintain payment process for its provided services without the control of third parties, and (iii) if IoT applications demand to preserve logs and traceability of sequential transactions, the blockchain can be one of the most effective solutions.

This chapter focuses on blockchain for IoT-based healthcare information systems. Specifically, it will review published works and identify existing and emerging challenges and potential research opportunities. After introducing blockchain technology, the chapter identifies several potential research opportunities and challenges. Finally, the chapter explained the future research direction and concluding remarks.

CHARACTERISTICS OF BLOCKCHAIN TECHNOLOGIES

Figure 2 outlines six blockchain features that can bring remarkable advances in existing healthcare systems, and additional itemized features are presented in the following subsections:

Decentralization

Most current healthcare facilities or institutions are based on centralized systems, resulting in overpowering a single entity. The centralized approach has several crucial limitations, e.g., a single point of failure stemming from natural disasters or bad intentions. Any unintentional or deliberate malfunctioning at the top of the hierarchy can negatively impact the entire healthcare system. Blockchain allows decentralization that leads to distributing and dispersing power away from a single or central authority, thereby making blockchain more resilient, efficient, and democratic technology. Blockchain can help improve health data access and security of patient information through decentralized principles and thus can overturn the healthcare hierarchy by enabling the development of new systems in which patients can manage their data (Pal, 2020) (Pal & Yasar, 2020) (Pal, 2021) (Pal, 2022).

Transparency

It is one of the most appealing features of blockchain technology. Enabling transparency of the health data can help to provide a fully auditable and valid ledger of transactions. Unfortunately, the current healthcare data management systems cannot provide privacy, security, and transparency at the same time together. Blockchain enforces a higher level of transparency, ensures privacy, and similarly provides authorized control over healthcare data. All the health-related transactions performed on the public blockchain are searchable and traceable. The level of transparency offered by blockchain technology can empower healthcare institutions to have complete knowledge of ingredients used to make a medicine, circumstances under which it was manufactured, the workflow between wholesalers, distributors, resellers, and customers. Greater transparency can undoubtedly make healthcare services more efficient. Blockchain achieves transparency through encryptions and control mechanisms.

Immutability

One of the main difficulties the current centralized healthcare systems raises is healthcare data immutability, as they are prone to hacking and data theft. Immutability

Figure 2. Essential characteristics of blockchain technology for healthcare application

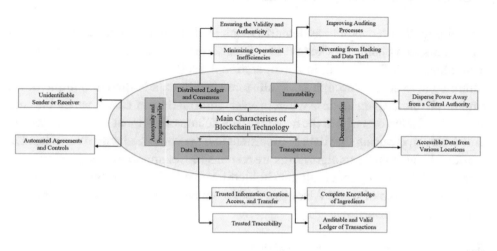

is another striking feature of blockchain technology. It refers to the ability of a blockchain ledger to remain unaltered and untamable. This striking feature has the potential to reshape and transform the auditing process into a fast, efficient, and cost-effective procedure. Also, it can enforce more trust and provide integrity of the health data, which is used and shared by medical institutions. Blockchain achieves immutability through cryptographic hashing. All transactions are registered on digital blocks, wherein each blockchain contains a hash created based on the previous block's hash, and the new information entered the new block.

Data Provenance

Data provenance is essential for healthcare to establish a certain level of trust in health data by providing complete information about its creation, access, and transfer. Blockchain ensures health data provenance by enabling track changes to data from its origin to the current form. For example, storing historical health records on the blockchain can enhance trustworthiness for data validation and audit purposes. Blockchain can provide secure health data provenance by preventing unauthorized access and alteration of healthcare systems. Also, it enables trusted traceability in healthcare industries. Finally, blockchain uses a timestamping process that involves computing hash values of the provenance record, which are transferred to consensus nodes that ensure a consistent ledger of all valid transactions.

Distributed Ledger and Consensus

Combining vital technological features, such as distributed ledger and consensus algorithms, can enable blockchain to offer a series of benefits. Distributed ledger technology (DLT) can minimize operational inefficiencies, resulting to save administrative costs. Through DLT, all stored health data is shared multiple times among all blockchain nodes, wherein each information is easily verifiable and accessible for anyone within the network. Blockchains self-update within a specific time interval, ensuring that data is consistent and synchronized with other files. On the other hand, consensus algorithms are responsible for approving transactions on a chain. In addition, they enable all stakeholders involved in healthcare systems to agree on a single source of truth. Also, they help to ensure the validity and authenticity of blockchain transactions.

Anonymity and Programmability

Anonymity and programmability are some essential features of public blockchains. Anonymity ensures that the identities of senders or receivers participating in transactions remain unidentifiable. The programmability feature enables the automation of new transactions and controls through smart contracts. Smart contracts contain self-executable codes that are based on the agreements between buyers and sellers. These codes help to control the execution of traceable and irreversible transactions.

Layered Structure of Blockchain Technology in Healthcare

Blockchain is one of the technologies getting massive attention within the healthcare industry. This section defines a simple description, characteristics and mechanisms generally used in industrial applications deployment purposes. For example, the simplified function of blockchain is a method for digital computer storage that exists as an extra layer on top of current computer storage technologies.

However, standardization of blockchain lacks the clarification, classification and categorization of which technologies make up core elements of blockchain technology and which can be separated as independent technologies attributed to blockchain technologies. This section presents a five-layer application, data, consensus, network, and execution layer as shown in Figure 3.

Figure 3. The layered structure of blockchain technology

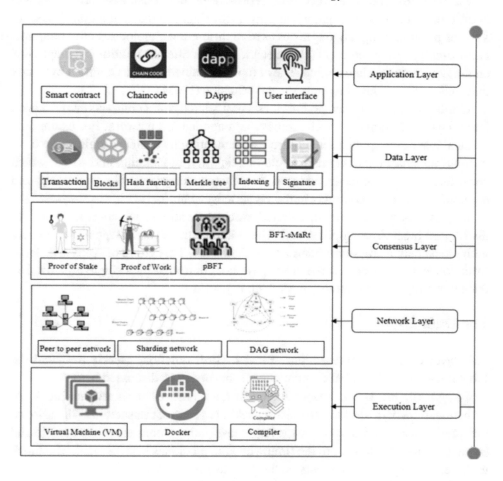

Application Layer

Blockchain-based healthcare service development begins on the application layer. This layer consists of smart contracts, chaincode, and dApps development facilities. This layer comprises two sub-layers: (i) the presentation layer and (ii) the execution layer. The presentation layer provides scripts, application programming interface (API), and user interface design. The execution layer includes smart contracts, chaincode and underlying logical rules. The presentation layer sends instructions to the execution layer that runs transactions. The components of the application layer are briefly described below:

Smart Contract: A smart contract represents a set of business operations logic in different functions executed when a transaction against those functions is issued. Various programming languages are used in different technological environments. For example, a smart contract (Hewa et al., 2020) written in Solidity language runs on the Ethereum runtime engine. The compiler produces a smart contract bytecode that runs faster on the Ethereum Virtual Machine (EVM).

Chaincode: In Hyperledger Fabric, several related smart contracts are packaged into a chaincode deployed in the blockchain application network. For example, a medical insurance application requires implementing its business logic in the form of multiple smart contracts named claims, liability, processing, and so on, which constitute a chain code. In addition, the chaincode governs the packaging and deployment of smart contracts in the Hyperledger Fabric.

dApps: dApps refer to distributed web applications, which run on top of distributed blockchain applications. These applications (i.e., dApps) can interact with blockchain using smart contracts or chaincode. This group of Apps is differed from conventional Apps, where dApps are not controlled by a single organization once they are deployed on the blockchain network.

The Data Layer

This layer consists of transactions, Blocks, Hash function, Merkle tree, and the Digital signature. Essential components of this layer are discussed below:

In general, the Block header includes: (i) a hash of the previous block for authentication, (ii) a Merkle tree root for packing a group of transactions, (iii) a Nonce that produces a hash value below the target level using a consensus mechanism and (iv) a Timestamp referring to the time when the block has been created. The block is shared among the participants on the peer-to-peer network, and each participant links the block to the existing chain of Blocks only if the block is approved by the consensus mechanism described in the later section. Thus, a decentralized ledger is formed on the blockchain and each node stores one copy of that ledger. This eliminates the need for the central control point, resulting in a high level of equity among the Blockchain participants. In addition, each block in the distributed ledger always has a distinctive cryptographic signature associated with a timestamp which makes the ledger auditable and unchangeable.

The Consensus Layer

No centralized body is commissioned to monitor the transaction or prevent attackers from manipulating or altering data when a node exchanges data on the blockchain network. To avoid fraud-related activities such as double-spending attacks, the trustworthiness of the block must be checked, and the data flow should be controlled to ensure the smooth exchange of information. These requirements are met using validation protocols known as consensus algorithms.

A consensus algorithm agrees between multiple insecure nodes on a single data block in the Blockchain context. Several consensus mechanisms from the literature are described below and presented in Figure 8, which shows five categorizations of consensus mechanism: Proof of Work(Pow), Proof of Stake(PoS), Byzantine Fault Tolerance(BFT), Proof of Authority(PoA) and Proof of Elapsed Time(PoET).

The Network Layer

The data communication network layer establishes communication between nodes, also known as the P2P network. The P2P network ensures that all nodes can discover and connect each other to propagate blocks throughout the network and synchronize the valid, current state of the blockchain.

The Execution Layer

This section describes the execution (or infrastructure) layer of Blockchain technology for two enterprise BCs: Ethereum (Aggarwal & Kumar, 2021) and Hyperledger Fabric (HF) (Androulaki et al., 2018). A user's computer can participate in Ethereum blockchain by running a client software such as Geth, Parity or Pantheon. Ethereum maintains two kinds of nodes: light node and full node. The light node runs the client software stores the cache and the state of the Ethereum. Further, the light node engages in verifying the execution of transactions while the full nodes download the entire ledger in their local storage, participate in full consensus enforcement, verify the signature, transactions, and Block formats, and check double spending. The Ethereum nodes execute the Ethereum Virtual Machine (EVM) like Java Virtual Machines (JVMs) running byte code, and EVM acting as sandboxes offers an execution environment for a smart contract.

The Hyperledger Fabric blockchain (Androulaki et al., 2018) is comprised of three types of nodes: (i) endorsers, (ii) orders, and (iii) peer nodes. The peer nodes host ledgers and chain codes known as smart contracts. Using Fabric Software Development Kit (SDK) APIs, the applications and administrators can always communicate with peer nodes to access the chaincode or distributed ledger. The Hyperledger Fabric manages multiple channels that refer to different private subnetworks with several peers(member). Each channel maintains its separate ledger, stored in each peer on the channel. A specific set of applications and peers can communicate to HF via channels.

Figure 4. The structure of a block

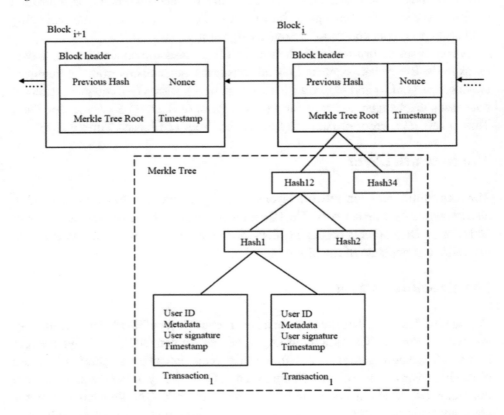

Figure 5. The taxonomy of consensus mechanism

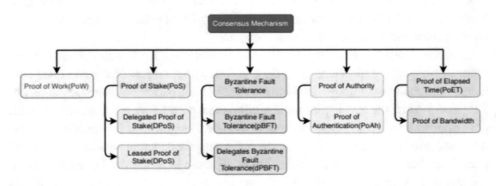

Table 1.The different types of blockchain in IoT literature

Acronym	Explication	Interpretation
PuB	Public Blockchain	Each of the transactions in a public blockchain is open for the public to verify. Anyone can download BC protocols and read, write, or participate in the network.
B	Private Blockchain	The private blockchain allows only trusted parties to participate in the network to verify and validate transactions.
CoB	Consortium Blockchain	The consortium blockchain is a semi-private which is controlled by a group of users across different organizations.
WEB	Enterprise Ethereum Blockchain	Ethereum is the second-largest enterprise open-source blockchain which is used for general purposes. Ethereum facilitates smart contracts and Distributed Applications (DApps) to be built and run without the requirements of a third party, any fraud and downtime.
B	Private Ethereum Blockchain	Ethereum Blockchain network describes a set of nodes connected to each other to create a network. For example, developers can build a private Ethereum network rather than the public network to make transactions and build smart contracts without real Ether.
EHF	Enterprise Hyperledger Fabric	Hyperledger Fabric refers to an open-source, permissioned distributed ledger developed by the Linux Foundation-hosted Hyperledger consortium. The client application uses Hyperledger Fabric SDK or REST web service to interact with the Hyperledger Fabric network.
PB	Public Permissioned Blockchain	A Public-Permissioned Blockchain network is defined as a new kind of network that bridges the gap between the Public-Permissionless networks (such as Bitcoin or Ethereum) and the Private Consortium networks.
PrPB	Private Permissioned Blockchain	This blockchain is permissioned and private, so only selected participants can join the network. (e.g., Hyperledger Fabric, R3's Corda).
CuB	Customized Blockchain	Developers or researchers use popular programming languages like C++, Java, Python, Go language to build their own private or public blockchain to analyze their applications' performance.
EPB	Enterprise Permission Blockchain	This is industry level Blockchain such as Hyperledger Fabric, where users require permission to participate in the network.
CB	Cloud Blockchain	Third-party cloud such as AWS provides resources for building and operating Blockchain operations.

Types of Blockchain Technology

Table 1 shows a classification of decentralized ledger technology (DTL). The forms of DTL in the literature differ concerning data structure and accessibility.

In chain structured DTL, blocks are interlinked in linear sequential orders while graph structured DTL stores transactions in a Distributed Acyclic Graph (DAG) (Huang et al., 2019). Individual DAG transactions are directly connected rather than joined together and processed in blocks. Depending on the accessibility, blockchain can be further categorized into two major types: public blockchain (or permission-less) and private blockchain (or permitted). A public Blockchain is a non-restrictive, permission-less distributed ledger system that allows anyone to join the network, make transactions, and engage in the consensus process (Griggs et al., 2018). Bitcoin and Ethereum, with open-source nature and smart contracts, are the most prominent public blockchains. Public blockchains are primarily reliable if the users strictly abide by the rules and regulations of the blockchain. On the other hand, a private Blockchain is an invitation-only network operated by a central authority, and a validation process would allow participants to confirm transactions in the blockchain.

Public Blockchains require no infrastructure costs to set up a network, while private Blockchains need widescale deployment and operational costs (Yang et al., 2020). Rimba and fellow researchers (Rimba et al., 2020) compared a Blockchain process's computation and storage cost with a traditional Cloud system. They run two business process instances from two different kinds of infrastructure: Ethereum blockchain and Amazon Simple Workflow (SWF) services to estimate their business process logic costs. Rimba et al. (Rimba et al., 2020) reported that the cost of execution of the business process on Ethereum Blockchain could be two orders of magnitude greater than on Amazon SWF service.

OBJECTIVES OF BLOCKCHAIN TECHNOLOGY IN IoT

The flexibility of blockchain technology has brought many benefits across various industries in trustless environments (Frizzo-Barker et al., 2019). In this section, several advantages and objectives of the blockchain in IoT are shown in Figure 6 and described below.

Decentralization

With its decentralized nature, blockchain is a promising technique for effectively solving bottleneck and one-point failure problems by eliminating the need for a trusted third party in the IoT network (Yu et al., 2018). The disruption of a blockchain node does not affect the operation of the BCIoT network. Blockchain data is usually stored in multiple nodes on the peer-to-peer network, and the system is highly resistant to technological failures and malicious attacks.

Figure 6. The objectives of blockchain

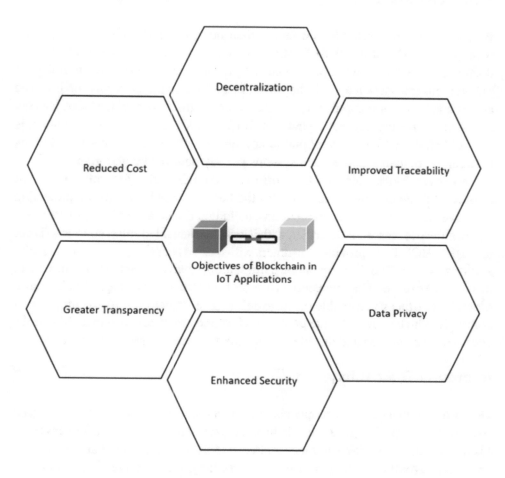

Enhanced Security

Blockchain is more reliable and secure than other record-keeping systems from several aspects (Yu et al., 2018). First, transactions must be agreed upon before being documented by the network participants. A transaction is encrypted and linked to the previous transaction upon its approval. In addition to that, information is stored across a network of computers rather than on a single server, which stops hackers from compromising transaction data. In Blockchains, the main security element is the utilization of PKI (private/ public key infrastructure). To secure transactions between participants, blockchain systems use asymmetrical cryptography.

Enhanced Security

Blockchain is more reliable and secure than other record-keeping systems from several aspects (Yu et al., 2018). First, transactions must be agreed upon before being documented by the network participants. A transaction is encrypted and linked to the previous transaction upon its approval. In addition to that, information is stored across a network of computers rather than on a single server, which stops hackers from compromising transaction data. In Blockchains, the main security element is the utilization of PKI (private/ public key infrastructure). To secure transactions between participants, Blockchain systems use asymmetrical cryptography.

Moreover, blockchain can transform how confidential information is shared to prevent fraud and illegal activities in the healthcare industry, where protecting sensitive data from different applications, including financial services, government, and healthcare, is essential. Further, with Blockchain-enabled smart contracts (Hu et al., 2018), BCIoT can provide consumers with trusted access control, automatically authorizing all IoT devices' operations. In addition, smart contract services offer data provenance to users. This enables data owners to control the exchange of their data on blockchain. Blockchain enables users to define access rules for self-executing smart contracts, which guarantees the privacy and ownership of personal data. Malicious access can be verified and disabled using smart contract-based authorization.

Improved Traceability

Goods traded in a complex supply chain using a traditional ledger cannot be traced back to their point of origin as quickly in other systems as in blockchain. For example, historical data transactions in blockchain can assist in checking the authenticity of assets and avoiding fraudulent activities. Similarly, the blockchain can store and track a patient's records that are important for patient's care.

Greater Transparency

The transaction histories in blockchain are more transparent since these histories are available to all network users. Blockchain is a distributed network in which all participants share the same documents instead of individual copies in the standard network. This shared document can be modified only using a consensus, meaning that all blockchain users have fair rights over the network to link, verify and track transaction activities.

Data Privacy

Thanks to blockchain's immutable and trustworthy features, storage systems are highly efficient to protect IoT data from alteration (Dwivedi et al., 2019). Blockchain archives data transactions and events in an integrity-preserved, authenticity-guaranteed manner by means of immutable hash chains and digital signatures. Essentially, the blockchain allows users to monitor transactions across the network so that computer and data rights are retained.

Reduced Cost

Cost reduction is one of the main aims for many businesses. Blockchain does not require third parties or intermediaries and infrastructure's deployment cost for public BC to guarantee business operations, reducing operating business costs (Bodkhe et al., 2020). Blockchain users do not need to review too much paperwork to complete a transaction, as each party has access to a single and unchangeable ledger.

Immutability

Transaction data on the blockchain remains immutable over time. Technically, transactions are timestamped after being checked by the Blockchain network and then inserted into a cryptographically protected Block by a hashing method. Hash mechanisms link Blocks together and construct a sequential chain. For example, one field of a new Block's header always holds the hash value of metadata of the previous block, which makes the chain strongly immutable (Tanwar et al., 2020).

TECHNICAL LIMITATIONS OF BLOCKCHAIN

While blockchain is increasingly committed to providing disrupting infrastructure for the Internet of Things, its implementation remains a series of critical challenges that need to be addressed in terms of scalability, computational cost, security, and privacy (Biswas et al., 2019).

Scalability Limitations

Current blockchain platforms have some bottlenecks that result in poor scalability with restricted throughput, efficiency, and high computational cost. Due to Block size constraints, many blockchains have lengthy processing periods for transactions to be written into the chain of previously confirmed blocks. Consequently, block time increases rapidly, reducing the overall system performance. If all transactions are saved on the chain, the ledger will become extremely large (Lin & Qiang, 2018). Given complex IoT scenarios such as eHealth, IoT data is enormous. Thus, the magnitude of IoT data would proliferate, complicating the processing of high volumes of data in the blockchain. Due to these limitations, many applications developers do not see blockchain technology as an alternative solution to the existing systems for large IoT systems (Kim et al., 2018).

High Computational Cost

Gavin Wood (Wood, 2014) reported the cost of completing a transaction as the computational cost of a Blockchain. The transaction processing involves various steps, including defining heavy security, mining, validating, and storing it across multiple participants (Jabbar & Dani, 2020). These steps combinedly consume considerable computing power. There are various mining techniques such as PoW, PoS, pBFT described above that require various levels of energy. For instance, pow, the most decentralized mining process, solves a complicated mathematical puzzle that requires powerful computational hardware to perform transaction validation. Due to the resource constraints of IoT systems, it is difficult for them to meet the resource requirements of PoW for qualifying the most decentralized nature. Even for IoT devices with significant computational capabilities, the sophistication of the Blockchain system will demand heavy technical and human resources. This would trigger consumers' concerns about high running costs that would limit the large-scale implementation of Blockchain-based systems.

Security and Privacy Issues

Blockchain can withstand major security attacks such as Sybil, DDoS, selfish mining, and Ransomware attacks; the existing blockchain has some inherent security flaws. For example, if more than half of the blockchain machines can control computing resources, they can alter consensus processes and stop confirming new transactions for malicious purposes.

Without robust monitoring of transactions, blockchain can be at risk of data loss and network disruption. For example, in a Sybil attack, the malicious nodes create several identities to flood the network with transactions or make false statements. Distributed service denial (DDoS) attacks are brutal to conduct on a network of blockchains. Still, blockchain technology is susceptible to message hijack and DDoS attacks, and these attacks are the most common on blockchain networks (Alladi et al., 2019). In addition, DDoS attackers attempt to disrupt the network's mining process, e-wallets, crypto exchanges, and other financial services. Selfish mining is a bitcoin mining strategy in which miners collaborate to increase their earnings. For example, a miner (or group of miners) tends to increase their revenue through selfish mining by strategically withholding and releasing Blocks into the network (Kang et al., 2019). Although BCIoT can support safe data sharing, storing all genres of health data on a Blockchain causes a delay in committing transactions and risks data leakage and disclosure of patients' sensitive information.

RESEARCH OF BLOCKCHAIN ASSISTED
IoT BASED HEALTH CARE SYSTEM

Leveraging the advantages of integrating blockchain in IoT, academics and practitioners have investigated how to handle different issues in the healthcare industry.

A group of researchers (Jamil et al., 2020) developed a Blockchain-based vital sign monitoring platform for hospital facilities. The patients equipped with wearable sensors in the hospital transmit vital signs to the authorized nodes on the BC networks. The architecture was advanced based on a Cloud-driven model. An intelligent contract supported controlled access to the BC ledger to ensure that patient vital sign information is confidential and consistent with data and hosted BC ledger functions across the proposed network. Further, the access control policy was implemented to allow system participants and users to access authorized content and transactions.

The nodes on the BC P2P network installed a couch database to hold the vital sign transactions. A benchmark tool known as Hyperledger Caliper (Hyperledger Caliper, 2021) was utilized to evaluate the system's performance in terms of several metrics, including Transaction Read Latency (TRL), Transaction Read Throughput (TRT), Transaction Latency (TL), and Read Throughput (RT).

Celesti co-researchers (Celesti et al., 2020) also proposed an eHealth system that connected the Clouds of a federated hospital using an Ethereum Blockchain to build a telemedical laboratory. Although the authors described the healthcare workflow for the proposed system, extensive performance analysis has not been carried out to demonstrate the system's feasibility.

Malpractice within healthcare, such as compelling patients to perform tests and purchases medicines from physician's preferred clinics or hospitals, arises in many countries from a lack of adequate national policies and regulations (Rathee et al., 2019). Healthcare professionals often manage patients' health data, and medical tests are under their oversight and control where patients cannot access those documents. Consequently, patients need to perform the same test twice when they switch to different physicians. To tackle these issues raised in the traditional healthcare system, Rathee et al.(Rathee et al., 2019) proposed a Blockchain-based hybrid system for processing multimedia produced from IoT healthcare. The Blockchain network applied in the framework consists of authenticating or miner nodes and executing nodes. The role of the executing node is to scrutinize whether the transactions that miners accumulate in the block is legitimate or not. The proposed scheme was simulated using NS2 to analyze its security strength.

BC has an enormous potential to secure pharmaceutical supply chains. BC can provide an integrated solution for avoiding counterfeited drugs by making the entire drug distribution network traceable to all stakeholders at any point in the supply chain. Haq et al.(Haq & Esuka, 2018) adopted BC in a drug delivery system to prevent counterfeit drugs. In this system, every transaction generated from drug production to distribution was recorded in a permission BC where only trusted authorities could join. As a result, the system can guarantee transparency and facilitates traceability while trading drugs.

Nguyen et al. (Nguyen et al., 2019) presented a conceptual, clinical assessment and control framework by integrating Blockchain, Cloud and IoT. They combined the data management system with a data-sharing platform using a decentralized mobile Blockchain network. Data integrity and privacy are ensured using a smart access-based authentication approach on the access control layer. However, the scalability and communication cost issues of the blockchain were not investigated.

Researchers have been of tremendous interest to apply Blockchain technologies to provide secure and stable data storage for healthcare. However, only a few countries, including Estonia, Peru, have already adopted Blockchain health management in practice. A Blockchain-based private health purchase management system (Celiz et al., 2018) was recently introduced in Peru. The Amazon Cloud implemented the blockchain to control the medical supply chain, ensuring secure communication between sales managers, manufacturers, and clients. Smart contracts are developed for storing medical sensor data to prevent data from malicious alternations or modifications.

BLOCKCHAIN FOR PRIVACY-PRESERVING IN HEALTHCARE

Preserving privacy in the eHealth system can make contact efficient between physician and patient, which is crucial for quality treatment, improved autonomy and tackling economic damage, embarrassment, and discrimination (Nass et al., 2009).

In (Kaur et al., 2018), BC was undertaken to build a privacy-preserved Cloud health data platform. Smart contract regulated encrypted health records are stored on the Cloud BC ledger. The vulnerabilities to data confidentiality are effectively tackled by encrypting data before inserting into the blockchain, which improves the transparency and security of cloud data storage. The limitation of the work is that comparisons have not been made between smart contract-based schemes and traditional schemes, and the model was not implemented to analyze performances.

Similar work in (Al-Omar et al., 2019) advanced a stable Cloud-based Blockchain EHR platform with four entities: (i) a key generation centre, (ii) healthcare professionals, (iii) Cloud patients, and (iv) data customers such as insurance firms. The timestamped medical data is stored in the blockchain, which increases the validity and traceability of health records. The weakness of the article is that a smart contract for managing data storage has not been implemented. The BC ledger is transparent to all the entities on the BC peer to peer network. Miners verify the contents of the block before writing it in the distributed BC ledger.

RESEARCH CHALLENGES AND SOLUTIONS

IoT technologies have promoted a huge promise for business process automation and digitization in the health care industries. Further research and development in IoT apps have enhanced the quality, flexibility, and scalability of the healthcare infrastructure, and thus it has minimized error, save cost, and enhanced performance and security in the healthcare business. Most existing IoT architecture maintains a centralized data centre for storing and processing Radio Frequency Identification (RFID) tags and sensors' data, which can be at risk of breaching security, single-point failure and malicious attacks (e.g., DDoS, Sybil). This results in the unavailability of service and the deluge of sensor data and thus outweighs the essential benefits of the IoT based information system. In addition, data interception can occur when IoT devices transfer data between them which questions the reliability of the collected data. The notion of integrating blockchain and IoT has recently gained significant popularity among researchers to exploit such hybrid architectures to address the issues. However, adopting blockchain technology into IoT applications poses various challenges (e.g., different mining rates, imbalanced resources capacity between IoT devices and the blockchain nodes). To meet these challenges, researchers (Ozyilmaz & Yurdakul, 2017) (Calvaresi et al., 2018) (Tom et al., 2020) (Qayumi, 2015) (Luo et al., 2018) suggested that autonomous agents adopt blockchain technology to solve different IoT applications for healthcare administration.

Hence, autonomous entities must track and analyze data while streaming the data from different types of IoT devices. The autonomous agent is a proactive body, which can decide the appropriate sensor data actions and automatically trigger action without the human user's intervention (Tom et., al., 2020). Machine learning and artificially intelligent technology typically form a basis for creating an autonomous agent to process and automatically identify action on the data streaming from sensors or online sources (Calvaresi et al., 2018).

Nonetheless, most of these proposals (Cha et al., 2018) are conceptual, and the notion of an agent in continuously monitoring patients' health has not been studied to optimize Blockchain algorithm and IoT eHealth data management. Health data is always regarded as a lucrative target for hackers, and researchers are highly motivated to exploit the secure transmission and storage of protected health information (PHI). Recent proposals to build secure eHealth systems adopt smart agents in the form of smart Gateway and smart contract to integrate Blockchain technologies in Body Area Sensor Networks (BASN).

For example, Griggs et al. (Griggs et al., 2018) integrated WBAN (Wireless Body Area Sensor Network) with a blockchain network. Smart contracts executed on the blockchain can automatically analyze health data based on threshold values and record logs of transactions in an immutable blockchain ledger for generating automatic reminders for caregivers. However, in the existing research of IoT eHealth and blockchain, little is known about the storage management of health data, mining management for the blockchain, and the security and privacy of the patient end's devices.

To bridge this research gap, Uddin et al.(Uddin et al., 2018) proposed a Patient Agent assisted End to End decentralized Blockchain leveraged eHealth framework. The patient agent can provide high performance by integrating blockchain, artificial intelligence and machine learning technology. The agent can address the challenges raised while merging body area sensors with blockchain.

IoT devices are manufactured with limited computational power and memory capacities, while Blockchain technology requires excessive storage and power (Atlam et al., 2018). The resource requirements for mining Blocks on the P2P Blockchain network outweigh resource constrained IoT devices' capabilities. For example, the Patient-Centric Agent introduced in (Uddin et al., 2020) (Uddin et al., 2018) running on Edge and Cloud server can handle Blockchain operations on behalf of the IoT devices. The Patient-Centric Agent (Uddin et al., 2018) runs a consensus mechanism and manages multiple Blockchains for IoT data.

Information processing on the blockchain nodes encounters the risk of data leakage as plaintext data is shared and accessed with many nodes. In the BC computing model, the implementation of homomorphic encryption technology has promising potential to secure user data and can allow mining to preserve users' privacy (Shrestha & Kim, 2019). The homomorphic encryption method allows any third-party service providers such as Cloud servers to conduct certain forms of operations on the ciphertext without first decrypting encrypted data while preserving data privacy at the same time. In addition, the integration of homomorphic encryption with Blockchain-based eHealth can potentially protect a patient's privacy in a decentralized model (Shrestha & Kim, 2019).

A consensus method that will be consistent with the homomorphic encryption technique must be designed. The current global health crisis due to COVID-19 involves tracking positive COVID-19 patients without centralized authority, tamper-proof sharing of COVID-19 related data, and maintaining privacy while collecting individual and healthcare centre COVID-19 datasets. In nature, the essence of the COVID-19 pandemic itself is distributed (Chamola, 2020). To cope with COVID-19 issues, distributed ledger technology, such as blockchain, can be highly advantageous, but this technology cannot guarantee users' privacy. However, the combination of Blockchain technology and federated machine learning can facilitate decentralized COVID-19 tracing applications without the need for centralized authority that can collect and share users' information with privacy and security. Federated learning (Xie et al., 2018) is a machine learning technique that trains an algorithm across several decentralized nodes or servers that do not exchange their local data samples with any centralized server.

FUTURE RESEARCH DIRECTION

There is a tremendous growth of IoT applications in smart healthcare applications. However, there may be a challenge in IoT technologies commercializing: (i) computing resources to provide appropriate interconnectivity, (ii) interoperability related technical issues when there is no standard application processing interface (API) and (iii) data collection, storage, and processing (Chan, 2017). Service-Oriented Computing (SOC) has been used to solve some of these problems. Also, data privacy and security issues are playing a dominating role in commercial applications to handle sensitive data. For example, IoT technology solutions and data privacy, security, and policy have been significant research themes (Pal, 2021). In addition, some of the data security issues that are attracting attention from scientific communities: (i) access to the commercial data with inappropriate access mechanisms, (ii) data breach and data loss relates to unauthorized access to sensitive data by the hackers, and (iii) as a result industry is facing data inconsistency problems, which are stopping timely decision making for the business operations.

Academics and practitioners investigate different aspects of IoT data breach-related issues and solutions. In recent years, a group of researchers (Gope & Sikdar, 2018) presented a multi-factor authentication technique to preserve the security of IoT data. This chapter's research theme will review IoT data breach-related issues in detail in the future.

CONCLUSION

Recent years have seen unprecedented progress in coronavirus treatment in therapeutic and technological domains. This chapter has advocated the opportunity to integrate these accomplishments by creating a new data-driven smart healthcare system using a hybrid information system architecture (i.e., IoT and blockchain technology). At the same time, technology allows closer virtual contact with patients outside of the clinical encounter to facilitate healthy lifestyle behaviours, symptoms assessment, and medication dose management. Moreover, there are still many technological, analytic, and workflow challenges that need to be overcome.

The current healthcare industry operating environment has been scrutinized to determine the primary needs of the enterprise information system's architecture. It is encouraging that the emerging IoT infrastructure can appropriately support information systems of next-generation healthcare enterprises. Anywhere and anytime, data collection systems are more than appropriate for gathering and sharing data among healthcare services.

This chapter briefly discussed some of the background information of electronic healthcare records (EHR), the evolution of IT architectures for EHR services, highlighted the constituent parts of a blockchain and IoT technology. Blockchain technology is gaining significant attention from academics, practitioners for smart healthcare applications; it can transform traditional healthcare applications with persistency and audibility features. In addition, the chapter reviewed research for some of the issues in the healthcare industries, which embedded blockchain-based information system architecture to find a solution for IoT systems' security and privacy issues.

REFERENCES

Aggarwal, S., & Kumar, N. (2021). Blockchain 2.0: Smart contracts, The Blockchain Technology for Secure and Smart Applications across Industry Verticals, Shubhani Aggarwal, Neeraj Kumar, and Pethuru Raj (Ed.), Volume 121 Advances in Computers, 2021.

Al Omar, A. (2019). Bhuiyan, Md Zakirul Alam Bhuiyan, Basu, A., Kiyomoto, S. & Rahman M. S. (2019). Privacy-friendly platform for healthcare data in cloud-based on blockchain environment. Future Generation Computer Systems, 95, 511–521.

Alladi, T., Chamola, V., Parizi, R. M., & Choo, K. R. (2019). Blockchain applications for industry 4.0 and industrial IoT: A review. IEEE Access : Practical Innovations, Open Solutions, 7, 176935–176951.

Androulaki, E., Barger, A., Bortnikov, V., Cachin, C., Christidis, K., Caro, A. D., Enyeart, D., Ferris, C., Laventman, G., & Manevich, Y. (2018). Hyperledger fabric: a distributed operating system for permissioned blockchains. In Proceedings of the thirteenth EuroSys conference, 1–15, 2018.

Azaria, A., & Ekblaw, A. (2016). MedRec: Using Blockchain for Medical Data Access and Permission Management, In 2nd International Conference on Open and Big Data (OBD), IEEE, 25-30, 2016.

Bahga, A., & Madisetti, V. K. (2013). A cloud-based approach for interoperable electronic health records (EHRs). IEEE Journal of Biomedical and Health Informatics, 17(5), 894–906.

Biswas, S. (2019). Sharif, K., Li, F., Maharjan, S., Mohanty, S. P., & Yu Wang. (2019). Post: A lightweight consensus algorithm for scalable IoT business blockchain. IEEE Internet of Things Journal, 7(3), 2343–2355.

Bodkhe, U., Tanwar, S., Parekh, K., Khanpara, P., Tyagi, S., Kumar, N., & Alazab, M. (2020). Blockchain for industry 4.0: A comprehensive review. IEEE Access : Practical Innovations, Open Solutions, 8, 79764–79800.

Calvaresi, D., Dubovitskaya, A., Calbimonte, J. P., Taveter, K., & Schumacher, M. (2018). Multi-agent systems and blockchain: Results from a systematic literature review. In International Conference on Practical Applications of Agents and Multi-Agent Systems, 10–126. Springer, 2018.

Celesti, A., Ruggeri, A., Fazio, M., Galletta, A., Villari, M., & Romano, A. (2020). Blockchain-based healthcare workflow for telemedical laboratory in federated hospital iot clouds. Sensors (Basel), 20(9), 2590.

Cha, S., Chen, J., Su, C., & Yeh, K. (2018). A blockchain connected gateway for ble-based devices in the internet of things. IEEE Access : Practical Innovations, Open Solutions, 6, 24639–24649.

Chamola, V., Hassija, V., Gupta, V., & Guizani, M. (2020). A Comprehensive Review of the COVID-19 Pandemic and the Role of IoT, Drones, AI, Blockchain, and 5G in Managing its Impact. May 2020. IEEE Access : Practical Innovations, Open Solutions, 8, 90225–90265.

Chan, M., 2017. Why Cloud Computing Is the Foundation of the Internet of Things.

Crameri, K.A., Mather, L., Van Dam, P., Prior, S. (2020). Personal Electronic Healthcare Records: What Influences Consumers to Engage with their Clinical Data Online? a Literature Review, Journal of Health Information Management, 2020.

Cubas Celiz, R. C., Escriba, Y., Cruz, D. L., & Sanchez, D. M. (2018). Cloud model for purchase management in health sector of Peru based on IoT and blockchain. In 2018 IEEE 9th Annual Information Technology, Electronics and Mobile Communication Conference (ICON), 328–334. IEEE, 2018.

Dwivedi, A. D., Malina, L., Dzurenda, P., & Srivastava, G. (2019). Optimized blockchain model for internet of things-based healthcare applications. In 2019 42nd International Conference on Telecommunications and Signal Processing (TSP), pages 135–139. IEEE, 2019.

Frizzo-Barker, J., Chow-White, P. A., Adams, P. R., Mentanko, J., Ha, D., & Green, S. (2019). Blockchain as a disruptive technology for business: A systematic review. International Journal of Information Management, ●●●, 2019.

Gope, P., & Sikdar, B. (2018). Lightweight and privacy-preserving two-factor authentication scheme for IoT devices. IEEE Internet Things.

Grant, R. W., Wald, J. S., Poon, E. G., Schnipper, J. L., Gandhi, T. K., Volk, L. A., & Middleton, B. (2006). Design and implementation of a web-based patient portal linked to an ambulatory care electronic health record: Patient gateway for diabetes collaborative care. Diabetes Technology & Therapeutics, 8(5), 576–586.

Griggs, K. N., Osipova, O., Kohlios, C. P., Baccarini, A. N., Howson, E. A., & Hayajneh, T. (2018). Healthcare blockchain system using smart contracts for secure automated remote patient monitoring. Journal of Medical Systems, 42(7), 130.

HL7. (2018). FHIR: Fast healthcare interoperability resources. https://hl7.org/fhir

Hewa, T., Ylianttila, M. & Liyanage. M. (2020). Survey on blockchain-based smart contracts: Applications, opportunities and challenges. Journal of Network and Computer Applications, page 102857, 2020.

Hu, Y., Liyanage, M., Mansoor, A., Thilakarathna, K., Jourjon, G., & Seneviratne, A. (2018). Blockchain-based smart contracts-applications and challenges. arXiv preprint arXiv:1810.04699, 2018.

Huang, J., Kong, L., Chen, G., Wu, M. Y., Liu, X., & Zeng, P. (2019). Towards secure industrial IoT: Blockchain system with credit-based consensus mechanism. IEEE Transactions on Industrial Informatics, 15(6), 3680–3689.

Hyperledger caliper (2021). https://www.hyperledger.org/, July 2021.

IHaq I. & Esuka. (2018). O. M. (2018). Blockchain technology in the pharmaceutical industry to prevent counterfeit drugs. International Journal of Computers and Applications, 180(25), 8–12.

IHE. (2019). The IHE IT Infrastructure (ITI) Technical Framework, Volume 1, Technical Report IHE. https://www.ihe.net/uploadedFiles/

Jabbar, A., & Dani, S. (2020). Investigating the link between transaction and computational costs in a blockchain environment. International Journal of Production Research, 58(11), 3423–3436.

Jamil, F., Ahmad, S., Iqbal, N., & Kim, D. (2020). Towards a remote monitoring of patient vital signs based on IoT-based blockchain integrity management platforms in smart hospitals. Sensors (Basel), 20(8), 2195.

Kang, J., Xiong, Z., Niyato, D., Ye, D., Kim, D. I., & Zhao, J. (2019). Toward secure blockchain-enabled internet of vehicles: Optimizing consensus management using reputation and contract theory. IEEE Transactions on Vehicular Technology, 68(3), 2906–2920.

Kaur, H., Afshar, M., Roshan A., J., Kumar A. M., & Chang, V. (2018). A proposed solution and future direction for M.A Uddin et al.: Blockchain: Research and Applications Page 72 of 80 Journal Pre-proof Blockchain Adoption in IoT: A Survey, Challenges and Solutions blockchain-based heterogeneous medicare data in cloud environment. Journal of medical systems, 42(8):156, 2018.

Kim, E., Rubinstein, S. M., Nead, K. T., Wojcieszynski, A. P., Gabriel, P. E., & Warner, J. L. (2019). The evolving use of electronic health recirds (HER) for research, Seminars in Radiation Oncology, 29(4), 354-361, ISSN: 1053-4296.

Kim, S., Kwon, Y., & Cho, S. (2018). A survey of scalability solutions on blockchain. In 2018 International Conference on Information and Communication Technology Convergence (ICTC), pages 1204–1207. IEEE, 2018.

Lin, F., & Qiang, M. (2018). The challenges of existence, status, and value for improving blockchain. IEEE Access : Practical Innovations, Open Solutions, 7, 7747–7758.

Liu, J., & Li, X., Ye, Lin., Y., Zhang, H., Du, X., & Guizani, M. (2018). Beds: A blockchain-based privacy-preserving data sharing for electronic medical records. In 2018 IEEE Global Communications Conference (GLOBECOM), 1–6. IEEE, 2018.

Luo, F., Dong, Z. Y., Liang, G., Murata, J., & Xu, Z. (2018). A distributed electricity trading system in active distribution networks based on multi-agent coalition and blockchain. IEEE Transactions on Power Systems, 34(5), 4097–4108.

Mettler, M. (2016). Blockchain technology in healthcare: The revolution starts here, in 18th International Conference on e-Health Networking, Applications and Services, IEEE Publication, 1-3, 14-16 September 2016.

Nguyen, D. C., Nguyen, K. D., & Pathirana, P. N. (2019). A mobile cloud-based iomt framework for automated health assessment and management. In 2019 41st Annual International Conference of the IEEE Engineering in Medicine and Biology Society (EMBC), 6517–6520. IEEE, 2019.

Official Website of The Office of the National Coordinator for Health Information Technology. (2020). Appendix I – source of security standards and security patterns. http://www.healthit.gov/isa/ISA_Document/Appendix_I

Pal, K. (2020). In I. Williams (Ed.), Information sharing for manufacturing supply chain management based on blockchain technology, in cross-Industry Use of Blockchain Technology and Opportunities for the Future (pp. 1–17). IGI Global.

Pal, K. (2021). Applications of Secured Blockchain Technology in Manufacturing Industry, in Blockchain and AI Technology in the Industrial Internet of Things, Subhendu Kumar Pani, Biju Patnaik, Sian Lun Lau, & Xingcheng Liu (Edited), Chapter 10, January 2021, IGI Global Publication, 701 E Chocolate Avenue, Hershey, PA, USA 17033.

Pal, K. (2022). Blockchain Integrated Internet of Things Architecture in Privacy Preserving for Large Scale Healthcare Supply Chain Data, in Blockchain Technology and Computational Excellence for Society 5.0, S Khan, H. Syed, R Hammad, & A Fouad Bushager (Edited), Chapter 6, January 2022, IGI Global Publication, 701 E Chocolate Avenue, Hershey, PA, USA 17033

Pal, K., & Yasar, A. (2020). Internet of Things and blockchain technology in apparel manufacturing supply chain data management. Procedia Computer Science, 170, 450–457.

Pianykh, O. S. (2012). Digital Imaging and Communications in Medicine (2nd ed.). Springer-Verlag.

Qayumi, K. (2015). Multi-agent-based intelligence generation from very large datasets. In 2015 IEEE International Conference on Cloud Engineering, 502–504. IEEE, 2015.

Rathee, G., Sharma, A., Saini, H., Kumar, R., & Iqbal, R. (2019). A hybrid framework for multimedia data processing in IoT-healthcare using blockchain technology. Multimedia Tools and Applications, ●●●, 1–23.

Reisman, M. (2017). EHRs: The Challenges of Making Electronic Data Usable and Interoperable. International Journal of Pharmacy and Therapeutics, 42(9), 572–575.

Rijo Jackson Tom. (2020). Suresh Sankaranarayanan, & Joel JPC Rodrigues. (2020). Agent negotiation in an IoT-fog based power distribution system for demand reduction. Sustainable Energy Technologies and Assessments, 38, 100653.

Rimba, P., Tran, A. B., Weber, I., Staples, M., Ponomarev, A., & Xu, X. (2020). Quantifying the cost of distrust: Comparing blockchain and cloud services for business process execution. Information Systems Frontiers, 22(2), 489–507.

Shrestha, R., & Kim, S. (2019). Integration of IoT with blockchain and homomorphic encryption: Challenging issues and opportunities. In Advances in Computers, 115, 293–331. Elsevier, 2019.

Tanwar, S., Parekh, K., & Evans, R. (2020). Blockchain-based electronic healthcare record system for healthcare 4.0 applications. Journal of Information Security and Applications, 50, 102407.

Tom, R. J., Sankaranarayanan, S., Joel, J. P. C., & Rodrigues, J. J. (2020). Agent negotiation in an iot-fog based power distribution system for demand reduction. Sustainable Energy Technology and Assessments, 38, 100653.

Uddin, M. A., Stranieri, A., Gondal, I., & Balasubramanian, V. (2018). Continuous patient monitoring with a patient-centric agent: A block architecture. IEEE Access : Practical Innovations, Open Solutions, 6, 32700–32726.

Uddin, M. A., Stranieri, A., Gondal, I., & Balasubramanian, V. (2020). Blockchain leveraged decentralized IoT health framework. Internet of Things, 9, 100159.

Wood., G. (2014). Ethereum: A secure decentralized generalized transaction ledger. Ethereum project yellow paper, 151(2014):1–32, 2014.

World Health Organization. (2019). Recommendations on Digital Interventions for Health System Strengthening – https://www.who.int/reproductivehealth/publications/digital=interventions-health-system-strengthening/en/

Xie, J., Yu, F. R., Huang, T., Xie, R., Liu, J., Wang, C., & Liu, Y. (2018). A survey of machine learning techniques applied to software-defined networking (sdn): Research issues and challenges. IEEE Communications Surveys and Tutorials, 21(1), 393–430.

Yang, R., Wakefield, R., Lyu, S., Jayasuriya, S., Han, F., Yi, X., Yang, X., Amarasinghe, G., & Chen, S. (2020). Public and private blockchain in construction business process and information integration. Automation in Construction, 118, 103276.

Yu, Y., Li, Y., Tian, J., & Liu, J. (2018). Blockchain-based solutions to security and privacy issues in the internet of things. IEEE Wireless Communications, 25(6), 12–18.

KEY TERMS AND DEFINITIONS

Blockchain: In simple, a blockchain is just a data structure that can be shared by different users using computing data communication network (e.g., peer-to-peer or P2P). Blockchain is a distributed data structure comprising a chain of blocks. It can act as a global ledger that maintains records of all transactions on a blockchain network. The transactions are timestamped and bundled into blocks where each block is identified by its *cryptographic hash*.

Block: A block is a data structure used to communicate incremental changes to the local state of a node. It consists of a list of transactions, a reference to a previous block and a nonce.

Cryptography: Blockchain's transactions achieve validity, trust, and finality based on cryptographic proofs and underlying mathematical computations between various trading partners.

Immutability: This term refers to the fact that blockchain transactions cannot be deleted or altered.

Provenance: In a blockchain ledger, provenance is a way to trace the origin of every transaction such that there is no dispute about the origin and sequence of the transactions in the ledger.

Decentralized computing infrastructure: These computing infrastructures feature computing nodes that can make independent processing and computational decisions irrespective of what other peer computing nodes may decide.

Internet of Things (IoT): The Internet of Things (IoT), also called the Internet of Everything or the Industrial Internet, is now a technology paradigm envisioned as a global network of machines and devices capable of interacting with each other. The IoT is recognized as one of the most important areas of future technology and is gaining vast attention from a wide range of industries.

Chapter 9
Blockchain and Supply Chain Management:
Implementation of COVID Vaccines

Prachurjya Kashyap
*National Institute of Technology,
Silchar, India*

Boddu Venkateswarlu
*National Institute of Technology,
Silchar, India*

Syed Tafreed Numan
*National Institute of Technology,
Silchar, India*

Naresh Babu Muppalaneni
*National Institute of Technology,
Silchar, India*

Amit Kumar
*National Institute of Technology,
Silchar, India*

Malaya Dutta Borah
*National Institute of Technology,
Silchar, India*

Rohit Paul
*National Institute of Technology,
Silchar, India*

ABSTRACT

Supply chain is one of critical components of vaccination drive. A robust and efficient supply chain of vaccines would help increase the speed and efficiency of vaccination, therefore reducing vaccine wastage. This system uses centralised algorithms. They are prone to single point of failure in terms of transparency, trackability and traceability, immutability, audit, and trust. These issues stymie and slow the distribution of COVID-19 vaccinations, and they make it impossible to provide a safe, secure, transparent, and reliable distribution and delivery process of COVID-19 vaccines. The authors propose a blockchain-based approach to manage data linked to COVID-19 vaccines. To automate vaccination tracing, a smart contract for vaccine distribution is being created. The authors discuss and implement the proposed solution, as well as their implementation testing and validation; they evaluate the proposed solution

DOI: 10.4018/978-1-7998-9606-7.ch009

by performing cost and security analyses and comparing them to existing solutions, and they evaluate the proposed solution by performing cost and security analyses and comparing them to existing solutions.

1. INTRODUCTION

The quick spreading of a novel COVID-19(Corona virus) has resulted in the emergence of a worldwide epidemic. The WHO has declared it a pandemic (WHO). The world has witnessed unprecedented health and economic events as a result of the COVID-19 pandemic, the world has witnessed unprecedented health and economic events. Even in times of crisis, though, there is the opportunity for new ideas and insights to emerge. The COVID-19 epidemic has taught us a lot about supply chains, resource fragility and During the crises, there were shortages of goods, an inability to source products in a face-to-face transaction framework, and a mismatch between the sizes and quantities of things available and what was required. A worldwide vaccination drive is necessary to get out of this pandemic. The entire process from manufacturing to end user involves multiple stages like manufacturing delivery and administration. An efficient supply chain is fundamental to a fully-functional healthcare system. Thus, the health supply system must be designed to quickly and reliably deliver crucial health commodities such as medicines, vaccines, and PPE during infectious disease outbreaks. Blockchain technology offers a distributed, secure and transparent approach to in-formation exchange in the supply chain. Blockchain technology continues to prove its capabilities in various areas in the healthcare sector, such as managing patient healthcare records, simplifying clinical trial processes, tracking donations, and supplies. This is possible due to the advancement in blockchain technology since its first release in 2008 in the form of cryptocurrency (Nakamoto, 2008). However, with Ethereum, representing the second-generation blockchain technology, the use of blockchain in diverse settings has grown especially due to the introduction of smart contracts, which act as self-managing software in the network. Hence, blockchain can facilitate secure information exchanges among geographically dispersed stakeholders, improve global trade logistics such as transportation management, procurement, tracking and tracing shipments, and trade finance (Nandi et al., 2021).

Figure 1 illustrates the process of vaccine delivery. As seen, it involves multiple stages and a good supply chain management is important to provide secure, trustworthy and efficient vaccine delivery.

Figure 1. Rules of Blockchain- Supply chain Management [8]

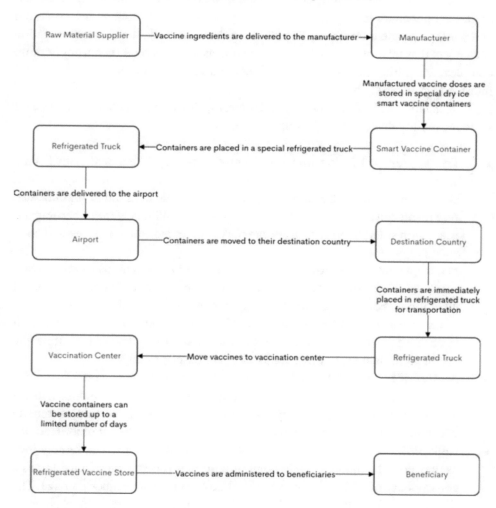

2. BACKGROUND

Blockchain is a web based technology that is valued for its ability to record, validate, and distribute transactions in immutable ledgers publicly. The technology was developed to support transactions in bitcoin, a decentralised digital currency. In essence, blockchain technology creates and distributes the ledger, or record, of every transaction to thousands or millions of computers connected to networks all over the world.

Blockchain is one of the most disruptive technologies that has transformed digital supply chain management. Over the past decade, blockchain has come out as a worthy opponent for untangling all of the documents, data and communication exchanges that take place inside supply chains as they become increasingly more complex, including a range of stakeholders and relying on a number of external intermediary ecosystems.

Blockchain is a highly applicable tool for utilization in supply chain management systems, mainly due to the following four reasons:

- **Transparency:** Blockchain has no central authority, like a bank. Blockchain based systems are extremely transparent because every participant in a blockchain is assigned a public key, which is visible to all other participants. As a result, anyone can view the transactions and holdings of every participant. Also, with smart contracts, users can make agreements in a risk-free and cost-effective manner.
- **Pre-approved transaction fees:** In the case of blockchain, users are already aware of the payment fees, which is not true for other kinds of financial institutions. For eg, when we make payment with Swift, only after completion of the transaction, is the commission of payment made aware to the users. It is because it has to run through several intermediary banks executing the transaction. Same is not true for blockchain based systems.
- **Auditability:** In blockchain based systems, no participant can modify, delete, or hide any information that has already been added to the blockchain (as a blockchain is immutable by nature). This makes blockchain extremely convenient to audit transactions as they are safe from external modification.
- **Reliability:** The risk of fraud in blockchain based systems is extremely low, as they do not contain a single point of failure, it is distributed in nature, as a consequence of which, a single node failing does not cause much damage. The risk of fraud is further reduced due to the immutable nature of blockchain.

Blockchains have a diverse set of applications, we describe the following points below:

- Procurement
- Provenance and traceability
- Digital payments and contracts
- Logistics

Manufacturing

2.1 Procurement

For all participants who conduct transactions on behalf of a user and negotiate terms with suppliers, such as partners and subsidiaries, blockchain acts as a primary source of truth. All the relevant data from all of a user's partners will be contained in the blockchain database, as a result of which, all the participants have a wide view of the full transactions, with no regards to who was actually in charge of the transactions. Audit completion is automated, minimising activities such as additional price verification that take up lots of time and resources. Consequently, individual participants will not be needed to exchange operational data and get it cross-checked by others (Nguyen et il., 2021).

For example, if a company wishes to negotiate an acquisition agreement based on the total amount of the ecosystem, which includes both your and your partners' purchase data. You may quickly calculate and mathematically establish the exact amount discount based on total purchases by storing the information in a blockchain-based system. What's the best part? You can do so without divulging the individual volumes of each organisation.

Furthermore, blockchain technology has the ability to change almost every part of the Procure-to-Pay (PTP) process.

2.2 Provenance and Improved Traceability

The supply chain of food will be the first one to make extensive use of blockchain technology, particularly in the distribution of fresh products. For many years, recalls have been a major and costly industry issue. As a result, many of the recent major food-related bacteria outbreaks in the United States are providing incentives for more and more organisations to study blockchain as a new method for increasing traceability and visibility of manufactured products (Lopez & Alvarez, 2020).

Costumers are also putting stress on businesses to produce more data about the origins, originality, and "life prior to arriving at the shelves" of goods. Most consumers are willing to pay a good price for goods that are made in a sustainable and ethical manner.

Walmart is a pioneer in this arena, having worked with IBM on a blockchain-based traceability solution for the company's food supply chain since 2016. The merchant was able to track incoming food supply in near store from "farm to store" using the tested method. In addition, the company is also investigating how blockchain technology can be applied to observing and putting a leash on the spread of illnesses related to food. In 2019, the food giant intends to implement a blockchain-based traceability programme that will be mandatory for all lettuce growers.

2.3 Payments and Digital Contracts

Smart contracts can be used to automate the process of invoicing and decrease the costly gaps in procure-to-pay. It is totally possible to codify payment terms, and cash can be paid immediately once the trade has been concluded and the logistics business has supplied proof of delivery.

Smart contracts in supply chain management will help to reduce redundancy of data among stakeholders and eliminating the costly errors. For example, if a seller sends a duplicate invoice, the blockchain based system will examine all contract elements – contract policy, open purchase orders, or previous invoices. If something is wrong the system will decline the invoice and it will bounce. If it is repeats, the system will reject the invoice and it will bounce back to the seller for additional verification.

Smart contracts on blockchain act as an independent third party, reviewing all aspects of contract and conditions and only accepting entries that match all pre-programmed values. This means that no false or erroneous invoices will come in the records. To summarize, smart contracts can do the following:

- Assist in ensuring data consistency among all supply chain actors and enforcing complete contract term execution.
- Maintaining the consistency among the transactions automatically and streamline the process of managing trading relationships.
- Provides high level security when compare to existing approaches.

2.4 Logistics

The logistics industry is still heavily reliant on a massive trail on paper, particularly in regards to customs. This significantly reduces companies' transparency into the status of shipments as they go through the supply chain. To address this issue, blockchain can do several things:

- Increase the amount of information exchanges among all stakeholders to improve logistics predictability and transparency.
- Reduce costs by enabling more automated, errorless and secure processes.
- Assist in the establishment of more sustainable and responsible supply chains on a large scale. Combining blockchain and IoT can aid logistics companies

obtain more insight into transportation conditions and implement further anti-counterfeiting actions.

2.5 Manufacturing

According to 63 percent of SAP survey respondents, the Internet of Things and blockchain are the most promising business opportunities in supply chain management. The combination of the two technologies provides several significant benefits to the manufacturing industry's supply chain:

- Improved data continuity IoT sensors can collect a wide range of information at production hubs and beyond, and then transmit it all to a centralized facility. Managers can obtain many insights about usage of material, transportation conditions, and so on, which they can then apply to planning and optimization.
- Detection of fraud is extremely effective. Systems based on blockchain are invulnerable to tampering. Any mishaps in the factories can be detected and addressed immediately. Companies that prioritise their reputation can decrease risks by being totally open about their process manufacturing and supply.

Producers who convert raw materials into finished goods can gain greater control over the flows incoming from suppliers, automate compliance to some extent, and gain better control over production. Because IoT sensors can be programmed to capture temperature, moisture levels, and other data during transportation via freight forwarders, it can be automatically ensured that the products are transported in the proper conditions. They can also gain a better understanding of the overall logistics.

3. LITERATURE SURVEY

4. SUPPLY CHAIN SYSTEM FOR COVID VACCINES

4.1 Overview

Author proposed solution models the material suppliers, manufacturer, farms etc as the actors, who have the authorization to make modifications on the chain. We include an off chain storage to store all less important data, which helps in reducing

Table 1. Literature Survey

Authors, Year	Approach/Methods/Technology used	Findings
Anshuman Kalla; TharakaHewa; Raaj Anand Mishra; Mika Ylianttila; Madhusanka Liyanage [1]	Contact tracing, Patient information sharing through blockchain, Supply chain management, automated surveillance	This paper discusses the use cases, applications, and service opportunities for covid-19 via blockchain. It proposes that smart contracts be established between patients and users to provide time-limited access to patients' data. It also suggests that directly uploading patient data to a blockchain-based system can eliminate issues like data forging and mutation.
DouniaMarbouh, Tayaba Abbasi, Fatema Maasmi, Ilhaam A. Omar, Mazin S. Debe, Khaled Salah, Raja Jayaraman & Samer Ellahham [2]	Implemented with Ethereum smart contracts and oracle network	This paper proposes, implements, and evaluates a blockchain-based system that uses Ethereum smart contracts and oracles to track reported data from trusted sources on the number of new cases, deaths, and recovered cases. It defines detailed algorithms for capturing the interactions between network stakeholders, security analysis, and the costs incurred by stakeholders and highlights the challenges and future directions of our work
Adnan Iftekhar, Xiaohui Cui [3]	Cold supply chain; meat supply chain; food safety; COVID-19; blockchain; hyperledger fabric	The purpose of this article is to discuss a blockchain-based supply chain architecture that ensures the availability of a tamper-proof audit trail. This tamper-proof audit trail ensures that all safety precautions are taken to reduce the risk of COVID-19 and other bacteria, fungi, and parasites in the frozen meat supply chain.
Ramirez Lopez, Leonardo Juan, Beltrán Álvarez, Nicolas (2020) [4]	Kardex digital or analog record, Ethereum	The paper outlines an approximate solution to the design of a secure blockchain-based supply chain surveillance design, with the goal of controlling the variables and critical points of the next vaccine distribution globally.
Nguyen, Dinh; Ding, Ming; Pathirana, Pubudu N.; Seneviratne, Aruna (2020) [5]	Machine Learning, Deep Learning, Bitcoin	This paper introduces a new conceptual architecture that combines blockchain and AI to fight COVID-19. It focuses on the key solutions that blockchain and AI can offer to combat the COVID-19 outbreak. The most recent research efforts on the use of blockchain and AI for COVD-19 combat in a variety of applications have been presented.
Fusco, A.; Dicuonzo, G.; Dell'Atti, V.; Tatullo, M. (2020) [6]	EHR Systems, Smart Contracts,	This paper proposes the use of blockchain to develop a generalizable predictive system that could aid in the containment of pandemic risk on national territory, as well as a trace-route for COVID19-safe clinical practise.
Pal, Kamalendu [7]	Decentralized Computing Infrastructure, Internet of Things	The paper explains how the Internet of Things (IoT) and blockchain technology-based information systems (IS) can be used to improve tracking of goods and services in offering and to create a collaborative operating environment among manufacturing industry business partners.

cost. We also include an on chain storage for storing all the critical data. Our solution employs ethereum smart contracts for the purpose of registration, traceability etc.

The main algorithm is as follows: The smart contract will first define the smart contract's owner that is manufacturer, the start time of deploying the smart contract, smart container contents, the Ethereum address of the smart container, the vaccination centre that will receive it, and the smart container's initial state. The delivery agent will pick the smart container and announce the start of the delivery. Once delivered to the location it will mark as the end point of the delivery. The smart contract will then announce the recipients of the vaccines. Any violation of the VVMs will let us know that the vaccine is not appropriate for consumption. The different entities in our system are manufacturers who will manufacture the medicine, distributors who will distribute the medicine to the vaccination centers, centers which will provide the vaccines to the patients, doctors who will prescribe the medicine and finally the nurses who will administer the dosage of the medicine given to the patients. Medicine is sold in the form of Lots and the buying of medicines lots/medicines boxes is handled by this smart contract. The lots to be delivered are stored in smart containers or VVMs (virtual vial monitors) which monitor the states the medicines containers are in. Medicines are sensitive to temperature, light etc. So this solution checks for such violations (Lopez & Álvarez, 2020).

Proposed Solution includes following elements:

- Actors – which includes material suppliers, manufacturers, VVMs, freezer farms etc. They have authorization to view the logs, transactions and violations on the chain.
- Off-chain storage – non-critical data is stored off chain to reduce cost. But it is less secure.
- On-chain storage is used to register actors, store logs, events generated by smart contracts, and record any violations that occur during the delivery process of the COVID-19 vaccine smart containers, ensuring reliability and providing real-time monitoring.
- Ethereum smart contracts - The Ethereum smart contract serves three functions: registration, traceability and monitoring of violations.

4.2 Implementation of COVID Vaccine Supply Chain System

- Smart contracts contain the mapping of the authorized distributors and various variables which includes addresses of manufacturers, vaccination centers and smart containers.

Figure 2. Vaccine Container Smart Contract

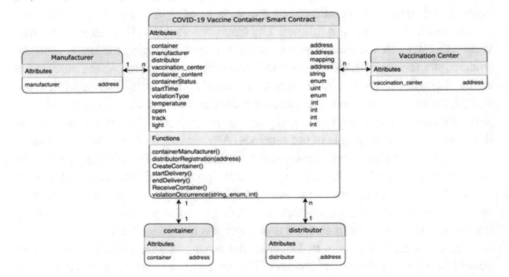

- "containerStatus" variable has many states such as "NotReady", "ReadyforDelivery", "StartDelivery", "onTrack" etc.
- The smart contract will first set the owner of smart contracts, which in this case is the manufacturer, the start time of deploying the smart contract, the contents of the smart container, the Ethereum address of the smart container, the vaccination centre that will receive it, and the smart container's initial state.
- The enumerate variable "violationType" contains actions for violations such as "Temp," which refers to a violation of the temperature range that is not acceptable, "Open," which indicates whether the container was opened unintentionally, "Light," which detects any violations of light exposure range, and "Route," which refers to a violation the smart container delivery track which is supposed to be follow.
- The delivery agent will pick the lot and report the start time of the delivery using the smart container.
- Once delivery is done to the destination it will mark as the end point of the delivery.
- The smart contract will then announce the recipients of the vaccines.
- Any violation of the VVMs will let us know that the vaccine is not appropriate for consumption.

4.3 Functions Used for The COVID Supply Chain System

1. containerManufacturer Function - does not take any input and is used to return the smart container manufacturer address.
2. CreateContainer Function – announces the creation of the smart containers. It can be only executed by the manufacturer and can be executed only when the status of the smart container is "NotReady".
3. DistributorRegistration Function – It describes the distributor's registration process in the smart contract in order to assign them their roles. Because the manufacturer is the only one who can modify this function, he or she is responsible for registering genuine distributors on the network.
4. ReceiveContainer Function – is executed by the vaccination center when the delivery process ends and the state of the smart container is "EndDelivery".
5. StartDelivery Function – represents the start of the delivery process by the distributor when the state of the smart container is "ReadyForDelivery".
6. EndDelivery Function – is executed by the distributor when the delivery ends and can only be executed when the state of the smart container is "OnTrack".
7. Smart Container - makes use of Lot and Registration contracts. The lots created are stored in smart containers to keep track of the state the medicines are in like NotReady, Ready, Delivered etc. Also keeps track of the amount of light, temperature etc on medicines. If any violation occurs the medicines are sent back to the vendor.
8. violationOccurrence Function – is executed by the smart container when any of the four main violations are triggered. They are temperature, light, open/close and route. They can be triggered only when the state of the smart container is "OnTrack".
9. Consumption - makes use of Registration contract has the prescription dates given by the doctor about the time and schedule of taking medicines and all other relevant things

4.4 Smart contracts used

4.4.1 Registration smart contract

WORKING – The different entities in our system are manufacturers who will manufacture the medicine, distributors who will distribute the medicine to the vaccination centers, centers which will provide the vaccines to the patients, doctors who will prescribe the medicine and finally the nurses who will administer the dosage of the medicine given to the patients. Registration is required so that only authorized entities can take part in our system.

The different functions used are

- manufacturerRegistration(address user) - The vaccines to be distributed are first made at the manufacturing centers. These centers are registered into our system through the registration smart contract by the system admin. This allows the manufacturers access to certain functions within the smart contracts like creation of lot, selling of lot etc. All other contracts in the system reference this smart contract to check if any entity claiming to be a manufacturer has the same address as any of the registered manufacturers or not.
- distributorRegistration(address user) - The addresses of the different distribution centers are stored here. The next point of destination of goods from the manufacturers is the distribution centers where the path or final destination of each vaccine is determined. Here, the vaccines are stored in the smart containers for path tracking. The smart container has several states which keep changing as the container moves along its path.
- centerRegistration(address user) - The patients can buy vaccines from the manufacturers which after reaching the distribution centers can be used by the patients. Only the vaccines which have not been violated with or damaged reach to this point.
- doctorRegistration(address user) - The doctors are consulted with by the patients. They assign a nurse for the patient and prescribe dosage for every individual patients according to his/her needs.
- nurseRegistration(address user) - The nurses administer the dosage of medicines given to the patient. For this they refer to the prescription details given by the doctor.

Events used -

- RegistrationInitiated(address indexed admin) - it can be run only by the initiator of the smart contract also known as the admin of the system.

Modifiers used -

- onlyAdmin()
- onlyCenter()

4.4.2. Lot smart contract

Medicine is sold in the form of Lots and the buying of medicines lots/medicines boxes is controlled by this smart contract. It makes use of the registration smart contract as "registrationcontract1" to check whether the entities participating in the selling of boxes have been registered.

Every lot is identified by a struct which contains -

- LotName – Name of the lot
- NumBoxes – amount of medicine boxes inside the lot
- LotPrice – Cost of the whole lot
- BoxPrice – Cost of the boxes inside the lot

Lots can be created by the registered manufacturer by mentioning the name, count of boxes in the lot and price of the lot. This is authorized for the manufacturer only. The customers or patients can buy the lot/boxes anytime they want to. They can also view the number of boxes bought under a particular customer address.

Functions used -

- currentOwner () - returns the ownerID of the contract who is the initiator of the contract who is the manufacturer but after buying the lot the buyer becomes the owner.
- lotDetails (string calldata _lotName, uint _lotPrice,uint _numBoxes, uint _boxPrice) - used to set the variables of the struct in the lot. Only the manufacturer can run this function.
- grantSale () - announces the start of a sale using the lotSale() event.
- buyLot () - lets the buyer buy the entire lot. The seller cannot buy the lot and checks whether the ethereum value sent by the buyer matches the price of the lot.
- buyBox (uint numboxes2buy) - same as the previous function but it let the buyer specific number of boxes from the lot instead of buying the entire lot.
- viewLot () - lets the user view all the details of the lot.
- viewBox (address _account) - lets the user see the number of boxes bought by the user.

Events used -

- newOwner (address oldownerID,addressnewownerID) - triggered whenever the owner of the lot is changed.
- lotManufactured (address manufacturer) - announces the completion of manufacturing of the lot.
- lotSale (string _lotName,uint _numBoxes, uint _lotPrice, uint _boxPrice) - report the commencement of a sale.
- lotSold (address newownerID) - announces that lot has been sold.

Figure 3. Lot smart Contract code

```
contract Lot{
    Registration public registrationcontract1;
    address payable internal ownerID;

    mapping(address => uint) public boxesPatient;

    struct lotdata{
        string lotName;
        uint numBoxes;
        uint lotPrice;
        uint boxPrice;
    }

    lotdata internal lot;

    // events
    event newOwner(address oldownerID,address newownerID);
    event lotManufactured(address manufacturer);
    event lotSale(string _lotName,uint _numBoxes, uint _lotPrice, uint _boxPrice);
    event lotSold(address newownerID);
    event boxesSold(uint _soldBoxes, address newownerID);

    constructor(address registrationaddress) public {

        registrationcontract1 = Registration(registrationaddress);
        ownerID = msg.sender;
        emit newOwner(address(0), ownerID);

    }

    function currentOwner() external view returns (address _currentOwner){
        return ownerID;
    }
}
```

- boxesSold (uint _soldBoxes, address newownerID) - announces the number of boxes sold.

Modifiers used -

- onlyManufacurer()
- onlyDistributor()
- onlyCenter()

Figure 4. Lot smart Contract code

```
function currentOwner() external view returns (address _currentOwner){
    return ownerID;
}

// modifiers
modifier onlyManufacurer() {
    require(registrationcontract1.manufacturer(msg.sender));
    _;
}

    modifier onlyDistributor() {
    require(registrationcontract1.distributor(msg.sender));
    _;
}

    modifier onlyCenter() {
    require(registrationcontract1.center(msg.sender));
    _;
}

function lotDetails(string calldata _lotName, uint _lotPrice,uint _numBoxes, uint _boxPrice) external onlyManufacurer() {

    lot.lotName = _lotName;
    lot.lotPrice = _lotPrice;
    lot.numBoxes = _numBoxes;
    lot.boxPrice = _boxPrice;

    //ownerID = msg.sender;

    emit lotManufactured(msg.sender);
}
```

4.4.3. SmartContainer smart contract

The lots to be delivered are stored in smart containers or VVMs (virtual vial monitors) which monitor the states the medicines containers are in. Medicines are sensitive to temperature, light etc. So it checks for such violations.

The containers may be in one of these states while it is on route to delivery:

{NotReady, ReadyforDelivery, StartDelivery, onTrack, EndDelivery, ContainerReceived, Violated}.

It uses the registration smart contract as "registration contact2" to check if the participating entities are registered and the lot smart contract as "lot contract" to identify the lot being delivered.

This smart contract creates containers to make them ready for the delivery process and has several functions to change the status of the container or initiate or terminate the delivery process. It also checks for several types of violations on the medicines like temperature, light, seal breaking etc. Damaged medicines are no longer fit for consumption and hence are sent back to where they came from.

Functions used -

Figure 5. Lot smart Contract code

```
function grantSale() external onlyManufacurer() onlyDistributor(){

    emit lotSale(lot.lotName,lot.numBoxes,lot.lotPrice,lot.boxPrice);

}


function buyLot () external onlyDistributor() onlyCenter() payable {
    address payable buyer = msg.sender;
    address payable seller = ownerID;
    require(buyer != seller, "The lot is already owned by the function caller");
    require(msg.value == lot.lotPrice, "insufficient payment");

    seller.transfer(lot.lotPrice);
    ownerID = buyer;

    emit lotSold(ownerID);



}

function buyBox (uint numboxes2buy) external payable {
    address payable buyer = msg.sender;
    address payable seller = ownerID;
    require(numboxes2buy <= lot.numBoxes, "The specified amount exceeds the limit");
    require(msg.value == lot.boxPrice*numboxes2buy, "incorrect payment");

    seller.transfer(lot.boxPrice*numboxes2buy);
    lot.numBoxes -= numboxes2buy;
    boxesPatient[buyer] = numboxes2buy;
```

- CreateContainer() - creates container and status is set to ReadyForDelivery.
- StartDelivery() - initiates the delivery process and status is set to onTrack.
- EndDelivery() - terminates a delivery process and status is set to EndDelivery.
- ReceiveContainer() - receives container by the center and status is set to ContainerReceived.
- ViolationOccurrence() - checks for violations like light, temperature, container opening, off track etc.

Events used -

- ContainerOwnership (address previous owner, address new owner)
- ContainerReadyForDelivery (address manufacturer)

Figure 6. Lot smart Contract code

```
function DrugReadyForDispensing(uint amount) public onlyHospital{
    require(drugstate == Drugstate.NotReady, "Other entities have already been made aware of this state of the drug");
    drugstate = Drugstate.ReadyForDispensing;
    availableAmount = amount;
    emit DrugReady(msg.sender, availableAmount);

}

function DrugPrescription(bytes32 _patientID, bytes32 _patientName, uint _patientAge, bytes32 _endorsements, bytes32 _prescriptionIPFShash) public onlyPrescriber{

    require(drugstate == Drugstate.ReadyForDispensing , "Can't prescribe controlled drug before it's ready");
    patientID = _patientID;
    patientName = _patientName;
    patientAge = _patientAge;
    endorsements = _endorsements;
    prescriptionIPFShash = _prescriptionIPFShash;
    drugstate = Drugstate.Prescribed;
    emit DrugPrescribed(msg.sender, patientID, patientName, patientAge, endorsements, prescriptionIPFShash);
}

function DrugAdministration(bytes32 _nurseName, uint _administrationDate, uint _dispensedAmount, bytes32 _sheetIPFShash) public onlyNurse{
    require(drugstate == Drugstate.Prescribed, "Controlled drugs must be prescribed first before administration");
    require(_dispensedAmount <= availableAmount , "The dispensed amount must be less than or equal to the available amount");
    nurseName = _nurseName;
    administrationDate = _administrationDate;
    dispensedAmount = _dispensedAmount;
    sheetIPFShash = _sheetIPFShash;
    availableAmount -= dispensedAmount;
    drugstate = Drugstate.Administered;
```

- DeliveryStart (address distributor)
- DeliveryEnd(address distributor)
- ContainerReception(address vaccination_center)
- TemperatureViolation(int v)
- ContainerOpening(int v)
- OffTrack (int v)
- LightExposure (int v)
- ErrorNoValidViolation ()

Modifiers used -

- onlyManufacturer ()
- onlyDistributor ()
- onlyCenter ()
- onlyContainer ()

Figure 7. Smart container smart contract code

```
contract SmartContainer{
    Registration public registrationcontract2;
    Lot public lotcontract;
    address public container;
    address public manufacturer;
    address vaccination_center;
    string container_content;
    enum containerStatus {NotReady, ReadyforDelivery, StartDelivery, onTrack, EndDelivery, ContainerReceived, Violated}
    containerStatus public state;
    uint startTime;
    enum violationType { None, Temp, Open, Light, Route}
    violationType public violation;
    int temperature;
    int open;
    int track;
    int light;

    // events
    event ContainerOwnership (address previousowner, address newowner);
    event ContainerReadyforDelivery (address manufacturer);
    event DeliveryStart (address distributor);
    event DeliveryEnd(address distributor);
    event ContainerReception(address vaccination_center);

    // violations
    event TemperatureViolation( int v);
    event ContainerOpening( int v);
    event OffTrack( int v);
    event LightExposure ( int v);
    event ErrorNoValidViolation();

    // modifiers
    modifier onlyManufacturer(){
        require(registrationcontract2.manufacturer(msg.sender), "Only authorised manufacturers can run this function.");
    _;
```

4.4.4. Consumption smart contract

This smart contains the prescription details prescribed by the doctor about the amount of medicine to be taken by the patient. The dosage of medicines given to the patient is administered by the nurses. Uses the registration smart contract to check if the distribution centres, doctors, nurses are authorised by the admin.

It is the final step in the entire process where the bought medicine is injected into the body of the patient by the nurses. The nurses consult the prescription given by the physician to regulate the dosage to be given to the patient.

Functions used -

- DrugReadyForDispensing (uint amount) - if the state of the drug is nt ready then it is set to ReadyForDispensing and the amount to be given is set.
- DrugPrescription (bytes32 _patientID, bytes32 _patientName, uint _ patientAge, bytes32 _endorsements, bytes32 _prescriptionIPFShash) - sets prescription details set by the prescriber. The drug state is set to prescribed.

Figure 8. Smart container smart contract code

```
// modifiers
modifier onlyManufacturer(){
    require(registrationcontract2.manufacturer(msg.sender), "Only authorised manufacturers can run this function.");
    _;
}

modifier onlyDistributor(){
    require(registrationcontract2.distributor(msg.sender), "Only authorised distributors can run this function.");
    _;
}

modifier onlyCenter(){
    require(registrationcontract2.center(msg.sender), "Only authorised centers can run this function.");
    _;
}

modifier onlyContainer(){
    require(container == msg.sender, "The sender is not eligible to run this function.");
    _;
}

// constructor
constructor(address lotaddress, address regaddress) public payable{
    lotcontract = Lot(lotaddress);
    registrationcontract2 = Registration(regaddress);
    manufacturer = msg.sender;
    startTime = block.timestamp;
    container = 0x4B209938c481177ec7E8F571ceCaE8A9e22C02db;
    vaccination_center = 0x78731D3Ca6bfE34aC0F824c42a7cC18A495cabaB;
    container_content = "This container contains X amount of Vaccine doses.";
    state = containerStatus.NotReady;// NotReady
    emit ContainerOwnership(address(0), manufacturer);
}
```

- DrugAdministration (bytes32 _nurseName, uint _administrationDate, uint _ dispensedAmount, bytes32 _sheetIPFShash) - administration of drug dosage by the nurses is carried out by this function. The drug state must be prescribed.
- DrugDisposal (bytes32 _nurseName, uint _disposalDate, uint _ disposedAmount, bytes32 _disposalsheetIPFShash) - unwanted drug is disposed of by the nurses once the state of the drug is administered.

Events used -

- ConsumptionSCDeployer (address indexed _address)
- DrugReady (address indexed _hospital, uint _amount)
- DrugPrescribed (address indexed prescriber, bytes32 patientID, bytes32 patientName, uintpatientAge, bytes32 endorsements, bytes32 prescriptionIPFShash)
- DrugAdministered (address indexed _nurse, bytes32 nurseName, uintadministrationDate, uintdispensedAmount, bytes32 sheetIPFShash)

Figure 9. Smart container smart contract code

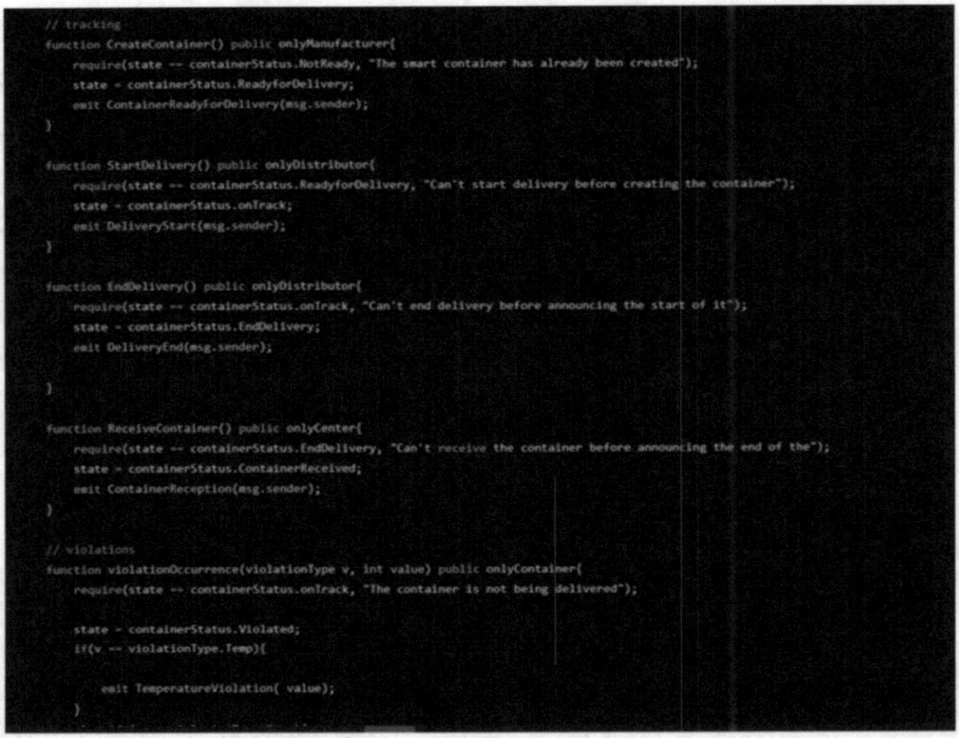

```
// tracking
function CreateContainer() public onlyManufacturer{
    require(state == containerStatus.NotReady, "The smart container has already been created");
    state = containerStatus.ReadyforDelivery;
    emit ContainerReadyForDelivery(msg.sender);
}

function StartDelivery() public onlyDistributor{
    require(state == containerStatus.ReadyforDelivery, "Can't start delivery before creating the container");
    state = containerStatus.onTrack;
    emit DeliveryStart(msg.sender);
}

function EndDelivery() public onlyDistributor{
    require(state == containerStatus.onTrack, "Can't end delivery before announcing the start of it");
    state = containerStatus.EndDelivery;
    emit DeliveryEnd(msg.sender);

}

function ReceiveContainer() public onlyCenter{
    require(state == containerStatus.EndDelivery, "Can't receive the container before announcing the end of the");
    state = containerStatus.ContainerReceived;
    emit ContainerReception(msg.sender);
}

// violations
function violationOccurrence(violationType v, int value) public onlyContainer{
    require(state == containerStatus.onTrack, "The container is not being delivered");

    state = containerStatus.Violated;
    if(v == violationType.Temp){

        emit TemperatureViolation( value);
    }
```

- DrugDisposed (address indexed nurse, bytes32 nurseName, uintdisposalDate, uintdisposedAmount, bytes32 disposalsheetIPFShash)

    Modifiers used -

- onlyHospital ()
- onlyPrescriber ()
- onlyNurse ()

5. SECURITY ANALYSIS OF THE BLOCKCHAIN-BASED COVID-19 VACCINE DELIVERY SOLUTION

- **Integrity:**

Figure 10. Smart container smart contract code

```
// violations
function violationOccurrence(violationType v, int value) public onlyContainer{
    require(state == containerStatus.onTrack, "The container is not being delivered");

    state = containerStatus.Violated;
    if(v == violationType.Temp){

        emit TemperatureViolation( value);
    }
    else if (v == violationType.Open){
        //either 1 or 0
        emit ContainerOpening ( value);
    }
    else if (v == violationType.Route){

        emit OffTrack( value);
    }
    else if (v == violationType.Light){

        emit LightExposure( value);
    }
    else
        emit ErrorNoValidViolation();
}
```

The implementation of the blockchain-based vaccine delivery solution provides a high level of integrity in the system. Smart containers are implemented in an event based approach where every transaction is recorded and logged on the chain, which makes it virtually impossible to break the system and thus maintains integrity.

From the buying of boxes by the customers to the delivery of vaccines by the distributor and the assignment of doses by the physicians, the entire process has been implemented in our model. Every patient can keep track of the number of boxes/lots bought by him/her. The VVMs tell us the exact state a particular lot is in at any given moment while making sure the medicines aren't damaged in any way.

- **Accountability and Authorization:**

Modifier feature of ethereum smart contract is used to assign different roles to different participants. Since every transaction is recorded on an immutable ledger, all the participants can be held accountable for their action. Hence, our implementation assures accountability and authorization.

Figure 11. Consumption smart contract code

```
contract Consumption{

    //Declaring variables

    Registration registrationcontract3;
    //Production schain;

    bytes32 public patientID;
    bytes32 public patientName;
    bytes32 public endorsements;
    bytes32 public prescriptionIPFShash;
    bytes32 public nurseName;
    bytes32 public sheetIPFShash;
    bytes32 public disposalsheetIPFShash;
    uint public patientAge;
    uint public prescriptionDate;
    uint public administrationDate;
    uint public availableAmount;
    uint public dispensedAmount;
    uint public disposedAmount;
    uint public disposalDate;


    enum Drugstate {NotReady, ReadyForDispensing, Prescribed, Administered, Disposed}
    Drugstate public drugstate; //refers to the state of the controlled drug after unboxing

    //Events

    event ConsumptionSCDeployer(address indexed _address);
    event DrugReady(address indexed _hospital, uint _amount);
    event DrugPrescribed (address indexed prescriber, bytes32 patientID, bytes32 patientName, uint patientAge, bytes32 endorsements, bytes32 prescriptionIPFShash);
    event DrugAdministered(address indexed _nurse, bytes32 nurseName, uint administrationDate, uint dispensedAmount, bytes32 sheetIPFShash);
    event DrugDisposed(address indexed nurse, bytes32 nurseName, uint disposalDate, uint disposedAmount, bytes32 disposalsheetIPFShash);
```

All the smart contracts used in our model refers to the authorised entities in the Registration smart contract to make sure that no unauthorized accesses have been made. The details of health records of the patient are confidential and only accessible by the doctor and the patient.

- **Availability:**

The nature of the vaccine delivery problem demands that the system be available at all times. The provided blockchain based solution is decentralized and distributed in nature. The decentralized nature of the solution makes it immune from single point failure, so even if a node fails the system would not fail in delivering vaccines. Hence, availability of the system at all times is ensured.

The drugs are made available by the manufacturing entities and appropriate events announce the availability of medicines. The system allows anyone to buy medicines anywhere at any time as long as there are boxes available to be sold.

Figure 12. Consumption smart contract code

```
modifier onlyHospital(){

    require(registrationcontract3.center(msg.sender), "Only the hospital is allowed to execute this function");
    _;
}

modifier onlyPrescriber(){

    require(registrationcontract3.doctor(msg.sender), "Only the prescriber is allowed to execute this function");
    _;
}

modifier onlyNurse(){

    require(registrationcontract3.nurse(msg.sender), "Only the nurse is allowed to execute this function");
    _;
}

//Constructor

constructor(address registrationaddress) public {

    registrationcontract3 = Registration(registrationaddress);
    //schain = Production(supplyaddress);
    emit ConsumptionSCDeployer(msg.sender); //Should be changed to msg.sender if someone else will deploy the SC other than the CDR

}


//Consumption contract Functions
```

6. CONCLUSION AND FUTURE WORK

Blockchain is gradually proving to be a viable "middleware" solution for enabling seamless interoperability across complex supply chains. Blockchain's technological nature enables secure, transparent, and fast data exchanges, as well as the creation of immutable record databases. In this chapter we discussed how the blockchain technology can be used to monitor covid 19 vaccines distribution and delivery. We propose a blockchain based approach to manage distribution and delivery of covid 19 vaccines. A vaccine distribution smart contract is developed to automate the traceability of vaccines. The proposed solution is implemented and their implementation testing and validation discussed. Our proposed solution was then compared against existing solutions by performing cost and security analysis and comparing it with existing solutions.

We discuss issues related to tracing and tracking of vaccines. We keep in mind features like traceable, transparent, reliable, auditable, secure, and trustworthy, which are achieved through the decentralized nature of blockchain.

An event-based approach has been taken in the implementation of the blockchain based solution, to ensure a high degree of integrity. Moreover, Ethereum's modifier feature has been fully utilized so that different roles can be assigned.

Figure 13. Consumption smart contract code

```
function DrugReadyForDispensing(uint amount) public onlyHospital{
    require(drugstate == Drugstate.NotReady, "Other entities have already been made aware of this state of the drug");
    drugstate = Drugstate.ReadyForDispensing;
    availableAmount = amount;
    emit DrugReady(msg.sender, availableAmount);

}

function DrugPrescription(bytes32 _patientID, bytes32 _patientName, uint _patientAge, bytes32 _endorsements, bytes32 _prescriptionIPFShash) public onlyPrescriber{

    require(drugstate == Drugstate.ReadyForDispensing , "Can't prescribe controlled drug before it's ready");
    patientID = _patientID;
    patientName = _patientName;
    patientAge = _patientAge;
    endorsements = _endorsements;
    prescriptionIPFShash = _prescriptionIPFShash;
    drugstate = Drugstate.Prescribed;
    emit DrugPrescribed(msg.sender, patientID, patientName, patientAge, endorsements, prescriptionIPFShash);
}

function DrugAdministration(bytes32 _nurseName, uint _administrationDate, uint _dispensedAmount, bytes32 _sheetIPFShash) public onlyNurse{
    require(drugstate == Drugstate.Prescribed, "Controlled drugs must be prescribed first before administration");
    require(_dispensedAmount <= availableAmount , "The dispensed amount must be less than or equal to the available amount");
    nurseName = _nurseName;
    administrationDate = _administrationDate;
    dispensedAmount = _dispensedAmount;
    sheetIPFShash = _sheetIPFShash;
    availableAmount -= dispensedAmount;
    drugstate = Drugstate.Administered;
```

Our proposed implementation is decentralized and distributed to make sure that the possibility of a single point of failure is eliminated. This also helps make sure that delivery of vaccines does not cease at any time.

The project is currently pushed into GitHub and further updates will be pushed in the future work.

GitHub Link - https://github.com/kirito39/Medicine-SupplyChain.git

Figure 14. Consumption smart contract code

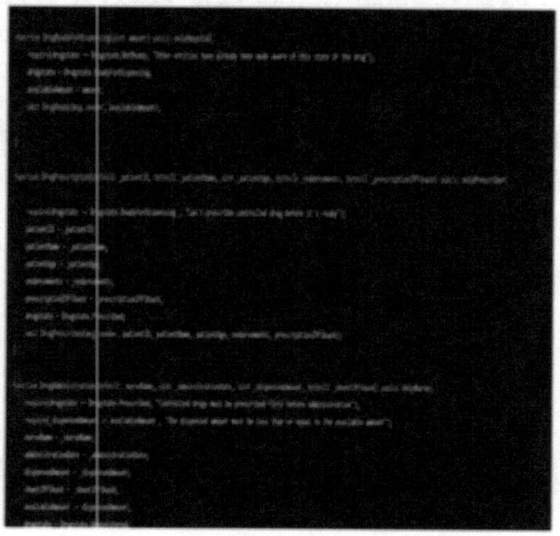

REFERENCES

C-19_Vaccine-Distribution_White-Paper_Stirling_Ultracold.pdf. (n.d.). Retrieved August 30, 2021, from https://www.stirlingultracold.com/wp-content/uploads/2020/12/C-19_Vaccine-Distribution_White-Paper_Stirling_Ultracold.pdf

Fusco, A., Dicuonzo, G., Dell'Atti, V., & Tatullo, M. (2020). Blockchain in Healthcare: Insights on COVID-19. *International Journal of Environmental Research and Public Health*, *17*(19), 7167. https://doi.org/10.3390/ijerph17197167

Idongesit, W. (2020). *Cross-Industry Use of Blockchain Technology and Opportunities for the Future*. IGI Global.

Iftekhar, A., & Cui, X. (2021). Blockchain-Based Traceability System That Ensures Food Safety Measures to Protect Consumer Safety and COVID-19 Free Supply Chains. *Foods*, *10*(6), 1289. https://doi.org/10.3390/foods10061289

Kalla, A., Hewa, T., Mishra, R. A., Ylianttila, M., & Liyanage, M. (2020). The Role of Blockchain to Fight Against COVID-19. *IEEE Engineering Management Review*, *48*(3), 85–96. https://doi.org/10.1109/EMR.2020.3014052

Marbouh, D., Abbasi, T., Maasmi, F., Omar, I. A., Debe, M. S., Salah, K., Jayaraman, R., & Ellahham, S. (2020). Blockchain for COVID-19: Review, Opportunities, and a Trusted Tracking System. *Arabian Journal for Science and Engineering*, *45*(12), 9895–9911. https://doi.org/10.1007/s13369-020-04950-4

Nguyen, D. C., Ding, M., Pathirana, P. N., & Seneviratne, A. (2021). Blockchain and AI-Based Solutions to Combat Coronavirus (COVID-19)-Like Epidemics: A Survey. *IEEE Access: Practical Innovations, Open Solutions*, 9, 95730–95753. https://doi.org/10.1109/ACCESS.2021.3093633

Ramirez Lopez, L. J., & Beltrán Álvarez, N. (2020). *Blockchain application in the distribution chain of the COVID-19 vaccine: A designing understudy.* doi:10.31124/advance.12274844.v1

Chapter 10
Scope and Application of Blockchain in an Ancient System of Indian Medicine, "Ayurveda":
Application of Blockchain in Ayurvedic Research and Ayurvedic Herbal Products

Amulya Murthy Aku
KAHER's KLE SBMK Ayurveda Mahavidyalaya, India

ABSTRACT

In a variety of ways, blockchain technology has the potential to enhance healthcare and well-being in the future. Products of high value but low volume such as pharmaceuticals, health food, cosmetics, and other things can all benefit from the potential applications of this technology in these niche sectors. In this chapter, the authors examine the breadth and applications of blockchain technology in the ancient Indian medical system, as well as the challenges and opportunities it presents. Ayurvedic science has been around for 5000 years and contains all of the principles, techniques, and treatments necessary to not only prevent and promote health but also to cure any underlying health concerns that may exist. This will improve the statistical reliability of clinical data in Ayurvedic medicine, as well as make it simpler to distinguish between false and accurate data while analyzing clinical data.

DOI: 10.4018/978-1-7998-9606-7.ch010

1. INTRODUCTION

The Ancient Indian System of Medicine is a great treasure of medical resources, which, for thousands of years, has provided a solid guarantee for people's health. Over the past century, with the rapid development of modern System of Medicine, there have been voices from the medical community questioning Ancient Indian System of Medicine mainly for the following reasons:

1. Although Ancient Indian System of Medicine can cure some disease, and even has better efficiency in treating some diseases compared with the western System of Medicine, it needs more solid proof in clinical practices to ensure its efficiency;

2. There are about several hundred formulations in clinical practices of Ancient Indian System of Medicine while doctors often modify the formula without validation support. These formulations are combination of herbs that work on different ailments synergistically as well as also increase the efficacy of each other to work for an ailment. This concept is quite new for western system of medicine as it is usually based on either active principle or single drug principle while Ancient system of Indian medicine believes in holistic nature of a herb or medicine.

3. The toxicity and side effects of Ancient Indian System of Medicine have long been the center of debate. At present, both prescribed and proprietary Indian System of Medicine lack observation, thus leading to doubts and questioning.

4. Over the past century, the rapid development of modern System of Medicine makes it the protagonist of the medical industry. Also, diseases were named based on modern System of Medicine while diagnosis and pathogenesis of Ancient Indian System of Medicine which are different then the names of diseases in ancient system of medicine (Ayurveda). Although it can be seen that Ayurvedic medicine is very efficient in chronic disorders or non communicable disorders like obesity, diabetes, stress, hypertention, musculo-skeletal-locomotory disorders (sciatica etc.) and it is also efficient in some of the communicable disorders. It is also seen that with holistic approach adapted by Indian government through Ayurveda has helped to tackle even the COVID-19 very efficiently. Still the problem arises or exits in the lack of big clinical data.

To summarise, the growth of the Ancient Indian System of Medicine requires the assistance of clinical big data. Thousands of years have passed without the help and verification of big data in the clinical diagnosis and treatment of Ancient Indian System of Medicine. Even now, hospitals and clinics using the Ancient Indian

System of Medicine lack a reliable data summary. The development of an Ayurvedic physician is founded on experience, namely on his own "clinical data." However, such data is not always and everywhere accessible, resulting in the "information island" issue. These information islands are dispersed throughout India, making them difficult to acquire through education alone. On the other hand, the Ancient Indian System of Medicine (Ayurveda) has some benefits in diagnosing and treating some diseases, which need to be proven using clinical big data and serve as a foundation for systematic diagnosis and therapy. Thus, practitioners practising Ancient Indian System of Medicine (Ayurveda) must link and record information islands, which will serve as the foundation for the system's strong and sustainable development (Ayurveda).

2. BACKGROUND

According to the Ministry of Industry and Information Technology's 2016 "White Paper on China's Blockchain Technology and Application Development," blockchain is a new application model for computer technologies such as distributed data storage, peer-to-peer transmission, consensus mechanism, and encryption algorithm, which is a decentralised and distrusted infrastructure and distributed computing paradigm. Blockchain technology is the outcome of the integration of numerous technologies, including database, cryptography, and network technology, and it possesses the properties of decentralisation, immutability, anonymity, and openness.

2.1 Characteristics of Blockchain Technology

1. The fundamental characteristic and primary advantage of blockchain is decentralisation. Decentralization is a dispersed structure in which the entire network is not reliant on third-party hardware or management agencies, and there is no central core system. Through distributed storage, any node failure will not result in network harm. As a result, significant intermediate expenses are avoided in practise. This is also one of the primary reasons for the widespread use of blockchain technology.
2. Confidentiality By utilising predefined algorithms, blockchain technology safeguards private information or data (generally asymmetric encryption algorithms). Only a pair of identical public and private keys can decrypt data. Unless needed by law, identity information between nodes does not have to be made public or confirmed. This innovation resolves the trust issue between nodes and enhances user privacy protection.

3.   Independence Autonomy is simply the move from "trusting people" to "trusting machines," the establishment of a trust network between machines in order to attain a greater degree of autonomy without human interference. The blockchain is built on open source software that is editable and adjustable by participating nodes. It is possible to monitor and track the operational rules and data.

4.   Transparency Except for private information, which is encrypted, all other data on the blockchain is public. Through an open interface, all nodes in the network can query data records. The information is assured to be highly transparent.

5.   Inability to tamper the data once validated and put to the blockchain, the information and data are permanently saved. They may be amended only if they control 51% of all data nodes, ensuring that they are not deliberately tampered with or removed. The consensus algorithm's overwhelming computer power protects the security of data.

6.   Reproducibility The blockchain utilises time stamp technology to give a temporal dimension to data and record the storage sequence, allowing for rapid tracking and traceability, while also ensuring the traceability and integrity of data.

3. METHOD TO USE BLOCKCHAIN IN AYURVEDA

As can be seen, many conventional medical systems across the world have now acknowledged the value of "Clinical Data" and the use of blockchain technology in data collection. In 2008, the introduction of blockchain technology, as described in Mr. Satoshi Nakamoto's bitcoin paper, presented a solution to the problem of data collecting and confirmation in Traditional Chinese medicine. Therefore, the concept of blockchain can be applied to even Ancient Indian medicine.

The Ayurvedic blockchain system must include the following parts:

1.   Computers of doctors for prescription should be connected to the Internet;

2.   For primary and secondary nodes of Ayurvedic block chain nodes, the primary nodes are composed of multiple servers connected to the Internet and the secondary nodes include the physician prescription computer of each medical institution;

3.   Patient-side network terminal;

4.   Timestamp server;

5.   P2P transmission based Ancient Indian Medicine block chain software that stores numerous nodes in the system, allowing information exchange through P2P data transmission technology.

This blockchain can be constructed and promoted by competent government departments. Electronic medical records created after Ancient Indian Medicine diagnosis and treatment will be received by computer, which would process doctor's prescription for data package, and then post it on the Internet by P2P technology. Over time, all the electronic medical records are uploaded into one block, which is timestamped by the system. A block is composed of the head and body. The body includes all the details of the block information packet while the head has the timestamp and the hash value of the block as well as hash value of the other blocks in the entire network. The hash value generated by hash algorithm create the body of a block, which will be recorded by other blocks in the network and stored in each node of the "Ancient Indian Medicine" chain of the blocks. All the blocks will be certified, and the electronic medical records will be coded to protect the privacy while the other information is accessible to the entire network. Once generated in a block, the information will be permanently sealed where modification is impossible. Any correction of data on a node would create differences between each node in the process of validation, where the system would carry out data rollback, restoring data to a level recognized by most data nodes. Unless the tamper controls most nodes of the whole network, the tampered data will be invalid. Therefore, electronic medical records based on blockchain have a high degree of authenticity. At the same time, the design of this system can trace the electronic medical records. The generation and connection of blockchain are shown in **Figure 1.**

Blocks are classified and managed by block head. For example: An Ancient Indian Medicine doctor recorded the diagnosis and treatment of a patient with Dysentry, who was identified as "Grahani Roga" as per Ayurvedic terminology with Vata and Pitta imbalance with vitiation of digestive fire (Agni Dushti). The doctor prescribed Medicated Herbal Buttermilk (Aushadhi Sadhita Takra). The block head recorded the key words of the electronic medical records (Medicated Herbal Buttermilk (Aushadhi Sadhita Takra), Grahani Roga, Vata-Pitta imbalance with vitiation of digestive fire) while the block body recorded details such as Indian and western diagnosis and examination (including imaging data). When the second electronic medical record of Vata-Pitta imbalance and Agni Dushti (vitiation of Digestive fire) is created in a chain block of the network, the system automatically would classify the "Grahani" as a block groups keyword, where all electronic medical records with "Grahini Roga" are classified into this block group and become related. Best part is each electronic medical record can be related by multiple block groups. For example, the above records can also relate to the "Dysentry" block group or Medicated Herbal Buttermilk (Aushadi Sadhita Takra).

Electronic medical records under the same block groups could form a block group, which doesn't record detailed diagnostic data but only keyword index. The existence of the group was recorded and certified by the nodes in the network,

Figure 1. Schematic diagram of Ancient Indian System of Medicine - Ayurvedic medicine Blockchain system

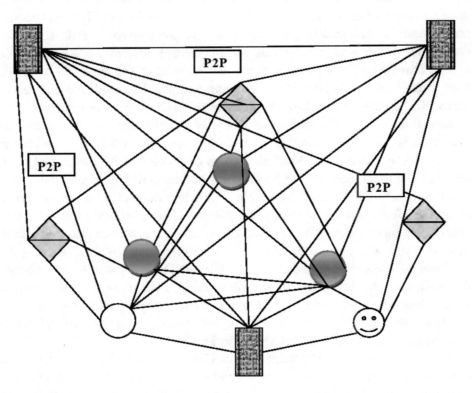

——————	Link
▢	Primary Nodes
◇	Secondary Nodes
☺	Patient Internet Client
◯	Block
◯	Block Group

which could be accessed for basic researches and statistics of Ancient Indian medicine. Patients can evaluate the effect of diagnosis and treatment through their own Internet client, which will be automatically recorded in the corresponding block by the system and nodes of the whole network forbidding modification. The evaluation of the curative effect of patients can be designed into an index system, which is composed of multiple evaluation indexes. When the study needs to read the clinical efficacy of a certain prescription, data extraction can be carried out in the blockchain to facilitate quick statistics. If any side effects or adverse reactions occur during the Ancient Indian Medicine diagnosis and treatment, the report shall be uploaded to the corresponding block of the electronic medical record. It can be uploaded via physician node or the patient node, or packaged by software in the patient or physician's system before being uploaded. When the entire network reaches a certain size, statistics of clinical Ancient Indian Medicine adverse reactions would be available to provide data support for the study of the side effects of Ancient Indian medicine. Records of patient evaluation and adverse reactions to the treatment is added to the corresponding block, where the system will regenerate the hash value of the block and broadcast it to the whole network, allowing synchronous updating and recording of the hash value to other blocks in the network.

4. PRIVACY PROTECTION

Private information (patient and physician privacy) in electronic medical records relating to each block will be coded in the blockchain technology. Such information could only be retrieved with the use of a key or with the key holder's authorisation. The remainder of the electronic records' information is made available to the whole network. The key is produced by the system software during the block generation process and is then stored in the relevant patient's and physician's network terminal in the electronic medical record.

Personal private data, such as electronic medical records, should be permitted by patients for use by other departments, but are now monopolised by a few of medical institutions. Patients have no right to know how their data is used, and there are even privacy breaches. It is impossible to assure that patients' data is transmitted safely and lawfully across multiple medical institutions during diagnosis; medical records data is still lost, attacked, and tampered with, posing a concealed threat. As a result, due to security and privacy considerations, it is difficult to create a summary electronic medical record for a single patient from several hospital databases.

The use of blockchain technology has effectively addressed the aforementioned privacy concerns. A consensus algorithm must be confirmed in the process of transferring or updating the patient's medical record data to the blockchain. The blockchain is based on open-source software, and each node may examine and track data changes, allowing it to be registered only once all nodes have verified it. Validated medical record data is encapsulated and stored by including a timestamp, which has legal standing and may be used as a voucher to safeguard the legality of patients, physicians, and medical institutions. Patients do not need to re-record past information when travelling to a different medical institution since the time and substance of the data are comprehensive and trustworthy. This reduces the occurrence of medical mishaps and dramatically improves the quality and efficiency of medical treatment. Provide the patient with a user ID or public key and store the patient's diagnosis and treatment information on the blockchain. Doctors and other institutions can access their medical behaviours with patients' permission, access dynamic icons, and even access various sections of the same medical information with separate permissions to avoid patient personal information from being leaked. Establish several encryption techniques to ensure the security of the management platform database, so that medical record data cannot be falsified or tampered with.

5. CLOUD SYSTEM

Wearable gadgets are becoming increasingly sophisticated and popular in recent years. If we apply cloud system in Ayurvedic Medicine (Ancient Indian System of Medicine) the system would collect data from patients and transfers it to a cloud server for storage and analysis using modern technology. Users and clinicians may query the analysis' results at any time, making it simple to follow patients and conduct condition research.

However, the largest issue is data security. The cloud server will conduct arithmetic and retrieval from the enormous data after collecting it. Due to the jumbled data, the computer may make a mistake, resulting in various data loss. And because many data in the human body are part of a nonlinear physiological complicated system, it's difficult to achieve reliable findings using current examination procedures, particularly with Ayurveda's individualized system of diagnosis methods, making this medicine feel subjective and erroneous.

The adoption of blockchain technology to safeguard medical data located in the cloud has enormous promise since it solves the above difficulties well. The data on the blockchain will not be removed maliciously. Any update will be recorded through its transparent processing system, and it can also be tracked back using timestamp technology, thereby avoiding doctor-patient disagreements.

Figure 2. The food-medicine interface: where to draw the line?

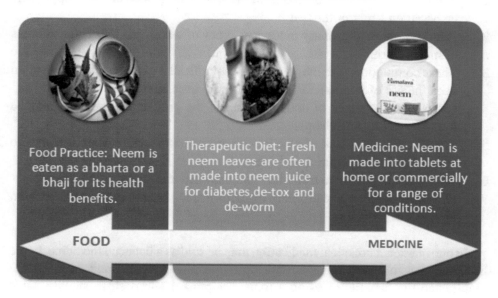

6. HERBAL PRODUCTS

Botanical material used in medicines and food has been a source of concern since the beginning of worldwide trading in such resources. This includes high-value foods, food supplements, cosmetics, and herbal medicines. Complex value chains are critical to the supply of raw materials for a wide range of goods, as shown in **Figure 2.**

Ethnopharmacology and medicinal plant research have been thrust into the heart of the worldwide commerce in high-value botanical goods because of the massive growth in global trade. There has been a tendency to concentrate either on fixing particular quality issues (such as adulteration and inefficient manufacturing processes) or on alleviating specific social or economic concerns. To solve these issues, a pharmacopoeia (for medicinal items) or an industrial Quality control (QC) standard were often used (esp. for food and cosmetic products). These supply chains also sparked a number of unique issues, including fair benefit-sharing/responsible sourcing and sustainable supply, especially in the context of protected or vulnerable areas. Since at least 2012, there has been a growing recognition of the importance of herbal materials' value chains in a worldwide market, which had previously been seen as a supply problem (Booker et al., 2012). This is in line with a number of the sector's fundamental features, which include:

1. The material may be collected from the wild or cultivated and the supply may be based on a mix of the two
2. A huge number of primary producers, many of whom generate little amounts of materia prima
3. These commodities are introduced into complicated value chains, which often need the use of intermediaries to connect to overseas suppliers.
4. Often, there is a lack of understanding of the product features that may be found in these value chains.
5. There is a general lack of understanding and bad practice when it comes to endangered and overharvested species.
6. A significant price rise from the main manufacturer to the end customer
7. Different markets have different regulatory statuses and, as a result, different business expectations.

In one market, a botanical medication may be sold as a licenced medicine, while in another, it is sold as an unregulated dietary supplement. While Booker et al. (2012) highlighted the benefits of using a trans-disciplinary approach to analyse value chains, more recent developments may offer a new solution – blockchain systems, a technology that is now widely viewed as a way to address the challenges posed by the rapidly changing socio-economic framework of how societies exchange information and goods (trade). A frontier in Blockchain, which was launched in September 2018 and publishes rigorously peer-reviewed research on the theory and applications of blockchain and blockchain-related technologies1, is an example of this. As a result, in this viewpoint it is important to look into the advantages of employing blockchain technologies in a multi-stakeholder industry, especially how they may help ensure fair rewards to producers, sustainable sourcing and manufacturing, and the highest quality of final goods.

7. THE CONCEPT OF BLOCKCHAIN IN HERBAL PRODUCTS/MEDICINES

Knowledge throughout a value chain of what is being transferred is critical in the interchange of goods and information, including precise needs pertaining to a product's composition, quality, source, and many other essential data, which was formerly held in analogue 'ledgers.' Blockchain (BC) is a decentralised data storage system constructed on a network of users, any of whom may become a node of the network, as opposed to the "Ancient" centralised system (Figorilli et al., 2018). Any new data (saved in blocks) is connected to prior data in other blocks, producing a chain of information and hence a history of interactions that is stored and duplicated in all nodes in the network. An important element is validation before to integration into the BC. As a result, each computer is in charge of one copy of the blockchain. The blockchain will include as many identical copies as there are computers in the network, enabling for more effective detection and management of damaged data. Data on the BC is unmodifiable since, in reality, all that can be changed is a single copy of the BC, which will then be different from all the other copies and can be readily identified and labelled as incorrect/corrupted. There seems to be no way to change many copies at once (Carson et al., 2018; Saberi et al., 2019). On the other hand, it's simple to see how data corruption occurs in a "Ancient" centralised system. When the main computer fails or data stored on it is corrupted, the error/modification spreads to all receivers linked to Central. As a result, data security is dependent on the central system's security. After that, blockchain becomes a revolutionary technique to move the problem of data security from external "security providers" to a free internal network of "trust." Galvez et al. (2016) argued persuasively in 2018 that blockchain techniques in the food industry provide great prospects (but also significant challenges). Their main emphasis is on the optimization of industrial processes and the potential of the blockchain system from the standpoint of big business. The early phases of manufacturing were not discussed in depth. They obviously did not address the added difficulty of ensuring that the finished goods would be therapeutically beneficial. Not only must a herbal medicinal product meet label claims, but it must also have a composition and quality that provide therapeutic effects. **Figure 3** discusses how BC systems in the food and herbal markets would assist a sector that relies on complicated transaction networks and often lacks confidence in its value chains.

The "trust" is built on the transparent exchange of immutable data, which is uploaded and securely kept on the blockchain, bypassing middlemen that act as "trust guarantors" between untrusting parties. Without the requirement for human trust, blockchain technology offers a safe/trusted platform for interactions between such parties. Smart contracts (SCs), which may be incorporated within the BC architecture, can help to reinforce this. SCs are a mechanism to quickly and securely authenticate a contract in the digital realm, resulting in a negotiation that is agreed to by all parties involved and whose requirements must be met in order to "release" the agreed-upon activities (Carson et al., 2018). To put it another way, if the entire contract's terms are satisfied, the payment to the relevant parties will be paid automatically, ensuring a fair and fraud-free transaction. The benefits of using this technology are:

1.   Increase in reliability even if the parties do not trust each other
2.   Increase of economic benefits, eliminating third party involvement for mediation, decreasing costs

3.   All records saved in the blockchain are available to see and can serve to promote the good practices of the parts
4.   On the small producer's side, this technology can help them to receive almost immediate benefits from the
5.   commercialization

Figure 3. A general overview of the various stages of value chains of botanical products and how these could be managed using blockchain systems. Levels of complexity range from low (*) to very high (****)

Botanical value chain	Blockchain (number of blocks connected)	Level of complexity of the Blockchain solution	Key challenges at each stage	Specific Benefits	General Benefits
Cultivation and collection	▪	★	• Costs of acquiring technology • Training for technology use	• Ensure best practice (GACP) and sustainability • Verifiable payment • Primary producers-benefits	
Primary processing	▪ ▪	★ ★ ★	• As above plus • The need to capture the technical complexities	• Ensure correct and clearly described procedures-SOP • Minimizing risk of contamination	Traceability and GxP Local Economic Benefits Transparency (along VCs) Increases Trustworthiness
Manufacturing	▪ ▪ ▪	★ ★ ★ ★ ★	• As above plus • Differences between regulated and unregulated market elements	• GMP – compliance and ascertaining Quality control • Understanding of the underlying supply system	
Retail	▪ ▪ ▪ ▪	★ ★	• The need for transparency towards consumers/patients	• Understanding of the underlying supply system ascertaining consumer trust	
Consumer	▪ ▪ ▪ ▪ ▪	★	• Understanding of benefits	• Obtaining high standard products • Certainty of sustainability and equitable benefits	

8. QUALITY CONSIDERATIONS IN HERBAL VALUE CHAINS

Herbal medicinal product quality assurance is a more involved procedure than pharmaceutical product quality assurance. Natural goods' chemical makeup is often very varied, and any quality evaluation must account for the long, diversified, and often complex value chains through which these products originate. Quality assurance cannot be ensured for poorly or uncontrolled medicines, even if they have a full pharmaceutical production licence and the quality standards are properly documented utilising pharmacopoeial methodologies. There are also food standards. The quality and safety of a product in a short chain, that is, when the plant is cultivated and utilised as a medication in close proximity or even by the same person, is relatively easy to control, analyse, and manage. When used as a pharmaceutical product or dietary supplement on the domestic market or as an export product, however, the same plant poses significantly larger hazards and, as a result, far bigger hurdles to overcome, necessitating the collection of complicated sets of data (Booker et al., 2012). Authenticity, purity, and compliance with the permissible maximum levels of contaminants (microbiological, heavy metals, and poisonous compounds) are often checked late in the process, and only a tiny percentage of botanical products are manufactured under strict pharmaceutical quality control. Contamination by Heavy Metal Heavy metal contamination is common in herbal products due to two factors: pollution and natural buildup. Heavy industry pollution is a particular challenge in fast-developing countries like India and India. Although some nations have begun to address this issue, the legacy of years of pollution making its way into agricultural land via rivers and streams will take a long time to repair, and contamination levels in individual places are frequently unknown. Second, certain plants naturally store heavy metals, such as cadmium and heavy metals are present in the subsoil in particular regions as well, such as cinnabar in rock formations, resulting in high mercury levels in specific species. These issues can only be mitigated by carefully selecting production locations and enforcing rigorous limits on wild harvesting. Pesticides are seldom needed in the short chain, but global supply and customer demands sometimes need intensively cultivated crops that require greater pesticide doses to generate large yields of the desired product at a cheap cost. Furthermore, several of these substances may be banned under European law. We can only expect to maintain pesticide residues within allowed limits by carefully managing the value chain and providing extensive instruction on which pesticides may be used and in what quantities.

8.1 Mycotoxin

Although aflatoxins (mycotoxins generated by Aspergillus spp.) are extremely dangerous and carcinogenic, they are frequently discovered in botanical materials, particularly in the food sector (Liu and Wu, 2010). Certain items are more vulnerable than others, and examination has revealed significant levels of aflatoxins in wheat, barley, maize, and nuts, for example, but nothing has been reported in the general media about the challenges experienced in herbal medicine production (Williams et al., 2004; Azziz-Baumgartner et al., 2005; Liu and Wu, 2010). This is partially owing to a lack of rigorous regulation in many importing nations, but it is also due to a lack of knowledge of these issues and their fatal potential within the value chain (Williams et al., 2004). Transportation, storage, and processing are all areas where blockchain management might assist reduce risk. In a short value chain, aflatoxins are unlikely to develop; however, issues occur when fungal moulds are given the correct circumstances to flourish, which is characteristic of worldwide complex value chains. Procedures used on a local level with modest amounts of products may be completely unsuited for the worldwide distribution of huge consignments, and it is critical to realise this and establish, execute, and control the appropriate processes and procedures.

8.2 Adulteration by Accident/for Profit

Often to obtain high yields and to meet the high demand from people the herbal companies opt to use adulterated version of the main herbal drug. For Example: "Guggulu" Commiphora wightii – is a widely used Ayurvedic drug that is used for a variety of variety of disorders, most notably arthritis, and as a weight-reducing agent in obesity. Other traditional uses have included treatment of liver problems, tumors, ulcers and sores, urinary complaints, intestinal worms, swelling, and seizures depending upon its combination with other drugs. The demand of drug is such that it is very difficult to fullfil this demand and it has been noted that many of the companies use fake or adulterated version of it. Although, laws like Good Manufacturing Practices and good agriculture and collection practises (GACP) are there but still strong monitoring is required that can be achieved by using blockchain technology.

9. SUSTAINABLE SOURCING

According to the Ethical Consumer Markets Report 2017, sustainability certification of items such as Certified Sustainable Seafood MSC and Rainforest Alliance (Ethical

Consumer Research Association [ECRA], 2017) accounted for the majority of the increase in consumer expenditure. First and foremost, the application of BC technology may help in the monitoring and processing of these materials, giving critical baseline data on what is actually harvested/ collected. This can help to promote sustainable manufacturing since all of the product's precise information will be available to all value chain participants. BC systems can certify the sourcing in these production systems if sustainable production systems are implemented. Geo tracking and information on the first processing can assist define better production processes and prevent overexploitation.

10. BENEFITS TO PRODUCERS OF THE MATERIA PRIMA

There is still a lot of dispute about the benefits for primary producers. Financial incentives are often limited. It is difficult for small farmers and farm laborers to enter into economic collaborations with herbal medicine producers and dealers in the industry. These things are a boon to producers as well as consumers if farmers and primary producers can create more complicated enterprises and international linkages. The ancient value chain where farmers sell their products at an auction house has long been recognized to have farmers with some degree of control over their crops and the ability to sell them for the highest price feasible. Farms generally hold onto their turmeric harvest instead of selling it, which necessitates insecticides and fungicides in order to protect it from degrading under adverse conditions. This has a significant impact on the final product's quality. By employing this technique, a pre-agreed-upon raw material price might be reached by both farmer and product maker. Due to the increased stability provided by the fixed price, farmers will be able to increase their profit margins over the normal market price by using this method of trading. In this way the firm would benefit from having more control over their supply chain and the ability to request customized needs (such as organic manufacturing or national norms) (Booker et al., 2012). Companies may leverage farmers' welfare advantages as part of a larger marketing and promotion plan, such as employment security, stable prices and premium prices. Better-quality goods that are also more socially responsible may be available to consumers. To ensure that all parties adhere to the terms of their contracts, protocols, and processes, there are presently just a few checks in place. A "me too" strategy that lacks the necessary skills and infrastructure to actually produce a product of quality and has little prospect for meaningful welfare benefits, despite the fact that some well-established companies have built trusting relationships with their partners over many years, does not have a barrier to prevent it. As a consequence of BC systems, it will be clear to both customers and producers what economic benefits and value there are. There may be direct ties between producers and manufacturers of finished items for domestic or foreign markets. It is possible to establish that a product's origins are organic and sustainable by using BC systems in the same way a finished product can be purchased with confidence knowing where it came from, what certifications (reliability) it has, and the environmental and social impact it has on society. Because BC-stored information is immutable, customers will have greater confidence in their purchases because they will not have to worry about information bias from businesses.

11. INDIAN MEDICINE MARKET: AN EXAMPLE OF ADDED COMPLEXITY WITHIN THE VALUE CHAIN

In many ways, the value chains of high-value botanical items are similar to those of ancient medicinal herbs utilised in traditions such as Indian, china, African, or American medical systems. Nevertheless, when applied to today's worldwide and linked markets, the very divergent ways to making use of these resources, each grounded in a distinct philosophical framework, creates some unique problems. There is a high probability that ancient techniques will be incorporated into modern value chains that produce internationally recognised items. To make matters worse, obtaining the necessary raw material might be difficult if the species or botanical medication in question isn't legal in the nation where it was discovered or is subject to various regulations. It is also common to need extensive processing of botanical material at an early stage of the value chain in order to enhance the medicinal use of the constituent. Ayurveda (Ancient Indian medicine) is used here to highlight some of the most pressing issues. The vast majority of herbal formula items in the Ayurveda herbal market are made up of three to ten components, and they are often prepared in methods that are unique to Ayurveda. As a result, there are a variety of complicated development, production, and retail issues. As a result, the danger of poor quality, adulteration, or other quality issues is greatly increased. For the future of Indian herbal formulae, for example, each raw ingredient utilised must be traceable, including a written record of its progression along the supply chain. It would be possible to record and verify that all primary processing was done in accordance with stated protocols, such as well-defined industry standards (i.e. SOPs – standard operating procedures), and that the right source material was utilised in the calculation. Outside of India, ancient Indian formula goods have struggled to acquire a stable and secure regulatory standing. Due to the fact that many of these items are made in Asia and sold in Asian markets, this problem has arisen. Legal restrictions of the countries in which they are sold are sometimes ignored or only partially considered when they become global products. Commercialization outside of the United States is sometimes sought through blurring the line between food and medication. "Dashmoola Kwatha or Ten-root decoction" consists of ten roots Indian medicinal plants. Ayurveda uses and cultivates all of these substances extensively. Materials for "Dashmoola Kwatha or Ten-root decoction" are sourced from a variety of places. Ayurvedic formulations frequently call for steaming or frying and other types of processing (Sanskara) as a means of improving/enhancing the activity of a component and to remove the impurities. Complex processes that may result in items utilised in an Ancient environment (India) or for a worldwide market may be accurately recorded using blockchain technologies, enabling transparency for suppliers, processors, and end users.

Innovative practises can be introduced through obtaining, integrating, evaluating, and exchanging medical data at various system levels. The start and end points of each traceability connection are kept in the blockchain using "smart contracts." As a result, the data included in the traceability system will not be deleted by the system or by other means of incursion. This information is given by the organisation in question and is intended to be accurate and dependable while remaining fully anonymous. The implementation of a traceability system for Indian medicines based on blockchain technology has the potential to open up the whole Ayurvedic medicine supply chain, increasing transparency and fostering the healthy growth of the Ancient Indian System of medicine. **Figure 4** explains it further.

12. INTELLECTUAL PROPERTY QUESTIONS

Any sensible development of a new herbal product must now adhere to international agreements and national legislation, which have grown increasingly contentious in the herbal (medical) product arena. Commercialization of genetic resources and indigenous knowledge without mutually agreed benefit sharing has resulted in exploitation and has frequently led to strained international relations. Biodiversity and genetic resources are seldom protected since the Convention on Biological Diversity (CBD) does not inevitably result in prosecution. A blockchain might help authorities in CBD-abiding nations prohibit the sale of unlawful items and help consumers make educated ethical purchases by providing the relevant information and making data about each stage transparent.

Figure 4. Hierarchical structure of Ayurvedic Medicine traceability

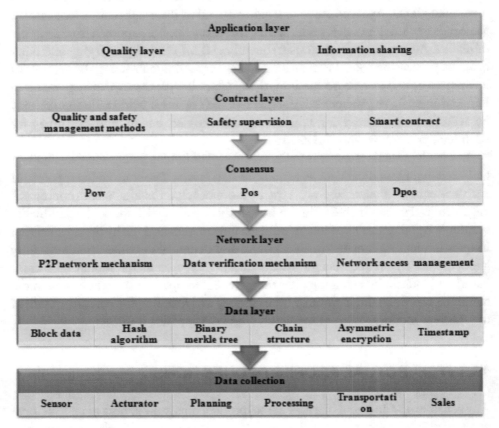

13. FUTURE PERSPECTIVES

13.1 Digital identity

Due to the fact that blockchain permits the consolidation of different data sets and electronic system interoperability, there are presently no feasible techniques for linking data for persons across data sets. (Zhang et al. 2018) emphasised that while healthcare institutions frequently utilise demographic data to associate individuals with other records, not all patients have (or are willing to supply) their social security numbers or other forms of identification. Complicating matters, names may be maintained in a variety of different forms or spellings, and patients may have similar names and other demographic information. Individuals, on the other hand, are often represented in research data sets by ID numbers rather than clearly identifiable information, which also eliminate information that may be used to link data across data sets. While some organisations are investigating the use of identity standards or identity management systems to control the identities of research participants (Jung and Pfister 2020), this poses a difficult trade-off between data value and privacy.

Additionally, this is true when it comes to illness diagnosis. For instance, in Ayurveda (Indian system of medicine), there are two types of sciatica: one caused by an imbalance of Vata-Pitta and another caused by an imbalance of Vata-Kapha. Therefore, it is critical to give these diseases distinct identities and to view them as distinct and distinct from one another.

In Ayurveda, each individual is thought to have a distinct identity and should be treated as such, but because to time constraints and a scarcity of data storage, this notion is compromised. In that regard, because blockchain technology may be used to store large amounts of data, it will be quite beneficial to successfully execute this idea.

13.2 Security

Electronic health record systems have become increasingly vulnerable to data breaches and ransomware attacks (Koczkodaj et al. 2019), and study participants express fear about unauthorised access to their private information. According to a 2019 poll by the Center for Information and Study on Clinical Research Participation (2020), 65 percent of potential research volunteers reported that confidentiality safeguards were a "very essential" factor in their decision to participate in research. While blockchain-based systems are very resistant to tampering, they are not immune to hacker attempts. (Saad et al. 2019) identify three primary areas of use for blockchains: mathematical/ cryptographic methodologies for producing the ledger, architectural distributions, and application contexts. While the majority of known attack methods are directed at crypto-currencies, generic risk principles such as domain name system assaults, consensus delays, and distributed denial of service attacks are applicable to all forms of distributed ledgers (Xu 2016). If study participants are required to engage with a blockchain, the biggest security problem is their occasionally lack of discernment when confronted with phishing assaults and key management (Radhakrishnan et al. 2019). Participants may be unable to recover their public/private key combination owing to unintentional loss or during an emergency or deterioration in health (Verde et al. 2019). If a blockchain-based user interface requires a password to access the system, weak passwords are easily guessable via a dictionary attack and when passwords are repeated (Takemiya and Vanieiev 2018). As a result, any solution to blockchain security must incorporate not only technology but also education, data governance, and risk management (Ballantyne 2020).

13.3 Slow adoption

It is very vital for any science to change according to the present times. This is believed in Ayurveda as well – According to Acharya Charaka (An Ancient Ayruvedic Scholar) the science should adapt to new ideas and subject to change according to the present times. Therefore, new technologies like blockchain, Design Thinking are need of the hour.

Including a blockchain technology in Ayurvedic Medicine will need some degree of cultural shift. This attempt is hampered by the fact that many suggested blockchain technologies are new and have not been implemented on a big enough scale to demonstrate benefit (Porsdam Mann et al. 2020). Porsdam Mann et al. (2020) advocate forming collaborations between health and technology divisions to educate stakeholders and dispel misconceptions about blockchain. These collaborations should foster an open and supportive conversation, with a particular emphasis on the key role that blockchain technology might play in research related to Ayurveda. A patient advocate may be able to give insight on patient-centric characteristics that may help to increase patient engagement. This cooperation must be ongoing, as the organization's rules, procedures, risk assessments, and monitoring all require revision (Kaye et al. 2015).

14. CONCLUSION

Once the Ancient Indian Medicine blockchain is established, a large number of blocks containing clinical electronic medical records will be generated, resulting in a wealth of data being stored in the Ancient Indian Medicine cloud. An enormous amount of clinical data will be available to support prescriptions compared to the sum of individual clinical experiences. Ancient Indian medicine's dialectical pathogenesis may be summarised by statistics when the blockchain data volume of the whole network reaches a certain scale, allowing for basic research into Ancient Indian medicine. As noted above, the problem of an information island in Ancient Indian medicine might be solved by a data sharing system that uses distributed storage. To guarantee that data is trustworthy and undamaged in the decentralisation of the blockchain, it is necessary to integrate patient input in the design of the block chain system, which includes the design of distributed storage, tech-oriented records and certification. Ancient Indian Medicine's potential to grow its blockchain system. An Ancient Indian Medicine cloud may be created with the help of a large blockchain database, which enables the introduction of AI algorithms for machine learning as an aid to Ancient Indian Medicine. To put it another way, by creating an Ancient Indian Medicine cloud and an AI auxiliary diagnostic and treatment system, a

Figure 5. Schematic diagram of the expansion of Blockchain system

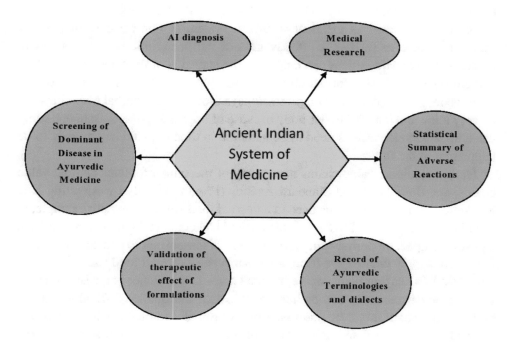

common Ancient Indian Medicine data system may be created using contemporary data technology, as shown in **Figure 5**.

Up to now, Ancient Indian medicine has been used in clinical treatments both in India and many other parts of the world. There are many kinds of prescriptions in Ancient Indian Medicine, most of which were handed down from ancient Indian Tradition. One thing need to be understood is a single drug in Ayurveda (Ancient System of Indian medicine) works on different ailments and purposes, when used with the combination with other drugs or certain type of prescribed food (Pathya) or water (temperature of consumed water) or the way the drug is processed (Sanskara) its mode of action changes. For example: Amalaki (Phyllanthus emblica) is an excellent source of Vitamin C rich in antioxidants and has been categorized under the category of the drugs that help in rejuvenation (Rasayana). Also, as it is a rich source of Vitamin C, in COVID-19 times it has been widely used for building up immunity and over all well being. When combined with Turmeric powder (Curcuma longa) it has an excellent effect on Diabetes Mellitus (Madhumeha). It is also categorized under the foods that should be consumed daily for balanced diet (Nitya Sevaniya Ahara). Since, in the blockchain technology each block is interconnected with each other it makes it an excellent tool for Ayurvedic Physicians and Researchers to use it as it gives them freedom to collect big data and organize the similar data in one block as well as compares the other blocks with similar keywords.

In short, we need an efficient statistical system of clinical data of Ancient Indian medicine to verify the effectiveness of the prescriptions. Ancient Indian medicine blockchain system can help with the statistics of the above information and eliminate the false information while reserving the true ones. It can also help us to record ADRs (Adverse Drug Reactions) as some Indian herbal medicines can be very toxic and harmful to our body because of improper dosage. Data regarding these toxic and side effects need to be gathered in time to avoid any tragedy to be happening in the future.

Herbal medicine value chains have many of the same problems as food value chains, and the UK's Food Standard Agency (FSA) is already investigating how blockchain technology may be used to construct food value chains (for example, in slaughterhouses) (FSA, 2018). It is clear that blockchain technologies might have a positive impact on herbal cultivation as well. It's important to consider what sets the herbal supply chain apart from any other type of farmed food (imported from outside). As a starting point, we've outlined a few common needs for BC systems, which aren't necessarily comprehensive. Most of the quality difficulties in the herbal value chain might be addressed by using a closed blockchain system that allows for easy upload and preservation of information. The raw materials source and transit, for example, may be tracked to ensure its traceability (e.g., indicating material cultivated in an area with heavy soil pollution). In order to ensure that it fulfills the norms of the nation in which it is being marketed, the local (end-market) authority would then put this material to particular and relevant testing, or it would be rejected at an early stage. Because it would eliminate the need for middlemen and make transactions more transparent, an open blockchain system would have a greater influence on the way these items are exchanged. Even if the recent push toward using Blockchain technology is simply another fad, the question of whether it will genuinely lead to a more sustainable and equal supply of high-quality botanicals must be asked very carefully. At this point, it is impossible to determine whether open or closed blockchain systems are better, and it is impossible to make a definitive decision. It's time to look at what's possible and what can't. Importantly, only if this becomes a sector-wide norm will we see a shift. Quality issues and adulterations will still occur, but the improved traceability will help all parties involved in the supply chain better detect and correct problems. At this point in time, the adoption of blockchain technology is being considered broadly, both in fields that are heavily controlled by the state (such as medical or particular ancient financial services) and in areas that are less regulated or self-regulated (e.g., bitcoinTrade). If proper tools are created, the trade in high-value botanical goods gives a perfect chance to study both the promise and the limitations of this technology. Even while it won't address every issue in the supply chain, it will provide a way for high-quality producers to prove that their efforts to ensure high quality are valid. The improved traceability provided by a Blockchain will not preclude issues, but it will make it simpler to handle them. It is also necessary to evaluate the impact on the system's functionality of incorrect entries into a BC. For the most part, blockchain technology will make it much simpler to track a product from "field to fork" (Figure 3). Offering a variety of items that have been certified to meet blockchain compliance criteria will benefit customers. A clearer picture will emerge of what constitutes best practise in the supply of botanicals of this calibre, making it easier for consumers to make informed decisions. Ethnopharmacology and natural product research will benefit from this viewpoint study on blockchains' potential, applications, and drawbacks.

REFERENCES

Azziz-Baumgartner, E., Lindblade, K., Gieseker, K., Rogers, H. S., Kieszak, S., Njapau, H., Schleicher, R., McCoy, L. F., Misore, A., DeCock, K., Rubin, C., & Slutsker, L. (2005). Case-control study of an acute aflatoxicosis outbreak, Kenya, 2004. *Environmental Health Perspectives*, *113*(12), 1779–1783. doi:10.1289/ehp.8384 PMID:16330363

Booker, A., Agapouda, A., Frommenwiler, D. A., Scotti, F., Reich, E., & Heinrich, M. (2018). St John's wort (Hypericum perforatum) products – an assessment of their authenticity and quality. *Phytomedicine*, *40*, 158–164. doi:10.1016/j.phymed.2017.12.012 PMID:29496168

Booker, A., Johnston, D., & Heinrich, M. (2012). Value chains of herbal medicines–research needs and key challenges in the context of ethnopharmacology. *Journal of Ethnopharmacology*, *140*(3), 624–633. doi:10.1016/j.jep.2012.01.039 PMID:22326378

Carson, B., Romanelli, G., Walsh, P., & Zhumaev, A. (2018). *Blockchain Beyond the Hype: What is the Strategic Business Value*. McKinsey&Company.

Esposito, C., De Santis, A., Tortora, G., Chang, H., & Choo, K. K. R. (2018). Blockchain: A Panacea for Healthcare Cloud-Based Data Security and Privacy? *IEEE Cloud Computing*, *5*(1), 31–37. doi:10.1109/MCC.2018.011791712

Ethical Consumer Research Association (ECRA). (2017). *Ethical Consumer Markets Report 2017*. Ethical Consumer Research Association.

Figorilli, S., Antonucci, F., Costa, C., Pallottino, F., Raso, L., Castiglione, M., Pinci, E., Del Vecchio, D., Colle, G., Proto, A., Sperandio, G., & Menesatti, P. (2018). A blockchain implementation prototype for the electronic open source traceability of wood along the whole supply chain. *Sensors (Basel)*, *18*(9), E3133. doi:10.339018093133 PMID:30227651

Frommenwiler, D. A., Reich, E., Sudberg, S., Sharaf, M. H. M., Bzhelyansky, A., & Lucas, B. (2016). St. John's Wort versus counterfeit St. John's Wort: An HPTLC study. *Journal of AOAC International*, *99*(5), 1204–1212. doi:10.5740/jaoacint.16-0170 PMID:27343017

FSA. (2018). *FSA Trials First Use of Blockchain*. Available at: https://www.food.gov.uk/news-alerts/news/fsa-trials-first-use-of-blockchain

Galvez, J. F., Mejuto, J. C., & Gandara, S. J. (2016). Future challenges on the use of blockchain for food traceability analysis. *Trends in Analytical Chemistry*, *107*, 222–232. doi:10.1016/j.trac.2018.08.011

Heinrich, M., & Hesketh, A. (2018). 25 years after the 'Rio Convention'–lessons learned in the context of sustainable development and protecting indigenous and local knowledge. *Phytomedicine*, *53*, 332–343. doi:10.1016/j.phymed.2018.04.061 PMID:30318154

Heinrich, M., Scotti, F., Booker, A., Fitzgerald, M., Kum, K. Y., & Löbel, K. (2019). Unblocking High-Value Botanical Value Chains: Is Therea Role for Blockchain Systems? *Frontiers in Pharmacology*, *10*, 396. doi:10.3389/fphar.2019.00396 PMID:31068810

Letsyo, E., Jerz, G., Winterhalter, P., Lindigkeit, R., & Beuerle, T. (2017). 'Incidence of pyrrolizidine Alkaloids in herbal medicines from German Retail markets: Risk assessments and implications to consumers.'. *Phytotherapy Research*, *31*(12), 1903–1909. doi:10.1002/ptr.5935 PMID:28960556

Saberi, S., Kouhizadeh, M., Sarkis, J., & Shen, L. (2019). Blockchain technology and its relationships to sustainable supply chain management. *International Journal of Production Research*, *57*(7), 2117–2135. doi:10.1080/00207543.2018.1533261

Zhou, S., Sheng, H., Ma, J., & Han, X. (2020). *Review of the Application of Blockchain Technology in Traditional Chinese Medicine Field*. doi:10.1145/3429889.3429932

Chapter 11
Analysis of Market Determinants Impacting the Blockchain Technology in the Healthcare Sector

Anusha Thakur
iD https://orcid.org/0000-0001-8761-2250
University of Petroleum and Energy Studies, India

ABSTRACT

Blockchain technology is paving its way from novel technology to leveraging its exclusive proficiencies. This technology refers to a platform that chronologically accounts and tracks the transactions and assets via distributed ledgers in a network. In today's scenario, the blockchain technology is gaining traction to completely revolutionize the healthcare services. This chapter discusses different competitive advantages offered by the healthcare sector on inclusion of blockchain technology in their strategic decisions and models. One of the key focus areas of the chapter includes market determinants impacting blockchain technology in the healthcare industry along with the market sizing and forecast analysis. Further, this chapter emphasizes how the blockchain concepts help in simplifying healthcare businesses amidst different challenges being faced by these industries in today's competitive scenario.

DOI: 10.4018/978-1-7998-9606-7.ch011

INTRODUCTION

With the spur in technological innovations, businesses in every sphere have been witnessing significant revolution over the years. In today's digitalized world, diversified systems interact with each other for various information and data exchange, wherein, reliability and security play a crucial role. Technologies such as blockchain offers a cost-effective, efficient, secure and reliable systems for directing and keeping a record of any transaction. Blockchain technology is increasingly gaining traction with its potentiality and increasing applications in the real-world scenario.

At its core, blockchain poses to be a suitable architecture for reserving and recording the transactional records. It is a public and distributed ledger, meant for tracking assets and recording transactions, wherein, stability is assured by a peer-to-peer system of computers (Yoon, 2019). The technology enables efficient management of electronic data with the potential to back up accountability and transparency features (OECD, December 2020). Blockchain is considered as an appropriate solution for transactions in businesses with a lighter digital footprint wherein, features such as immutability and transparency pose to be an advantage.

Enormous potential of blockchain extends to healthcare sector wherein, it represents another phase in the development of accurate, timely, as well as informed reviews on the basis of peer reviewed and updated guidelines. In the healthcare sector, blockchains are considered beneficial for management of pharmaceutical and medical supply chain processes, handling of dynamic patient consent, accessibility and data sharing permissions along with verification of identity. Data recorded on blockchain poses to be difficult to be modified or hacked, owing to the strong safety characteristics of the same. Blockchain permits the patients and clinicians to link the information related to critical healthcare in a secured manner, with transparency and privacy being maintained through codes and encryptions. The technology offers incredible prospects catering to the challenges existing in the industry, such as integrity, interoperability, traceability, accessibility and security.

Blockchain in the healthcare industry depends largely on the acceptance of new innovations and technology within the health care environment in order to generate technical structure. However, there are few assumptions and concerns regarding integration of blockchain with current healthcare systems and its adoption. The chapter outlines the market determinants impacting the implementation of blockchain technology in healthcare sector, with analysis of different challenges and trends in the market.

Research Questions

- Need for blockchain technology in the healthcare industry?

240

- What are the market estimates and forecasts for blockchain technology in healthcare sector in terms of revenue for the forecast period 2019 - 2028?
- What are the growth opportunities and trend analysis for the blockchain technology in the healthcare sector?
- Which outlook segment dominated the market?
- Which end-user segment accounted for the largest market share?
- What are the market share analysis and competitive strategies of different segments?

Purpose of the Article

This article illustrates the estimated and forecasted market size with global analysis of outlook type, end-user segments, and regional segments, and key emphasis on different factors bolstering and hindering the market growth of blockchain technologies in the healthcare sector. The paper also focuses on the key growth opportunities for the application of these technologies in the healthcare space. In addition to these, future implementations of this technology, with a brief description of competitive strategies adopted by the existing players and new entrants have also been illustrated.

Key Findings in the Research

Growing prevalence of data breach and leakage, along with the increasing need to control such issues, are expected to contribute favorably for the market growth. Different initiatives by major players, coupled with the growing need for effective health data management systems and the rising demand to minimize counterfeiting of drugs, are few of the factors expected to favorably impact the implementation of this technology. The study is a market research-based study which describes and analyses the blockchain technology application in healthcare market on the basis of outlook, regional segments and end-user segments. The article presents an in-depth description of market study and wide-range of statistics for each of each of these segments for the forecast period of 2019-2028.

LITERATURE REVIEW

The Blockchain technology is continuously witnessing a surge in businesses, with latest innovations in the sector. It was initially used as a pillar for the cryptocurrency, Bitcoin, however, in today's scenario, its applications and capabilities are prolonged beyond cryptocurrencies. Blockchain, a decentralized node system stores information and is proven to be an exceptional technology for protecting confidential data and information (Haleem, 2021). It is a ledger structure which controls data and their transactions with the help of time-stamped blocks via cryptography in a scattered way over computing system.

In the healthcare sector, blockchain is expected to serve as a substitute to the conventional distributed database management systems, which are generally client-server databases with relational ideas. Although the conventional distributed database networks are a recognized platform in the health-care systems, they have significant restrictions, such as absence of an immutable audit trail, vulnerability to outside adversaries, and inability to back-up the peer-to-peer sharing of data. Incorporation of blockchain technology in the sector, generates a decentralized health-care related information management network, and enables the formation of transactions recorded both on and outside the blockchain ledger (Ng, October 12, 2021).

The paper emphasizes on presenting a latest systematic literature review focusing on the trends, opportunities, and potential applications of the blockchain technologies in healthcare sector along with the market analysis.

NEED FOR BLOCKCHAIN IN HEALTHCARE INDUSTRY

Healthcare is an enormous market across the world. The health care expenditure across different regions in the world continue to escalate, thereby posing as an opportunity to the healthcare systems. For instance, the health care expenditure spending was approximately $7.72 trillion in the world, with $3.55 trillion in the United States in 2017 ((IET)).

As far as the healthcare industry is concerned, the urgency of advancement increases at an exponential speed. One of the major factors for growth lies in the implementation of latest technologies supported by quality health services in the industry.

The healthcare industry is under immense pressure to regulate the costs and offer high quality services to the patients. The industry is a multifaceted system of interrelated entities (Capgemini, 2017). With the evolution of health care industry along-with the market intrusive technologies, it poses to be difficult for businesses to minimize the costs while being competitive as well. Revolution of healthcare delivery has significantly led to the growth of participatory approach or patient-centricity concept in the healthcare industry. The finest quality of experience is expected to happen only when the patients are involved in different parts of the care-services delivery. Implementation of technologies such as blockchain in the healthcare space is expected to increase the security of different transactional activities, minimize manual inefficiencies, regularize patient related information and enhance the quality of care for the same (Arsene, 2021). This fast-developing and unique technological

Figure 1.Potential applications of Blockchain among the healthcare providers and shareholders
Source: (Team, October - 2019)

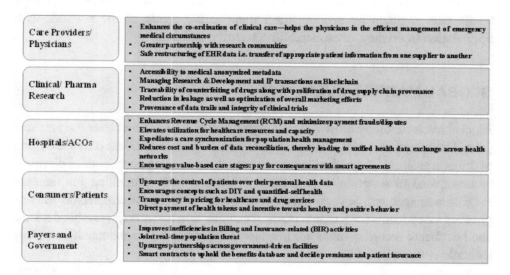

sector is projected to provide fertile ground for proof-of concept, investment, and exploration testing (Group, 2021). It offers an innovative model for Health Information Exchanges (HIE) by making electronic records more secure, disintermediated, as well as efficient, and further, preventing the spread of patient data across different geographical regions without settling on security and privacy factors. A blockchain driven HIE is projected to reveal the exact rate of interoperability. Various HIEs presently use a decentralized method for their information architecture, which helps in guaranteeing that the patient related sensitive health information can easily be scrutinized across various barricades, in spite of a single gateway (Team F., 2018).

In addition to these, blockchain technology in healthcare market helps in addressing the supply chain matters by offering a distributed ledger shared among all the shareholders in the supply chain processes. Records entered in the blockchain at every stage of the process are decentralized, permanent, and immutable, which in turn eradicates the susceptibility of fraud or errors. With this technological system in place, even the end users are expected to have all the information relevant to the product from its formation to the consumption (CitiusTech, May 2018).

The figure mentioned above illustrates the different potential applications of blockchain among the healthcare providers and shareholders.

Few uses of the technology includes Nationwide Interoperability Roadmap, Patient Care and Outcomes Research (PCOR), and Precision Medicine Initiative. It further supports continuous sharing of information thereby minimizing inconsistencies, duplication and errors happening due to centralized data storage.

Hence, the concept of Blockchain owes the potentiality to transform the overall health care segment by keeping the patient at the centre of the network with upgradation in privacy, interoperability, security, and data.

GLOBAL MARKET OVERVIEW

Blockchain technology has witnessed significant rise in demand over the past few years. Growing demand for effective clinical data management and avert counterfeiting of drugs is projected to bolster the market growth. Increasing prevalence of diseases, is anticipated to generate huge amount of data, thereby propelling the demand for data management. Several untapped avenues in the healthcare sector, such as growing investments for efficient medical examination networks, wearable devices, and healthcare record systems are few factors boosting the implementation of this technology over the forecast period.

The concept of "Blockchain" offers abundant prospects for the health care sector; but it is still not matured in today's scenario, nor a solution which can instantly applied. It is essential for several behavioural, organizational, and technical economic challenges to be addressed before the adoption of a health care blockchain by businesses across the world.

In order to stay competitive, there is an increasing need to enhance the synchronization among different shareholders and accordingly, implement legal aspects and current processes to better cater to the changing market scenario.

MARKET DRIVERS

Increasing Demand to Minimize Drug Counterfeiting

Counterfeiting has a wide-spread adverse impact, such as causing lawsuits, loss of sales, product recalls, long-term reputational damage, and loss of customer confidence. In the healthcare sector, counterfeiting of the prescription drugs leading to accidental overdoses is one of the prevalent issues. Implementation of blockchain technology in the healthcare sector helps to confront counterfeiting by recognizing provenance of any product. This can mainly be attributed to the fact that the technology helps to offer a trusted and secure tracking system through every step of the supply chain process.

Counterfeiting of the drugs is similar to the real drugs, with the packaging design and branding. However, fake drugs are ineffective or contaminated. For instance, with the (Food and Drug Administration) FDA's call in 2019 for the companies to generate experimental projects for testing automated inter-operable systems, nearly 2 dozen firms in the pharmaceutical industry, extending from drug makers (including Eli Lilly, Pfizer Inc. and Company), to retailers and distributors, established a blockchain platform named MediLedger Network, for tracking the prescription drugs to minimize counterfeiting issues across the different regions (Dreyfuss, 2020). Features of healthcare segment in blockchain such as auditable, immutable, and transparency, holds the potentiality to augment the functionality, integrity, security, and data provenance of supply chain process.

Implementation of blockchain in healthcare supply chain owes the capability to reduce theft and counterfeiting issues and manage inventory as well. Globally, firms such as Global Fund, USAID, and Red Cross, focuses on tracing back the supply of contributed medications across various regions. Hence, application of this technology permits clear perception of the product's drive from producer to the patients with digitized transactions. Consequently, it would also be possible to inspect susceptible facts in the supply chain thereby minimizing the probability of frauds and costs related to it (LeewayHertz, 2021).

Growing Need for Efficient Health Data Management Systems

As far as management of data is concerned, blockchain in healthcare enhances complete security of the electronic medical records of a patient, allows safe interoperability between the healthcare businesses, and solves the issues of traceability of drugs supply chain, as well as drug authenticity (Philip, 2021). The concept of blockchain, enables the healthcare providers to form an efficient and elaborate database management system. The system owes the capacity to house an extensive variety of data for different patient insurance and medical information, emergency contact information, test results and diagnostics, as well as variety of medicines. Transactions between the patients, wholesalers, doctors, and pharmaceutical companies creates a private blockchain system, wherein, the cryptographic encoding keeps the data safe and secure. In order to build such a huge database, a systematic approach is required. The technology enables easy and better performance of managerial tasks such as managing medicine inventories and scheduling a doctor's appointment. Overall, the technology not only offers a cost-effective model but also the functional efficiency model for data management. Hence, blockchain functionalities are of enormous help, in terms of maintaining databases related to medicines and drugs.

MARKET RESTRAINTS

Scalability Constraints for Blockchain Technology

In the world of blockchain, scalability has always been a major question for healthcare businesses. Scalability of blockchain technology, poses to be a challenge, as validation and verification with Distributed Ledger Technology (DLTs) requirement of high computing energy cannot be spread for more multifaceted healthcare information. Scalability has continually been a consideration in software executions. It is significantly one of the biggest problems faced by entrepreneurial firms manufactured across smaller set of clients, who require to integrate with a larger group of clients. This same situation can be repetitive in case of the blockchains for healthcare sector as well, for storing the healthcare information, wherein, businesses are looking for expansion (Healthcare Information and Management Systems Society, 2021). With the implementation of blockchain technology, the capacity to refactor all the data collected for the healthcare sector is expected to be difficult.

Further, blockchain driven healthcare system, including sensor-based products for patient care, is expected to face storage constraint issues, thereby, leading to heavy weight computation which needs to be resolved (Peters G. W., 2016). Implementation of blockchain system leads to slower execution of transactions and subsequently results in sluggish throughput as well (Lazar, 2017). In addition to these, transaction time of the technology is considerably lengthy, wherein, it executes nearly 7 transactions per second (1 MB block size) as per the protocol, when, compared to the Twitter and Visa networks, which performs approximately 5000 and 2000 transactions per second respectively. This speed problem is thereby, anticipated to substantially limit the scalability of blockchain systems.

Data Standardization and Scope

Standards are the key for growth of the blockchain technology. In the healthcare sector, it is very essential for the firms to consider the information stored off or on the blockchain. One of the concerns for healthcare information stored, includes size of the data to be stored on the blockchain. Giving-in information such as doctor's notes on blockchain, are anticipated to generate unreasonably larger transaction sizes which can unfavourably impact the overall technological performance.

It is thereby very crucial and essential for the regulators to recognize the characteristics of this latest technology, if they need to treat it considerately. Effectiveness of standards totally depends upon the understanding of stakeholders and their steps for implementing the same (Deshmukh, 2020). Hence, in order to manage performance and standardize the information stored, it is essential for the firms to align on a framework for defining which format, size and data needs to be submitted.

REGULATORY SCENARIO FOR BLOCKCHAIN IN HEALTHCARE INDUSTRY

Like any cutting-edge technology, usage of blockchain in the healthcare sector lacks formal and regulatory guidance. In today's scenario, consideration of collaboration in between the health care policy makers and industry plays a crucial role to understand and facilitate the growth of ecosystem within new policy objectives and existing regulatory framework. Few of these considerations includes consequence of the scattered storage nature of the blockchain, who takes the proprietorship of records and how is accessibility granted by using blockchain. Regulators across different regions in the world are anticipated to inspect these technologies in healthcare systematically, with security and privacy being the key points, over the next five years.

Health Insurance Portability and Accountability Act and General Data Protection Regulation

Health and Human Services (HHS), via Health Insurance Portability and Accountability Act (HIPAA) privacy rule, has launched standards to safeguard the medical record privacy of any individual. This rule enables protecting the privacy of personal health data and accordingly sets conditions and limits on its disclosures and usage without the authorization of patients.

In the US, the HIPAA offers security and privacy provisions for protecting medical-related data. General Data Protection Regulation (GDPR) is a law on privacy and protection of data for all the individual citizens of the European Economic Area (EEA) and the European Union. Both of the regulations offer a substantial motivation for the implementation of blockchain-powered usage in the healthcare sector (Network, 2020).

Interoperability and transparency have been the key barriers for the adoption and integration of Electronic Health Records (EHR) over the past few years, with blockchain technology proving to be a revolution which the business needs.

Drug Supply Chain Security Act

The FDA's, Drug Supply Chain Security Act (DSCSA) is proposed to boost the regulatory error of contaminated, stolen, and counterfeit, or harmful drugs. Few pilot projects under the DSCSA test enables how blockchain can protect information sharing across different healthcare enterprises. The aim of the act is to develop an interoperable and electronic system which will trace and identify prescription drugs when these are distributed within the US. For instance, KPMG, Walmart, Merck, and IBM have been selected for an experimental program which is anticipated to discover and enhance the security of drug distribution and supply with the help of blockchain technology.

FUTURE OPPORTUNITIES AND SCENARIO OF BLOCKCHAIN TECHNOLOGY IN HEALTHCARE INDUSTRY

Blockchain technology, still in its nascent stage, offers abundant opportunities. The technology generates exclusive prospects to minimize complexity, enable trustless alliance, and create immutable and secure information. HHS tracks this developing field to recognize and sense the trends and areas, wherein the government support might be required for the technology to comprehend its complete potential in health care. In order to shape the future of blockchain, it is essential for HHS to emphasize on convening and mapping the blockchain ecosystem, thereby developing a framework to synchronize the initial adopters, and backup a consortium for discovery and dialogue.

A blockchain trusted exchange of health information offers longitudinal opinions of patient's health, forms new visions about the population health, and supports the shift towards value-based care. With larger accessibility, trust, and transparency to information, HHS owes the capability to gather perceptions for better effectiveness, security, safety, and quality of vaccines, drugs, and medical devices. Blockchain has extensive consequences for shareholders in the health care ecosystem. Exploiting this technology has the possibility to link fragmented systems to create better understanding thereby, better assessing the value of care. Hence, for a long-term scenario, implementation of a blockchain system is anticipated to enhance the efficiencies and support improved health results for the patients.

IMPACT OF COVID-19 ON THE IMPLEMENTATION OF BLOCKCHAIN TECHNOLOGY IN THE MARKET

The COVID-19 crisis has largely impacted the healthcare sector, and has boosted the implementation of digital technology across different regions in the world. One of such technologies includes the blockchain technology, which possess unique characteristics such as decentralization, immutability and transparency, which have their usage across various domains such as mobile health, management of electronic medical records and few more.

Blockchain is considerably presenting abundant avenues in this pandemic situation, as it enables efficient monitoring and tracking solutions and guarantees a clear supply chain process of vital services and products. This can be attributed to the fact that blockchain consists of a chronologically well-organized list of encoded signatures, a safe scattered ledger comprising of permanent transactional records which can be shared by all the associates in the system (Marbouh, October 12, 2020).

RESEARCH METHODOLOGY

The study offers an analysis of market forces impacting the blockchain technology in healthcare sector, with key focus on market sizing and forecasts over the projected period. The research focuses on different market drivers, trends, challenges, opportunities, regulatory policies, and strategies impacting market growth over the forecast period. The forecast analysis will be in terms of revenue at the global, and regional levels, with the key trends varying for 2019-2028 (forecast period)

Research objectives

Objectives of the research study can be illustrated as:

- To study the evolution of blockchain technology, with major focus on recent technological trends in the market.
- To emphasize on the future aspects, challenges and implications of this technology in the market
- To examine competitive scenarios such as collaborations, mergers & acquisitions, R&D activities, and advanced developments in the global blockchain technology in healthcare market.
- To recognize the factors bolstering growth of blockchain technology in healthcare sector across different end-user verticals over the forecast period.
- Impact of COVID-19 on the implementation of this technology in the market

Inclusions

- Outlook type on the basis of Private and Public
- End-user segment by Hospitals, Drug and Medical Device Companies, Insurance providers, Others
- Regional segmentation based on North America, Europe, Asia Pacific, Latin America and Middle East & Africa

Scope of the Study

The article contemplates the current scenario of Global blockchain technology in healthcare market along with the key market forces for the forecast period of 2019 - 2028. The article emphasizes on anticipating market recast by assigning weightage to market forces (drivers, restraints, opportunities). Further, the study focuses on regional as well as segment revenue for assessing the overall market scenario. It further emphasizes on the competitive strategies and share analysis of the market as well.

Enclosed aspects comprise of market size and estimates of the blockchain technology in healthcare market in terms of revenue over the forecast period; as well as segmentation on the basis of region covering North America, Europe, Asia Pacific, and the Rest of the World (RoW). This helps in determining overall size of the market over the forecasted period in terms of revenue, get insights about the factors which are engaged in propelling the market growth and the factors which poses to be restraining its growth and development. The given statistics is consequently attained from secondary sources via various company annual reports, investor documents, journals and statistics published by various market leaders. The data can be analysed owing to the below mentioned factors:

- Demand and supply estimates
- Market developments and trends.
- Future aspects and opportunities offering insights on product commercialization as well as expansion in different regions.

The data has been categorized based on varied parameters such as region, outlook type, and end-user segment. Methodologies to study the gathered data can be illustrated as:

- **Top-Down Approach:** The data are collected for the global scenario and are then separated into different entities (which include outlook type/region/end-user, in this case it is based on regional analysis).
- **Bottom-Up Approach:** The data are collected and estimated for regional segments and are then combined to obtain the global numbers. The data are then forecasted on the basis of different market initiatives and trends for over the forecast period of 2019 to 2028. This helps to gain holistic information and understand current market scenario as well as future trends of the same, thereby enabling the companies to accordingly strategize their plans and policies.

Figure 2.Global Blockchain technology in healthcare market 2019-2028 ($ million)
Source: Secondary Sources

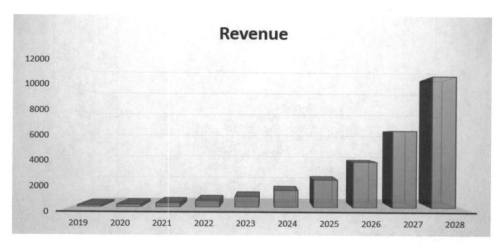

FINDINGS AND MARKET ANALYSIS

Global analysis

Blockchain technology in healthcare market was valued at $159.98 million in 2019, and is expected to witness a surge in its growth rate over the forecast period. The market was expected to be valued at $10999.99 million in 2028.

Type analysis

On the basis of type, the blockchain technology can be categorized into private and public types. Public system has wide-spread usage for the management of data. In today's scenario, Ethereum technology also known as "permission-less" system (a public network), is the most used in healthcare sector. Accessibility to a larger database and low-cost structure are considerably the major factors causing the the evolution of these networks.

Private blockchains are known as the permissioned systems. For instance, Hyperledger Fabric offers high security, fast transactions, and privacy. Hence, usage of these systems is mainly for specific enterprise requirements. Key factors leading to the growth of private blockchain system can be attributed to the rising demand for safety and security in the supply chain processes along with the recording and data management aspects.

Figure 3.Global Blockchain technology in healthcare market 2019-2028 ($ million)
Source: Secondary Sources

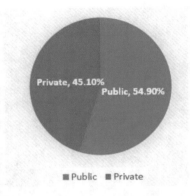

End-use analysis

On the basis of end-use, the market can be segmented into hospitals, insurance providers, drug and medical device companies and others. Hospitals accounted for the market share of nearly 33.99 per cent of the overall market. This can mainly be attributed to the fact that the hospitals nowadays are engaged in safeguarding the patient-centric information, thereby improving the overall efficiency of the system in the industry.

Drug and medical device company segment reported a share of 45.59 per cent in 2019, due to the rising traceability, and transparency in clinical trials, prevention of counterfeit of drugs coupled with the verification of the authenticity of the drugs.

Regional analysis

On the basis of geographies, the market can be segmented into regions of North America, Europe, Asia Pacific, Latin America, and Middle East & Africa. Europe accounted for the market share of nearly 46.79 per cent of the overall market. This can mainly be attributed to the increasing preferences among government and businesses to promote the usage of blockchain.

North America accounted for nearly 39.69 per cent of the total share in 2019, thereby witnessing a considerable growth along with the Asia Pacific regions as well. Presence of a large number of players and their strategic initiatives is expected to propel the market demand.

The Middle Eastern and Latin American regions are expected to witness considerable growth over the forecast period, owing to the increasing trends of identity detection solutions, and the development of new and efficient health-care system in the region.

Figure 4.End-use analysis of global Blockchain technology in healthcare market (in terms of market share)
Source: Secondary Sources

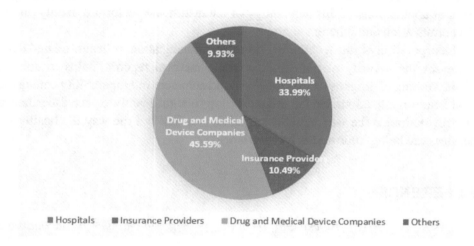

Figure 5.Geographical analysis of global Blockchain technology in healthcare market in 2020 ($ billion)
Source: Secondary Sources

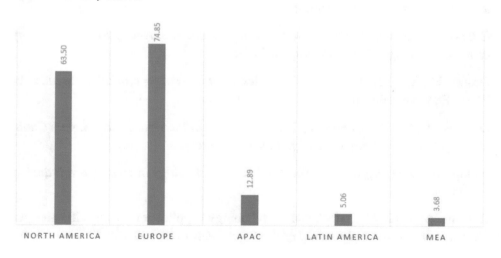

CONCLUSION

Blockchain technology is one of the emerging technologies and has an enormous potential to conduct and change the way businesses are done. Considering all the capabilities of this technology, blockchain offers several opportunities to become the next big technological innovation in the world. Adoption of blockchain technology in the healthcare sector is expected to witness a surge over the forecast period. Several applications of this technology in the healthcare sector are mainly due to decentralization and inherent encryption.

Incorporation of this technology promotes monetization of health-related data, increases the security of patient's electronic medical records, helps to combat counterfeiting of drugs as well as vaccines, and enhances interoperability among the healthcare organizations. Hence, this technology is significantly expected to enhance and revolutionize the way patients are taken care off and the way the healthcare services are being improved across the world.

REFERENCES

Anderson, N. (2016). *Blockchain Technology: A game-changer in accounting?* Deloitte.

Arsene, C. (2021, August 21). *Blockchain in Healthcare: An Executive's Guide for 2021*. Digital Authority Partners.

Capgemini. (2017). *Blockchain: A Healthcare Industry View*. Capgemini.

CenterSource. (n.d.). *How Blockchain Technology Can Impact Hospitality: 5 Steps to Prepare Your Business*. Author.

CitiusTech. (2018). *Blockchain for Healthcare: An opportunity to address many complex challenges in healthcare*. CitiusTech.

Deshmukh, S. P. (2020, October 27). *6 lessons for creating blockchain standards*. World Economic Forum.

Dreyfuss, G. C. (2020, February 21). *Companies in Pharmaceutical Supply Chain Develop System to Track Counterfeit Drugs*. Reuters.

Group, M. (2021, September 20). *Blockchain Technology in Healthcare Industry*. Academic Press.

Haleem, A. J. (2021). Blockchain Technology Applications in Healthcare: An Overview. *International Journal of Intelligent Networks*, 130-139.

Healthcare Information and Management Systems Society. (2021). *Blockchain in Healthcare*. Author.

IET. (n.d.). *Blockchain in Healthcare. The Institution of Engineering and Technology*. TheIET.

Lazar, M. A.-M. (2017). Digital revolution in depression: A technologies update for clinicians. *Personalized Medicine in Psychiatry*, *4*, 1–6.

LeewayHertz. (2021). *Blockchain in Pharma Supply Chain - Reucing Counterfeit Drugs*. Author.

Marbouh, D. A. (2020). *Blockchain for COVID-19: Review, Opportunities, and a Trusted Tracking System*. National Center for Biotechnology Information, U.S. National Library of Medicine.

Network MD. (2020, July 7). *Blockchain in Healthcare: Regulatory Themes*. Author.

Ng, W. Y.-E.-K.-H. (2021, October 12). Blockchain Applications in Health Care for COVID-19 and Beyond: A Systematic Review. *Lancet*.

OECD. (2020). *Blockchain Policy Series: Opportunities and Challenges of Blockchain Technologies in Health Care*. Policy Brief: Opportunities and Challenges of Blockchain in Healthcare.

Peters, G. W. (2016). Understanding modern banking ledgers through blockchain technologies: Future of transaction processing and smart contracts on the internet of money. In *Banking beyond banks and money* (pp. 239–278). Springer.

Philip. (2021). *Blockchain Technology in Healthcare in 2021*. The Block Box.

Team, F. (2018, October 22). *The Use of Blockchain in Healthcare – How Can Technology Keep Health Data Secure and Private?* Academic Press.

Team, G. T. (2019). *Global Blockchain Technology Market in the Healthcare Industry, 2018–2022*. Frost & Sullivan.

Yoon, H.-J. (2019). *Blockchain Technology and Healthcare*. National Center for Biotechnology Information, U.S. National Library of Medicine.

Compilation of References

Abdulsalam, Y., Alhuwail, D., & Schneller, E. S. (2020). Adopting identification standards in the medical device supply chain. *International Journal of Information Systems and Supply Chain Management*, *13*(1), 1–14. doi:10.4018/IJISSCM.2020010101

Abouelmehdi, K., Abderrahim, B., Khaloufi, H., & Saadi, M. (2017). Big data security and privacy in healthcare: A Review. *Procedia Computer Science*, *113*, 73-80. . doi:10.1016/j.procs.2017.08.292

Agbo, C. C., Mahmoud, Q. H., & Eklund, J. M. (2019, June). Blockchain technology in healthcare: a systematic review. In Healthcare (Vol. 7, No. 2, p. 56). Multidisciplinary Digital Publishing Institute. doi:10.3390/healthcare7020056

Aggarwal, S., & Kumar, N. (2021). Blockchain 2.0: Smart contracts, The Blockchain Technology for Secure and Smart Applications across Industry Verticals, Shubhani Aggarwal, Neeraj Kumar, and Pethuru Raj (Ed.), Volume 121 Advances in Computers, 2021.

Ahmad, R. W., Salah, K., Jayaraman, R., Yaqoob, I., Ellahham, S., & Omar, M. (2021). The role of blockchain technology in telehealth and telemedicine. *International Journal of Medical Informatics*, 104399.

Aich, S., Chakraborty, S., Sain, M., Lee, H. I., & Kim, H. C. (2019, February). A review on benefits of IoT integrated blockchain based supply chain management implementations across different sectors with case study. In *2019 21st international conference on advanced communication technology (ICACT)* (pp. 138-141). IEEE. 10.23919/ICACT.2019.8701910

Aithal, P. S., & Madhushree, L. M. (2019). Emerging Trends in ICCT as Universal Technology for Strategic Development of Industry Sectors. Chapter in a Book - IT and Computing for all the Domains and Professionals: The Emergence of Computer and Information Sciences, Edited by P.K. Paul, A. Bhuimali, K.S. Tiwary, and P. S. Aithal published by New Delhi Publishers, New Delhi. pp 1-26, ISBN: 978-93-88879-66-8.

Aithal, P. S., & Aithal, S. (2018). Study of various General-Purpose Technologies and Their Comparison towards developing Sustainable Society. [IJMTS]. *International Journal of Management, Technology, and Social Sciences*, *3*(2), 16–33.

Aithal, P. S., & Aithal, S. (2019). Management of ICCT underlying Technologies used for Digital Service Innovation. [IJMTS]. *International Journal of Management, Technology, and Social Sciences*, *4*(2), 110–136.

Aithal, P. S., & Aithal, S. (2019, October). Digital Service Innovation Using ICCT Underlying Technologies. In *Proceedings of International Conference on Emerging Trends in Management, IT and Education* (Vol. 1, No. 1, pp. 33-63).

Aithal, P. S., & Madhushree, L. M. (2019). Information Communication & Computation Technology (ICCT) as a Strategic Tool for Industry Sectors. [IJAEML]. *International Journal of Applied Engineering and Management Letters*, *3*(2), 65–80.

Akkaoui, R., Hei, X., & Cheng, W. (2020). EdgeMediChain: A Hybrid Edge Blockchain-Based Framework for Health Data Exchange. *Access IEEE*, *8*, 113467–113486.

Al Omar, A. (2019). Bhuiyan, Md Zakirul Alam Bhuiyan, Basu, A., Kiyomoto, S. & Rahman M. S. (2019). Privacy-friendly platform for healthcare data in cloud-based on blockchain environment. Future Generation Computer Systems, 95, 511–521.

Al Omar, A., Rahman, M. S., Basu, A., & Kiyomoto, S. (2017). Mainchain: a blockchain based privacy preserving platform for healthcare data. In *International Conference on Security, Privacy and Anonymity in Computation, Communication and Storage* (pp. 534–543) Springer. 10.1007/978-3-319-72395-2_49

Alladi, T., Chamola, V., Parizi, R. M., & Choo, K. R. (2019). Blockchain applications for industry 4.0 and industrial IoT: A review. IEEE Access : Practical Innovations, Open Solutions, 7, 176935–176951.

Alla, S., Soltanisehat, L., Tatar, U., & Keskin, O. (2018). Blockchain technology in electronic healthcare systems. *IISE Annual Conference and Expo 2018, May*, 901–906.

Alla, S., Soltanisehat, L., Tatar, U., & Keskin, O. (2018, May). Blockchain technology in electronic healthcare systems. In *Proceedings of the 2018 IISE Annual Conference* (pp. 1-6).

AlShamsi, M., Salloum, S. A., Alshurideh, M., & Abdallah, S. (2021). Artificial intelligence and blockchain for transparency in governance. In *Artificial Intelligence for Sustainable Development: Theory, Practice and Future Applications* (pp. 219–230). Springer.

Altman, E. (1999). Constrained Markov decision processes. CRC Press.

Anderson, N. (2016). *Blockchain Technology: A game-changer in accounting?* Deloitte.

Androulaki, E., Barger, A., Bortnikov, V., Cachin, C., Christidis, K., Caro, A. D., Enyeart, D., Ferris, C., Laventman, G., & Manevich, Y. (2018). Hyperledger fabric: a distributed operating system for permissioned blockchains. In Proceedings of the thirteenth EuroSys conference, 1–15, 2018.

Angeletti, F., Chatzigiannakis, I., & Vitaletti, A. (2017, September). The role of blockchain and IoT in recruiting participants for digital clinical trials. In *2017 25th International Conference on Software, Telecommunications and Computer Networks (SoftCOM)* (pp. 1-5). IEEE.

Angraal, S., Krumholz, H. M., & Schulz, W. L. (2017). Blockchain technology: Applications in health care. *Circulation: Cardiovascular Quality and Outcomes*, *10*(9), e003800.

Arsene, C. (2019). *Hyperledger Project Explores Fighting Counterfeit Drugs with Blockchain*. Available online: https://healthcareweekly.com/blockchain-in-healthcare- guide/

Arsene, C. (2021, August 21). *Blockchain in Healthcare: An Executive's Guide for 2021*. Digital Authority Partners.

Aste, T., Tasca, P., & Di Matteo, T. (2017). Blockchain technologies: The foreseeable impact on society and industry. *Computer*, *50*(9), 18–28.

Azaria, A., & Ekblaw, A. (2016). MedRec: Using Blockchain for Medical Data Access and Permission Management, In 2nd International Conference on Open and Big Data (OBD), IEEE, 25-30, 2016.

Azogu, I., Norta, A., Papper, I., Longo, J., & Draheim, D. (2019, April). A Framework for the Adoption of Blockchain Technology in Healthcare Information Management Systems: A Case Study of Nigeria. In *Proceedings of the 12th International Conference on Theory and Practice of Electronic Governance* (pp. 310-316).

Azzi, R., Chamoun, R. K., & Sokhn, M. (2019). The power of a blockchain-based supply chain. *Computers & Industrial Engineering*, *135*, 582–592. doi:10.1016/j.cie.2019.06.042

Azziz-Baumgartner, E., Lindblade, K., Gieseker, K., Rogers, H. S., Kieszak, S., Njapau, H., Schleicher, R., McCoy, L. F., Misore, A., DeCock, K., Rubin, C., & Slutsker, L. (2005). Case-control study of an acute aflatoxicosis outbreak, Kenya, 2004. *Environmental Health Perspectives*, *113*(12), 1779–1783. doi:10.1289/ehp.8384 PMID:16330363

Bader, L., Pennekamp, J., Matzutt, R., Hedderich, D., Kowalski, M., Lücken, V., & Wehrle, K. (2021). Blockchain-based privacy preservation for supply chains supporting lightweight multi-hop information accountability. *Information Processing & Management*, *58*(3), 102529. doi:10.1016/j.ipm.2021.102529

Bahga, A., & Madisetti, V. K. (2013). A cloud-based approach for interoperable electronic health records (EHRs). IEEE Journal of Biomedical and Health Informatics, 17(5), 894–906.

Bayrak, T., & Özdiler Çopur, F. (2017). Evaluation of the unique device identification system and an approach for medical device tracking. *Health Policy and Technology*, *6*(2), 234–241. doi:10.1016/j.hlpt.2017.04.003

Beckmann, H. (2012). *Prozessorientiertes Supply Chain Engineering: Strategien, Konzepte und Methoden zur modellbasierten Gestaltung*. Springer Fachmedien Wiesbaden. https://site.ebrary.com/lib/alltitles/docDetail.action?docID=10627905 doi:10.1007/978-3-658-00269-5

Begoyan, A. (2007). *An overview of interoperability standards for electronic health records*. Society for Design and Process Science.

Benchoufi, M., Porcher, R., & Ravaud, P. (2017). Blockchain protocols in clinical trials: Transparency and traceability of consent. *F1000 Research*, *6*(1), 1–66.

Benchoufi, M., & Ravaud, P. (2017). Blockchain technology for improving clinical research quality. *Trials*, *18*(1), 1–5.

Benčić, F. M., & Zarko, I. P. (2018). *Distributed ledger technology: Blockchain compared to directed acyclic graph*. https://www.researchgate.net/publication/326566509_Distributed_Ledger_Technology_Blockchain_Compared_to_Directed_Acyclic_Graph

Bernard, Z. (2018). *Everything you need to know about Bitcoin, its mysterious origins, and the many alleged identities of its creator*. Business Insider.

Bhattacharya, S., Singh, A., & Hossain, M. M. (2019). Strengthening public health surveillance through blockchain technology. *AIMS Public Health*, *6*(3), 326.

Bhawiyuga, A., Wardhana, A., Amron, K., & Kirana, A. P. (2019, December). Platform for Integrating Internet of Things Based Smart Healthcare System and Blockchain Network. In *2019 6th NAFOSTED Conference on Information and Computer Science (NICS)* (pp. 55-60). IEEE.

Bhuvana, R., & Aithal, P. S. (2020). Blockchain based Service: A Case Study on IBM Blockchain Services & Hyperledger Fabric. [IJCSBE]. *International Journal of Case Studies in Business, IT, and Education*, *4*(1), 94–102.

Bhuvana, R., & Aithal, P. S. (2020). RBI Distributed Ledger Technology and Blockchain-A Future of Decentralized India. [IJMTS]. *International Journal of Management, Technology, and Social Sciences*, *5*(1), 227–237.

Bhuvana, R., Madhushree, L. M., & Aithal, P. S. (2020). Blockchain as a Disruptive Technology in Healthcare and Financial Services-A Review based Analysis on Current Implementations. [IJAEML]. *International Journal of Applied Engineering and Management Letters*, *4*(1), 142–155.

Bhuvana, R., Madhushree, L., & Aithal, P. S. (2020). Comparative Study on RFID based Tracking and Blockchain based Tracking of Material Transactions. [IJAEML]. *International Journal of Applied Engineering and Management Letters*, *4*(2), 22–30.

Biais, B., Bisiere, C., Bouvard, M., & Casamatta, C. (2019). The blockchain folk theorem. Review of Financial Studies, 32(5), 1662–1715.

Biais, B., Bisiere, C., Bouvard, M., & Casamatta, C. (2019). The blockchain folk theorem. *Review of Financial Studies*, *32*(5), 1662–1715.

Bianchini, E., Francesconi, M., Testa, M., Tanase, M., & Gemignani, V. (2019). Unique device identification and traceability for medical software: A major challenge for manufacturers in an ever-evolving marketplace. *Journal of Biomedical Informatics*, *93*, 103150. doi:10.1016/j.jbi.2019.103150 PMID:30878617

Biswas, S. (2019). Sharif, K., Li, F., Maharjan, S., Mohanty, S. P., & Yu Wang. (2019). Post: A lightweight consensus algorithm for scalable IoT business blockchain. IEEE Internet of Things Journal, 7(3), 2343–2355.

Bocek, T., Rodrigues, B. B., Strasser, T., & Stiller, B. (2017, May). Blockchains everywhere-a use-case of blockchains in the pharma supply-chain. In *2017 IFIP/IEEE symposium on integrated network and service management (IM)* (pp. 772-777). IEEE.

Bodkhe, U., Tanwar, S., Parekh, K., Khanpara, P., Tyagi, S., Kumar, N., & Alazab, M. (2020). Blockchain for industry 4.0: A comprehensive review. IEEE Access : Practical Innovations, Open Solutions, 8, 79764–79800.

Booker, A., Agapouda, A., Frommenwiler, D. A., Scotti, F., Reich, E., & Heinrich, M. (2018). St John's wort (Hypericum perforatum) products – an assessment of their authenticity and quality. *Phytomedicine, 40*, 158–164. doi:10.1016/j.phymed.2017.12.012 PMID:29496168

Booker, A., Johnston, D., & Heinrich, M. (2012). Value chains of herbal medicines–research needs and key challenges in the context of ethnopharmacology. *Journal of Ethnopharmacology, 140*(3), 624–633. doi:10.1016/j.jep.2012.01.039 PMID:22326378

Borioli, G. S., & Couturier, J. (2018). How blockchain technology can improve the outcomes of clinical trials. *British Journal of Healthcare Management, 24*(3), 156–162.

Buterin, V. (2014). A next-generation smart contract and decentralized application platform. *white paper, 3*(1),1-36.

C-19_Vaccine-Distribution_White-Paper_Stirling_Ultracold.pdf. (n.d.). Retrieved August 30, 2021, from https://www.stirlingultracold.com/wp-content/uploads/2020/12/C-19_Vaccine-Distribution_White-Paper_Stirling_Ultracold.pdf

Calvaresi, D., Dubovitskaya, A., Calbimonte, J. P., Taveter, K., & Schumacher, M. (2018). Multi-agent systems and blockchain: Results from a systematic literature review. In International Conference on Practical Applications of Agents and Multi-Agent Systems, 10–126. Springer, 2018.

Capgemini. (2017). *Blockchain: A Healthcare Industry View*. Capgemini.

Carlisle, B., Kimmelman, J., Ramsay, T., & MacKinnon, N. J. C. T. (2015). Unsuccessful trial accrual and human subjects' protections: *An empirical analysis of recently closed trials. Clinical Trials, 12*(1), 77–83.

Carson, B., Romanelli, G., Walsh, P., & Zhumaev, A. (2018). *Blockchain Beyond the Hype: What is the Strategic Business Value*. McKinsey&Company.

Casey & Wong. (2017). Global supply chains are about to get better, thanks to blockchain. *Harvard Business Review.* https://hbr.org/2017/03/global-supply-chains-are-about-to-get-better-thanks-to-blockchain

Casino, F., Dasaklis, T. K., & Patsakis, C. (2019). A systematic literature review of blockchain-based applications: Current status, classification and open issues. *Telematics and Informatics*, *36*, 55–81. doi:10.1016/j.tele.2018.11.006

Castro, M., & Liskov, B. (2002). B. (2002). "Practical byzantine fault tolerance and proactive recovery. ACM Transactions on Computer Systems, 20(4), 398–461.

Čeke, D., & Kunosić, S. "Smart Contracts as a diploma anti-forgery system in higher education - a pilot project", *Information Communication and Electronic Technology (MIPRO) 2020 43rd International Convention on*, pp. 1662-1667, 2020.

Celesti, A., Ruggeri, A., Fazio, M., Galletta, A., Villari, M., & Romano, A. (2020). Blockchain-based healthcare workflow for telemedical laboratory in federated hospital iot clouds. Sensors (Basel), 20(9), 2590.

CenterSource. (n.d.). *How Blockchain Technology Can Impact Hospitality: 5 Steps to Prepare Your Business*. Author.

Cha, S., Chen, J., Su, C., & Yeh, K. (2018). A blockchain connected gateway for ble-based devices in the internet of things. IEEE Access : Practical Innovations, Open Solutions, 6, 24639–24649.

Chamola, V., Hassija, V., Gupta, V., & Guizani, M. (2020). A Comprehensive Review of the COVID-19 Pandemic and the Role of IoT, Drones, AI, Blockchain, and 5G in Managing its Impact. May 2020. IEEE Access : Practical Innovations, Open Solutions, 8, 90225–90265.

Chan, M., 2017. Why Cloud Computing Is the Foundation of the Internet of Things.

Chatterjee, K., Goharshady, A. K., Ibsen-Jensen, R. & Velner, Y. (2018). Ergodic mean-payoff games for the analysis of attacks in cryptocurrencies. *CONCUR 2018*, 11:1 – 11:17.

Chatterjee, R., & Chatterjee, R. (2017, October). An overview of the emerging technology: Blockchain. In 2017 3rd International Conference on Computational Intelligence and Networks (CINE) (pp. 126-127). IEEE.

Chattu, V. K., Nanda, A., Chattu, S. K., Kadri, S. M., & Knight, A. W. (2019). The emerging role of blockchain technology applications in routine disease surveillance systems to strengthen global health security. *Big Data and Cognitive Computing*, *3*(2), 25.

Chen, Y., Li, H., Li, K., & Zhang, J. An improved P2P file system scheme based on IPFS and Blockchain. In Proceedings of the 2017 IEEE International Conference on Big Data (Big Data), Boston, MA, USA, 11–14 December 2017; pp. 2652–2657. [**Google Scholar**]

Chenthara, S., Ahmed, K., Wang, H., & Whittaker, F. (2020, October). A Novel Blockchain Based Smart Contract System for eReferral in Healthcare: HealthChain. *International Conference on Health Information Science* (pp. 91-102). Springer, Cham.

Chen, Y., Ding, S., Xu, Z., Zheng, H., & Yang, S. (2019). Blockchain-based medical records secure storage and medical service framework. *Journal of Medical Systems*, *43*(1), 1–9.

Choudhury, O., Fairoza, N., Sylla, I., & Das, A. (2019). A blockchain framework for managing and monitoring data in multi-site clinical trials. *arXiv preprint arXiv:1902.03975.*, 1-13.

Chowdhury, M. J. M., Colman, A., Kabir, M. A., Han, J., & Sarda, P. (2018, August). Blockchain versus database: a critical analysis. In *2018 17th IEEE International Conference on Trust, Security and Privacy in Computing and Communications/12th IEEE International Conference on Big Data Science and Engineering (TrustCom/BigDataSE)* (pp. 1348-1353). IEEE.

Christidis, K., & Devetsikiotis, M. (2016). Blockchains and smart contracts for the internet of things. *IEEE Access : Practical Innovations, Open Solutions, 4*(1), 2292–2303.

CitiusTech. (2018). *Blockchain for Healthcare: An opportunity to address many complex challenges in healthcare.* CitiusTech.

Conti, M., Kumar, S., Lal, C., & Ruj, S. (2018). A survey on security and privacy issues of bitcoin. IEEE Communications Surveys and Tutorials.

Courtois, T. (2014). On The Longest Chain Rule and Programmed Self-Destruction of Crypto Currencies. *CoRR: Computing Research Repository.*

Crameri, K.A., Mather, L., Van Dam, P., Prior, S. (2020). Personal Electronic Healthcare Records: What Influences Consumers to Engage with their Clinical Data Online? a Literature Review, Journal of Health Information Management, 2020.

Cubas Celiz, R. C., Escriba, Y., Cruz, D. L., & Sanchez, D. M. (2018). Cloud model for purchase management in health sector of Peru based on IoT and blockchain. In 2018 IEEE 9th Annual Information Technology, Electronics and Mobile Communication Conference (ICON), 328–334. IEEE, 2018.

Dai, M., Zhang, S., Wang, H., & Jin, S. (2018). A low storage room requirement framework for distributed ledger in blockchain. *IEEE Access : Practical Innovations, Open Solutions, 6,* 22970–22975.Google ScholarCrossRef

Daley, S. (2021). *How using blockchain in healthcare is reviving the industry's capabilities.* Builtin. https://builtin.com/blockchain/blockchain-healthcare-applications-companies

Deloitte. (2019). *Deloitte's 2019 Global Blockchain Survey: Blockchain Gets Down to Business.* https://www2.deloitte.com/content/dam/Deloitte/se/Documents/risk/DI_2019-global-blockchainsurvey.pdf

Demirkan, H. (2013). A Smart Healthcare Systems Framework. *IT Professional, 15*(5), 38–45.

Deshmukh, S. P. (2020, October 27). *6 lessons for creating blockchain standards.* World Economic Forum.

Dhamal, S., Chahed, T., Ben-Ameur, W., Altman, E., Sunny, A., & Poojary, S. (2018). *A stochastic game framework for analyzing computational investment strategies in distributed computing with application to blockchain mining.* Academic Press.

Dhiran, A., Kumar, D., & Abhishek, A. A. "Video Fraud Detection using Blockchain", *Inventive Research in Computing Applications (ICIRCA) 2020 Second International Conference on*, pp. 102-107, 2020.

Di Pierro, M. (2017). What is the blockchain? *Computing in Science & Engineering, 19*(5), 92–95.

Dimitrov, D. V. (2019). Blockchain Applications for Healthcare Data Management. *Healthcare Informatics Research, 25*(1), 51–56. doi:10.4258/hir.2019.25.1.51 PMID:30788182

Do, H. G., & Ng, W. K. (2017, June). Blockchain-based system for secure data storage with private keyword search. *IEEE World Congress on Services (SERVICES), 1*(1), 90-93.

Dreyfuss, G. C. (2020, February 21). *Companies in Pharmaceutical Supply Chain Develop System to Track Counterfeit Drugs*. Reuters.

Dubovitskaya, A., Xu, Z., Ryu, S., Schumacher, M., & Wang, F. (2017). Secure and trustable electronic medical records sharing using blockchain. *AMIA Annual Symposium Proceedings American Medical Informatics Association,* 650-659.

Düdder, B., Fomin, V., Gürpinar, T., Henke, M., Iqbal, M., Janavičienė, V., Matulevičius, R., Straub, N., & Wu, H. (2021). *Interdisciplinary blockchain education: Utilizing blockchain technology from various perspectives.* . doi:10.3389/fbloc.2020.578022

Dutta, P., Choi, T. M., Somani, S., & Butala, R. (2020). Blockchain technology in supply chain operations: Applications, challenges and research opportunities. *Transportation Research Part E, Logistics and Transportation Review, 142*, 102067. doi:10.1016/j.tre.2020.102067 PMID:33013183

Dwivedi, A. D., Malina, L., Dzurenda, P., & Srivastava, G. (2019). Optimized blockchain model for internet of things-based healthcare applications. In 2019 42nd International Conference on Telecommunications and Signal Processing (TSP), pages 135–139. IEEE, 2019.

El Rifai, O., Biotteau, M., de Boissezon, X., Megdiche, I., Ravat, F., & Teste, O. (2020, September). Blockchain-Based Personal Health Records for Patients' Empowerment. In *International Conference on Research Challenges in Information Science* (pp. 455-471). Springer, Cham.

Esposito, C., De Santis, A., Tortora, G., Chang, H., & Choo, K. K. R. (2018). Blockchain: A Panacea for Healthcare Cloud-Based Data Security and Privacy? *IEEE Cloud Computing, 5*(1), 31–37. doi:10.1109/MCC.2018.011791712

Ethical Consumer Research Association (ECRA). (2017). *Ethical Consumer Markets Report 2017*. Ethical Consumer Research Association.

EU Health Programme. (2017). *Unique device identification (udi) system under the eu medical devices regulations 2017/745 and 2017/746*. https://ec.europa.eu/health/sites/default/files/md_topics-interest/docs/md_faq_udi_en.pdf

European Parliament. (2017, April 5). *Regulation (eu) 2017/745 of the European parliament and of the council of 5 April 2017 on medical devices, amending directive 2001/83 / ec, regulation (ec) no. 178/2002 and regulation (ec) no. 1223 / 2009 and repealing council directives 90/385 / eec and 93/42 / eec.*

Evangelatos, N., Özdemir, V., & Brand, A. (2020). Blockchain for digital health: Prospects and challenges. *OMICS: A Journal of Integrative Biology, 24*(5), 237–240.

Eyal, I. (2015). The miner's dilemma. In *Security and Privacy (SP), 2015 IEEE Symposium on.* IEEE.

Eyal, I., & Sirer, E. G. (2014). Majority is not enough: Bitcoin mining is vulnerable. *Proc. of the International Financial Cryptography and Data Security Conference.*

Farhin, F., Kaiser, M. S., & Mahmud, M. (2021). Secured Smart Healthcare System: Blockchain and Bayesian Inference Based Approach. In *Proceedings of International Conference on Trends in Computational and Cognitive Engineering* (pp. 455-465). Springer, Singapore.

FDA. (2013). *Unique device identification system.* https://www.federalregister.gov/documents/2013/09/24/2013-23059/unique-device-identification-system

FDA. (2019). *Udi basics.* https://www.fda.gov/medical-devices/unique-device-identification-system-udi-system/udi-basics#recognize

Fedkenhauer, T., Fritzsche-sterr, Y., Nagel. I., Pauer, A., & Resetko, A. (2017). *Datenaustausch als wesentlicher Bestandteil der Digitalisierung.* Academic Press.

Fernandez-Alemán, J. L., Señor, I. C., Lozoya, P. Á. O., & Toval, A. (2013). Security and privacy in electronic health records: A systematic literature review. *Journal of Biomedical Informatics, 246*(3), 541–562. doi:10.1016/j.jbi.2012.12.003 PMID:23305810

Fiaidhi, J., Mohammed, S., & Mohammed, S. (2018). EDI with blockchain as an enabler for extreme automation. *IT Professional, 20*(4), 66–72.

Figorilli, S., Antonucci, F., Costa, C., Pallottino, F., Raso, L., Castiglione, M., Pinci, E., Del Vecchio, D., Colle, G., Proto, A., Sperandio, G., & Menesatti, P. (2018). A blockchain implementation prototype for the electronic open source traceability of wood along the whole supply chain. *Sensors (Basel), 18*(9), E3133. doi:10.339018093133 PMID:30227651

Fill, H.-G., Haerer, F., & Meier, A. (2020). Wie funktioniert die blockchain? In Blockchain. Grundlagen, anwendungsszenarien und nutzungspotenziale. doi:10.1007/978-3-658-28006-2_1

Foroglou, G., & Tsilidou, A. L. (2015). Further applications of the blockchain. *Abgerufen Am., 3*(1), 1–9.

Francisco, K., & Swanson, D. (2018). The supply chain has no clothes: Technology adoption of blockchain for supply chain transparency. *Logistics, 2*(1), 1–13.

Frommenwiler, D. A., Reich, E., Sudberg, S., Sharaf, M. H. M., Bzhelyansky, A., & Lucas, B. (2016). St. John's Wort versus counterfeit St. John's Wort: An HPTLC study. *Journal of AOAC International, 99*(5), 1204–1212. doi:10.5740/jaoacint.16-0170 PMID:27343017

FSA. (2018). *FSA Trials First Use of Blockchain.* Available at: https://www.food.gov.uk/news-alerts/news/fsa-trials-first-use-of-blockchain

Fusco, A., Dicuonzo, G., Dell'Atti, V., & Tatullo, M. (2020). Blockchain in Healthcare: Insights on COVID-19. *International Journal of Environmental Research and Public Health, 17*(19), 7167. https://doi.org/10.3390/ijerph17197167

Gade, Dipak S.&Aithal, P. S. (2020). Blockchain Technology: A Driving Force in Smart Cities Development. [IJAEML]. *International Journal of Applied Engineering and Management Letters, 4*(2), 237–252.

Galvez, J. F., Mejuto, J. C., & Gandara, S. J. (2016). Future challenges on the use of blockchain for food traceability analysis. *Trends in Analytical Chemistry, 107*, 222–232. doi:10.1016/j.trac.2018.08.011

Gao, Z., Xu, L., Chen, L., Zhao, X., Lu, Y., & Shi, W. (2018). Coc: A unified distributed ledger based supply chain management system. *Journal of Computer Science and Technology, 33*(2), 237–248. doi:10.100711390-018-1816-5

Gatteschi, V., Lamberti, F., Demartini, C., Pranteda, C., & Santamaria, V. (2018). To blockchain or not to blockchain: That is the question. *IT Professional, 20*(2), 62–74.

Gope, P., & Sikdar, B. (2018). Lightweight and privacy-preserving two-factor authentication scheme for IoT devices. IEEE Internet Things.

Gordon, W. J., & Catalini, C. (2018). Blockchain technology for healthcare: Facilitating the transition to patient-driven interoperability. *Computational and Structural Biotechnology Journal, 16*(1), 224–230.

Górski, T., & Bednarski, J. (2020). Applying Model-Driven Engineering to Distributed Ledger Deployment. *Access IEEE, 8*, 118245–118261.

Grant, R. W., Wald, J. S., Poon, E. G., Schnipper, J. L., Gandhi, T. K., Volk, L. A., & Middleton, B. (2006). Design and implementation of a web-based patient portal linked to an ambulatory care electronic health record: Patient gateway for diabetes collaborative care. Diabetes Technology & Therapeutics, 8(5), 576–586.

Griggs, K. N., Osipova, O., Kohlios, C. P., Baccarini, A. N., Howson, E. A., & Hayajneh, T. (2018). Healthcare blockchain system using smart contracts for secure automated remote patient monitoring. Journal of Medical Systems, 42(7), 130.

Große, N., Leisen, D., Gürpinar, T., Forsthövel, R. S., Henke, M., & ten Hompel, M. (2020). *Evaluation of (De-)Centralized IT technologies in the fields of Cyber-Physical Production Systems.* Institutionelles Repositorium der Leibniz Universität Hannover. https://www.repo.uni-hannover.de/handle/123456789/9736 doi:10.15488/9680

Group, M. (2021, September 20). *Blockchain Technology in Healthcare Industry.* Academic Press.

Gul, M. J., Subramanian, B., Paul, A., & Kim, J. (2021). Blockchain for public health care in smart society. *Microprocessors and Microsystems, 80,* 103524.

Gürpinar, T., Harre, S., Henke, M., & Saleh, F. (2020). *Blockchain technology – integration in supply chain processes.* doi:10.15480/882.3117

Gürpinar, T., Straub, N., Kaczmarek, S., & Henke, M. (2019). *Blockchain-technologie im interdisziplinären umfeld.* Academic Press.

Gurtu, A., & Johny, J. (2019). Potential of blockchain technology in supply chain management: A literature review. *International Journal of Physical Distribution & Logistics Management, 49*(9), 881–900. doi:10.1108/IJPDLM-11-2018-0371

Hafid, A., Hafid, A. S., & Samih, M. (2020). Scaling Blockchains: A Comprehensive Survey. *Access IEEE, 8,* 125244–125262.

Halamka, J. D., Alterovitz, G., Buchanan, W. J., Cenaj, T., Clauson, K. A., Dhillon, V., Hudson, F. D., Mokhtari, M., Porto, D. A., Rutschman, A., & Ngo, A. L. (2020). *Top 10 Blockchain Predictions for the (Near) Future of Healthcare.* Blockchain in Healthcare Today. doi:10.30953/bhty.v2.106

Haleem, A. J. (2021). Blockchain Technology Applications in Healthcare: An Overview. *International Journal of Intelligent Networks,* 130-139.

Han, Z., Niyato, D., Saad, W., Basar, T., & Hjørungnes, A. (2012). Game theory in wireless and communication networks: theory, models, and applications. Cambridge University Press.

Haque, A. B., Muniat, A., Ullah, P. R., & Mushsharat, S. (2021, February). An Automated Approach towards Smart Healthcare with Blockchain and Smart Contracts. In *2021 International Conference on Computing, Communication, and Intelligent Systems (ICCCIS)* (pp. 250-255). IEEE.

Hasan, H. R., & Salah, K. (2018). Proof of delivery of digital assets using blockchain and smart contracts. *IEEE Access : Practical Innovations, Open Solutions, 6,* 65439–65448. Google ScholarCrossRef

Hasselgren, A., Kralevska, K., Gligoroski, D., Pedersen, S. A., & Faxvaag, A. (2020). Blockchain in healthcare and health sciences—A scoping review. International Journal of Medical Informatics, 134. doi:10.1016/j.ijmedinf.2019.104040

Hathaliya, J., Sharma, P., Tanwar, S., & Gupta, R. (2019, December). Blockchain-based remote patient monitoring in healthcare 4.0. In *2019 IEEE 9th International Conference on Advanced Computing (IACC)* (pp. 87-91). IEEE.

He, X., Dai, H., Ning, P., & Dutta, D. (2016). Zero-determinant strategies for multi-player multi-action iterated games. IEEE Signal Processing Letters, 23(3), 311–315.

Healthcare Information and Management Systems Society. (2021). *Blockchain in Healthcare.* Author.

Heinrich, M., & Hesketh, A. (2018). 25 years after the 'Rio Convention'–lessons learned in the context of sustainable development and protecting indigenous and local knowledge. *Phytomedicine*, *53*, 332–343. doi:10.1016/j.phymed.2018.04.061 PMID:30318154

Heinrich, M., Scotti, F., Booker, A., Fitzgerald, M., Kum, K. Y., & Löbel, K. (2019). Unblocking High-Value Botanical Value Chains: Is Therea Role for Blockchain Systems? *Frontiers in Pharmacology*, *10*, 396. doi:10.3389/fphar.2019.00396 PMID:31068810

Helo, P., & Shamsuzzoha, A. H. M. (2020). Real-time supply chain—A blockchain architecture for project deliveries. *Robotics and Computer-integrated Manufacturing*, *63*, 101909. doi:10.1016/j.rcim.2019.101909

Hewa, T., Ylianttila, M. & Liyanage. M. (2020). Survey on blockchain-based smart contracts: Applications, opportunities and challenges. Journal of Network and Computer Applications, page 102857, 2020.

Hinckeldeyn, J. (2019). *Blockchain-technologie in der supply chain: Einführung und anwendungsbeispiele.* Https://doi.Org/10.1007/978-3-658-26440-6

HL7. (2018). FHIR: Fast healthcare interoperability resources. https://hl7.org/fhir

HonarPajooh, H., Rashid, M., Alam, F., & Demidenko, S. (2021). Multi-layer blockchain-based security architecture for internet of things. *Sensors (Basel)*, *21*(3), 1–26.

Hu, Y., Liyanage, M., Mansoor, A., Thilakarathna, K., Jourjon, G., & Seneviratne, A. (2018). Blockchain-based smart contracts-applications and challenges. arXiv preprint arXiv:1810.04699, 2018.

Huang, J., Kong, L., Chen, G., Wu, M. Y., Liu, X., & Zeng, P. (2019). Towards secure industrial IoT: Blockchain system with credit-based consensus mechanism. IEEE Transactions on Industrial Informatics, 15(6), 3680–3689.

Huillet, M. (2019). *Blockchain not understood by almost 70% of firms in asiapacific.* Academic Press.

Huillet, M. (2019). China's State-Run Media: Bitcoin Is Blockchain's First Success. *Cointelegraph.* https://cointelegraph.com

Hyperledger caliper (2021). https://www.hyperledger.org/, July 2021.

Iansiti, M., & Lakhani, K. R. (2017). The Truth About Blockchain. *Harvard Business Review.* https://hbr.org/2017/01/the-truth-about-blockchain

Idongesit, W. (2020). *Cross-Industry Use of Blockchain Technology and Opportunities for the Future.* IGI Global.

IEEE. (2021). *How Blockchain Can Transform Healthcare.* IEEE. https://innovationatwork.ieee.org/how-blockchain-can-transform-healthcare/

IET. (n.d.). *Blockchain in Healthcare. The Institution of Engineering and Technology.* TheIET.

Iftekhar, A., & Cui, X. (2021). Blockchain-Based Traceability System That Ensures Food Safety Measures to Protect Consumer Safety and COVID-19 Free Supply Chains. *Foods*, *10*(6), 1289. https://doi.org/10.3390/foods10061289

IHaq I. & Esuka. (2018). O. M. (2018). Blockchain technology in the pharmaceutical industry to prevent counterfeit drugs. International Journal of Computers and Applications, 180(25), 8–12.

IHE. (2019). The IHE IT Infrastructure (ITI) Technical Framework, Volume 1, Technical Report IHE. https://www.ihe.net/uploadedFiles/

ildebrandt, A., & Landhäußer, W. (Eds.). (2017). *Management-Reihe Corporate Social Responsibility. CSR und Digitalisierung: Der digitale Wandel als Chance und Herausforderung für Wirtschaft und Gesellschaft.* Springer Berlin Heidelberg., doi:10.1007/978-3-662-53202-7

Ismail, L., Materwala, H., & Zeadally, S. (2019). Lightweight Blockchain for Healthcare. *IEEE Access: Practical Innovations, Open Solutions*, *7*, 149935–149951. doi:10.1109/ACCESS.2019.2947613

Jabbar, A., & Dani, S. (2020). Investigating the link between transaction and computational costs in a blockchain environment. International Journal of Production Research, 58(11), 3423–3436.

Jakob, S., Schulte, A. T., Sparer, D., Koller, R., & Henke, M. (2018). *Blockchain und smart contracts: Effiziente und sichere wertschöpfungsnetzwerke.* Academic Press.

Jamil, F., Ahmad, S., Iqbal, N., & Kim, D. (2020). Towards a remote monitoring of patient vital signs based on IoT-based blockchain integrity management platforms in smart hospitals. Sensors (Basel), 20(8), 2195.

Jenkinson, G. (2019) Can Blockchain Become an Integral Part of Autonomous Vehicles? *Cointelegraph. 2019.* https://cointelegraph.com/news/can-blockchain-become-an-integral-part-of-autonomous-vehicles

Jung, H. H., & Pfister, F. M. (2020). Blockchain-enabled clinical study consent management. *Technology Innovation Management Review*, *10*(2), 14–24.

Kalla, A., Hewa, T., Mishra, R. A., Ylianttila, M., & Liyanage, M. (2020). The Role of Blockchain to Fight Against COVID-19. *IEEE Engineering Management Review*, *48*(3), 85–96. https://doi.org/10.1109/EMR.2020.3014052

Kang, J., Xiong, Z., Niyato, D., Ye, D., Kim, D. I., & Zhao, J. (2019). Toward secure blockchain-enabled internet of vehicles: Optimizing consensus management using reputation and contract theory. IEEE Transactions on Vehicular Technology, 68(3), 2906–2920.

Katuwal, G. J., Pandey, S., Hennessey, M., & Lamichhane, B. (2018). Applications of blockchain in healthcare: current landscape & challenges. arXiv preprint arXiv:1812.02776.

Kaur, H., Afshar, M., Roshan A., J., Kumar A. M., & Chang, V. (2018). A proposed solution and future direction for M.A Uddin et al.: Blockchain: Research and Applications Page 72 of 80 Journal Pre-proof Blockchain Adoption in IoT: A Survey, Challenges and Solutions blockchain-based heterogeneous medicare data in cloud environment. Journal of medical systems, 42(8):156, 2018.

Khalilov, M. C. K., & Levi, A. (2018). A survey on anonymity and privacy in bitcoin-like digital cash systems. IEEE Communications Surveys and Tutorials.

Khubrani, M. M. (2021). A Framework for Blockchain-based Smart Health System. [TURCOMAT]. *Turkish Journal of Computer and Mathematics Education*, *12*(9), 2609–2614.

Kim, E., Rubinstein, S. M., Nead, K. T., Wojcieszynski, A. P., Gabriel, P. E., & Warner, J. L. (2019). The evolving use of electronic health recirds (HER) for research, Seminars in Radiation Oncology, 29(4), 354-361, ISSN: 1053-4296.

Kim, S. K. (2019). The Trailer of Blockchain Governance Game. Computers & Industrial Engineering, 136, 373–380.

Kim, S., Kwon, Y., & Cho, S. (2018). A survey of scalability solutions on blockchain. In 2018 International Conference on Information and Communication Technology Convergence (ICTC), pages 1204–1207. IEEE, 2018.

Kim, K.-W. (2006). Measuring international research collaborationof peripheral countries: Taking the contextinto consideration. *Scientometrics*, *66*(2), 231–240. doi:10.100711192-006-0017-0

Kirmse, G. (2016). Rückverfolgung der Aufbereitung. *OP*, *6*(2), 75–80. doi:10.1055-0041-109841

Koens, T., & Poll, E. (2018). What blockchain alternative do you need? In *Data Privacy Management, Cryptocurrencies and Blockchain Technology* (pp. 113–129). Springer. doi:10.1007/978-3-030-00305-0_9

Kohli, R., Garg, A., Phutela, S., Kumar, Y., & Jain, S. (2021). An Improvised Model for Securing Cloud-Based E-Healthcare Systems. In *IoT in Healthcare and Ambient Assisted Living* (pp. 293–310). Springer.

Ko, M., Tiwari, A., & Mehnen, J. (2010). A review of soft computing applications in supply chain management. *Applied Soft Computing*, *10*(3), 661–674. doi:10.1016/j.asoc.2009.09.004

Koptyra, K., & Ogiela, M. R. (2021). Imagechain—Application of Blockchain Technology for Images. *Sensors (Basel)*, *21*(1), 82.

Kroll, J. A., Davey, I. C., & Felten, E. W. (2013). The economics of bitcoin mining, or bitcoin in the presence of adversaries. *Proceedings of WEIS, 11*.

Kumar, A., Krishnamurthi, R., Nayyar, A., Sharma, K., Grover, V., & Hossain, E. (2020). A Novel Smart Healthcare Design, Simulation, and Implementation Using Healthcare 4.0 Processes. *IEEE Access : Practical Innovations, Open Solutions*, *8*(1), 118433–118471.

Kumar, A., Liu, R., & Shan, Z. (2020). Is Blockchain a Silver Bullet for Supply Chain Management? Technical Challenges and Research Opportunities. *Decision Sciences*, *51*(1), 8–37. doi:10.1111/deci.12396

Kumar, N. M., & Mallick, P. K. (2018). Blockchain technology for security issues and challenges in IoT. *Procedia Computer Science*, *132*, 1815–1823.

Kumar, R., & Tripathi, R. (2021). Building an IPFS and Blockchain-Based Decentralized Storage Model for Medical Imaging. In *Advancements in Security and Privacy Initiatives for Multimedia Images* (pp. 19–40). IGI Global.

Kumar, R., Wang, W., Kumar, J., Yang, T., Khan, A., Ali, W., & Ali, I. (2021). An Integration of Blockchain and AI for Secure Data Sharing and Detection of CT images for the Hospitals. *Computerized Medical Imaging and Graphics*, *87*, 101812.

Kuo, T. T., & Ohno-Machado, L. (2018). Model Chain: Decentralized privacy-preserving healthcare predictive 154 modelling framework on private blockchain networks. arXiv preprint arXiv:1802.01746.

Laraki, R. (2002). The splitting game and applications. International Journal of Game Theory, 30(3), 359–376.

Lazar, M. A.-M. (2017). Digital revolution in depression: A technologies update for clinicians. *Personalized Medicine in Psychiatry*, *4*, 1–6.

Le Nguyen, T. (2018, August). Blockchain in healthcare: A new technology benefit for both patients and doctors. In *2018 Portland International Conference on Management of Engineering and Technology (PICMET)* (pp. 1-6). IEEE.

Lee, H. A., Kung, H. H., Udayasankaran, J. G., Kijsanayotin, B., Marcelo, A. B., Chao, L. R., & Hsu, C. Y. (2020). An architecture and management platform for blockchain-based personal health record exchange: Development and usability study. *Journal of Medical Internet Research*, *22*(6), e16748.

Lee, S. H., & Yang, C. S. (2018). Fingernail analysis management system using microscopy sensor and blockchain technology. *International Journal of Distributed Sensor Networks*, *14*(3), 1–13. doi:10.1177/1550147718767044

LeewayHertz. (2021). *Blockchain in Pharma Supply Chain - Reucing Counterfeit Drugs*. Author.

Leino-kilpi, H., Välimäki, M., Dassen, T., Gasull, M., Lemonidou, C., Schopp, A., Scott, P. A., Arndt, M., & Kaljonen, A. (2003). *Perceptions of Autonomy, Privacy and Informed Consent in The Care of Elderly People in Five European Countries: Comparison and Implications for The Future*. Academic Press.

Leng, M., & Parlar, M. (2005). Game theoretic applications in supply chain management: A review. *INFOR*, *43*(3), 187–220. doi:10.1080/03155986.2005.11732725

Compilation of References

Letsyo, E., Jerz, G., Winterhalter, P., Lindigkeit, R., & Beuerle, T. (2017). 'Incidence of pyrrolizidine Alkaloids in herbal medicines from German Retail markets: Risk assessments and implications to consumers.'. *Phytotherapy Research*, *31*(12), 1903–1909. doi:10.1002/ptr.5935 PMID:28960556

Li, H., Zhu, L., Shen, M., Gao, F., Tao, X., & Liu, S. (2018). Blockchain-Based Data Preservation System for Medical Data. Journal of Medical Systems, 42(8). doi:10.100710916-018-0997-3

Liang, X., Zhao, J., Shetty, S., Liu, J., & Li, D. (2017, October). Integrating blockchain for data sharing and collaboration in mobile healthcare applications. In 2017 IEEE 28th Annual International Symposium on Personal, Indoor, and Mobile Radio Communications (PIMRC) (pp. 1-5).

Lin, F., & Qiang, M. (2018). The challenges of existence, status, and value for improving blockchain. IEEE Access : Practical Innovations, Open Solutions, 7, 7747–7758.

Lin, I. C., & Liao, T. C. (2017). A survey of blockchain security issues and challenges. *International Journal of Network Security*, *19*(5), 653–659.

Lipsey, R., Carlaw, K. I., & Bekhar, C. T. (2005). *Economic Transformations: General Purpose Technologies and Long-Term Economic Growth*. Oxford University Press.

Liu, J., & Li, X., Ye, Lin., Y., Zhang, H., Du, X., & Guizani, M. (2018). Beds: A blockchain-based privacy-preserving data sharing for electronic medical records. In 2018 IEEE Global Communications Conference (GLOBECOM), 1–6. IEEE, 2018.

Lopez, E. (2017). *Big Pharma builds blockchain prototype to stop counterfeits*. Supply Chain Dive. https://www.supplychaindive.com/news/big-pharma-blockchain-experiment-returns/525689

Lorenz, J. T., Münstermann, B., Higginson, M., Olesen, P. B., Bohlken, N., & Ricciardi, V. (2017). Blockchain in Insurance–Opportunity or Threat? McKinsey & Company. http://www.mckinsey.com/~/media/McKinsey/Industries/Financial Services/Our Insights/Blockchain in insurance opportunity or threat/Blockchain-in-insurance-opportunity-or-threat.ashx. Accessed April 20, 2020.

Luo, F., Dong, Z. Y., Liang, G., Murata, J., & Xu, Z. (2018). A distributed electricity trading system in active distribution networks based on multi-agent coalition and blockchain. IEEE Transactions on Power Systems, 34(5), 4097–4108.

Luu, L., & Teutsch, J., Kulkarni., & Saxena, P. (2015). Demystifying incentives in the consensus computer. *Proceedings of the 22nd ACM SIGSAC Conference on Computer and Communications Security, 1*(1), 706-719.

Luu, L., Narayanan, V., Baweja, K., Zheng, C., Gilbert, S., & Saxena, P. (2015). *Scp: A computationally scalable byzantine consensus protocol for blockchains*. Cryptology ePrint Archive, Report 2015/1168, 2015. http://eprint.iacr.org/

Luu, L., Chu, D. H., Olickel, H., Saxena, P., & Hobor, A. (2016). Making smart contracts smarter. In *Proceedings of the 2016 ACM SIGSAC conference on computer and communications security* (pp. 254- 269).

MacKenzie, D. (2019). Pick a nonce and try a hash. *London Review of Books*, *41*(8), 35–38.

Manish, V. (2021, April). Building predictive model owned and operated by public infrastructure that uses blockchain technology. *International Journal for Science and Advance Research in Technology*, *7*(4), 20.

Marbouh, D. A. (2020). *Blockchain for COVID-19: Review, Opportunities, and a Trusted Tracking System*. National Center for Biotechnology Information, U.S. National Library of Medicine.

Marbouh, D., Abbasi, T., Maasmi, F., Omar, I. A., Debe, M. S., Salah, K., ... Ellahham, S. (2020). Blockchain for COVID-19: Review, Opportunities, and a Trusted Tracking System. *Arabian Journal for Science and Engineering*, *45*(1), 9895–9911.

Maseleno, A., Hashim, W., Perumal, E., Ilayaraja, M., & Shankar, K. (2020). Access control and classifier-based blockchain technology in e-healthcare applications. In *Intelligent Data Security Solutions for e-Health Applications* (pp. 151–167). Academic Press.

Maull, R., Godsiff, P., Mulligan, C., Brown, A., & Kewell, B. (2017). Distributed ledger technology: Applications and implications. *Strategic Change*, *26*(5), 481–489.

McBee, M. P., & Wilcox, C. (2020). Blockchain technology: Principles and applications in medical imaging. *Journal of Digital Imaging*, *33*(3), 726–734.

McConaghy, T., Marques, R., Müller, A., De Jonghe, D., McConaghy, T., & McMullen, G. ... &Granzotto, A. (2016). Bigchaindb: a scalable blockchain database. white paper, BigChainDB, 1-70.

Mettler, M. (2016). Blockchain technology in healthcare: The revolution starts here, in 18th International Conference on e-Health Networking, Applications and Services, IEEE Publication, 1-3, 14-16 September 2016.

Mettler, M. (2016, September). Blockchain technology in healthcare: The revolution starts here. In *2016 IEEE 18th international conference on e-health networking, applications and services (Healthcom)* (pp. 1-3). IEEE.

Miller, D. (2018). Blockchain and the internet of things in the industrial sector. *IT Professional*, *20*(3), 15–18. doi:10.1109/MITP.2018.032501742

Monrat, A. A., Schelén, O., & Andersson, K. (2019). A survey of blockchain from the perspectives of applications, challenges, and opportunities. *IEEE Access: Practical Innovations, Open Solutions*, *7*, 117134–117151. doi:10.1109/ACCESS.2019.2936094

Mukherjee, P., & Singh, D. (2020). The Opportunities of Blockchain in Health 4.0. In Blockchain Technology for Industry 4.0 (pp. 149–164). Springer. doi:10.1007/978-981-15-1137-0_8

Mukherji, A., & Ganguli, N. "Efficient and Scalable Electronic Health Record Management using Permissioned Blockchain Technology", *Electronics Materials Engineering & Nano-Technology (IEMENTech) 2020 4th International Conference on*, pp. 1-6, 2020.

Compilation of References

Myerson, R. B. (2013). Game theory. Harvard University Press.

Nakamoto, S. (2008). *Bitcoin: A peer-to-peer electronic cash system.* Selfpublished Paper.

Nakamoto, S. (2008). Bitcoin: A Peer-to-Peer Electronic Cash System. SSRN *Electronic Journal.* doi:10.2139/ssrn.3440802

Naz, M., Al-zahrani, F. A., Khalid, R., Javaid, N., Qamar, A. M., Afzal, M. K., & Shafiq, M. (2019). A Secure Data Sharing Platform Using Blockchain and Interplanetary File System. *Sustainability*, *11*, 7054. https://doi.org/10.3390/su11247054

Neto, M. M., Coutinho, E. F., Moreira, L. O., & de Souza, J. N. (2019, October). Toward blockchain technology in IoT applications: an analysis for e-health applications. In *IFIP International Internet of Things Conference* (pp. 36-50). Springer, Cham.

Neto, M. M., Marinho, C. S. D. S., Coutinho, E. F., Moreira, L. O., Machado, J. D. C., & de Souza, J. N. (2020, March). Research Opportunities for E-health Applications with DNA Sequence Data using Blockchain Technology. In *2020 IEEE International Conference on Software Architecture Companion (ICSA-C)* (pp. 95-102). IEEE.

Network MD. (2020, July 7). *Blockchain in Healthcare: Regulatory Themes.* Author.

Neumann, J. V. (1928). Zur Theorie der Gesellschaftsspiele. *Mathematische Annalen, 100*, 295–300. doi:10.1007/bf01448847

New Age TechSci Research Pvt Ltd. (2020). *Blockchain in Healthcare Market to Grow at Staggering 70% CAGR until 2027.* New Age TechSci Research Pvt Ltd. https://www.einnews.com/pr_news/510619051/blockchain-in-healthcare-market-to-grow-at-staggering-70-cagr-until-2027-techsci-research

Nguyen, D. C., Nguyen, K. D., & Pathirana, P. N. (2019). A mobile cloud-based iomt framework for automated health assessment and management. In 2019 41st Annual International Conference of the IEEE Engineering in Medicine and Biology Society (EMBC), 6517–6520. IEEE, 2019.

Nguyen, J. (2021). *Blockchains are the building blocks of better healthcare.* MedCity News. https://medcitynews.com/2021/03/blockchains-are-the-building-blocks-of-better-healthcare/?rf=1

Nguyen, D. C., Ding, M., Pathirana, P. N., & Seneviratne, A. (2021). Blockchain and AI-Based Solutions to Combat Coronavirus (COVID-19)-Like Epidemics: A Survey. *IEEE Access: Practical Innovations, Open Solutions*, *9*, 95730–95753. https://doi.org/10.1109/ACCESS.2021.3093633

Nguyen, D. C., Pathirana, P. N., Ding, M., & Seneviratne, A. (2019). A. Blockchain for secure hrs sharing of mobile cloud based e-health systems. *IEEE Access : Practical Innovations, Open Solutions*, *7*, 66792–66806. doi:10.1109/ACCESS.2019.2917555

Ng, W. Y.-E.-K.-H. (2021, October 12). Blockchain Applications in Health Care for COVID-19 and Beyond: A Systematic Review. *Lancet.*

Niederman, F., Mathieu, R. G., Morley, R., & Kwon, I. W. (2007). Examining RFID applications in supply chain management. *Communications of the ACM*, *50*(7), 92–101. doi:10.1145/1272516.1272520

Nizamuddin, N., Hasan, H., Salah, K., & Iqbal, R. (2019). Blockchain-Based Framework for Protecting Author Royalty of Digital Assets. *Arabian Journal for Science and Engineering*, *44*, 3849–3866.Google ScholarCrossRef

Normand, S.-L. T., Hatfield, L., Drozda, J., & Resnic, F. S. (2012). Postmarket surveillance for medical devices: America's new strategy. *BMJ, 345*(2), e6848. doi:10.1136/bmj.e6848

Nugent, T., Upton, D., & Cimpoesu, M. (2016). Improving data transparency in clinical trials using blockchain smart contracts. *F1000 Research*, *5*(2541), 1–7.

OECD. (2020). *Blockchain Policy Series: Opportunities and Challenges of Blockchain Technologies in Health Care*. Policy Brief: Opportunities and Challenges of Blockchain in Healthcare.

Official Website of The Office of the National Coordinator for Health Information Technology. (2020). Appendix I – source of security standards and security patterns. http://www.healthit.gov/isa/ISA_Document/Appendix_I

Oluyisola, O. E., Strandhagen, J. W., & Buer, S.-V. (2018). Rfid technology in the manufacture of customized drainage and piping systems: A case study. *IFAC-PapersOnLine*, *51*(11), 364–369. doi:10.1016/j.ifacol.2018.08.320

Omar, I. A., Jayaraman, R., Salah, K., Simsekler, M. C. E., Yaqoob, I., & Ellahham, S. (2020). Ensuring protocol compliance and data transparency in clinical trials using Blockchain smart contracts. *BMC Medical Research Methodology*, *20*(1), 1–17.

Pal, K. (2020). In I. Williams (Ed.), Information sharing for manufacturing supply chain management based on blockchain technology, in cross-Industry Use of Blockchain Technology and Opportunities for the Future (pp. 1–17). IGI Global.

Pal, K. (2020). Information sharing for manufacturing supply chain management based on blockchain technology. In I. Williams (Ed.), Cross-Industry Use of Blockchain Technology and Opportunities for the Future (pp. 1–17). IGI Global.

Pal, K. (2021). Applications of Secured Blockchain Technology in Manufacturing Industry, in Blockchain and AI Technology in the Industrial Internet of Things, Subhendu Kumar Pani, Biju Patnaik, Sian Lun Lau, & Xingcheng Liu (Edited), Chapter 10, January 2021, IGI Global Publication, 701 E Chocolate Avenue, Hershey, PA, USA 17033.

Pal, K. (2021). Applications of Secured Blockchain Technology in Manufacturing Industry. In Blockchain and AI Technology in the Industrial Internet of Things. IGI Global.

Pal, K. (2022). Blockchain Integrated Internet of Things Architecture in Privacy Preserving for Large Scale Healthcare Supply Chain Data, in Blockchain Technology and Computational Excellence for Society 5.0, S Khan, H. Syed, R Hammad, & A Fouad Bushager (Edited), Chapter 6, January 2022, IGI Global Publication, 701 E Chocolate Avenue, Hershey, PA, USA 17033

Pal, K. (2022). Blockchain Integrated Internet of Things Architecture in Privacy Preserving for Large Scale Healthcare Supply Chain Data. In Blockchain Technology and Computational Excellence for Society 5.0. IGI Global.

Pal, K., & Yasar, A. (2020). Internet of Things and blockchain technology in apparel manufacturing supply chain data management. Procedia Computer Science, 170, 450–457.

Pandey, P., & Litoriya, R. (2020). Securing and authenticating healthcare records through blockchain technology. *Cryptologia*, *44*(4), 341–356.

Park, J. S., Youn, T. Y., Kim, H. B., Rhee, K. H., & Shin, S. U. (2018). Smart contract-based review system for an IoT data marketplace. *Sensors (Basel)*, *18*, 3577.Google ScholarCrossRef

Patel, V. (2019). A framework for secure and decentralized sharing of medical imaging data via blockchain consensus. *Health Informatics Journal*, *25*(4), 1398–1411.

Patil, K. H., & Seshadri, R. (2014). Big Data Security and Privacy Issues in Healthcare. In Proceedings IEEE International Congress on Big Data (pp. 762-765). IEEE.

Pavitra Haveri, U. B. Rashmi, D.G. Narayan, K. Nagaratna, K. Shivaraj, "EduBlock: Securing Educational Documents using Blockchain Technology", *Computing Communication and Networking Technologies (ICCCNT) 2020 11th International Conference on*, pp. 1-7, 2020.

Peters, G. W. (2016). Understanding modern banking ledgers through blockchain technologies: Future of transaction processing and smart contracts on the internet of money. In *Banking beyond banks and money* (pp. 239–278). Springer.

Peters, G., Panayi, E., & Chapelle, A. (2015). Trends in cryptocurrencies and blockchain technologies: A monetary theory and regulation perspective. *Journal of Financial Perspectives*, *3*(3), 1–46.

Peterson, K., Deeduvanu, R., Kanjamala, P., & Boles, K. (2016). A blockchain-based approach to health information exchange networks. *Proc. NIST Workshop Blockchain Healthcare*.

Philip. (2021). *Blockchain Technology in Healthcare in 2021*. The Block Box.

Pianykh, O. S. (2012). Digital Imaging and Communications in Medicine (2nd ed.). Springer-Verlag.

Pollock, D. (2018). The Fourth Industrial Revolution Built on Blockchain and Advanced with AI. *Forbes*. https://www.forbes.com/sites/darrynpollock/2018/11/30/the-fourth-industrial-revolutionbuilt-on-blockchain-and-advanced-with-ai/#7ce023c24242

Premkumar, A., & Srimathi, C. (2020, March). Application of Blockchain and IoT towards Pharmaceutical Industry. In *2020 6th International Conference on Advanced Computing and Communication Systems (ICACCS)* (pp. 729-733). IEEE.

Pustokhin, D. A., Pustokhina, I. V., & Shankar, K. (2021). Challenges and Future Work Directions in Healthcare Data Management Using Blockchain Technology. In *Applications of Blockchain in Healthcare* (pp. 253–267). Springer.

Qayumi, K. (2015). Multi-agent-based intelligence generation from very large datasets. In 2015 IEEE International Conference on Cloud Engineering, 502–504. IEEE, 2015.

Qiu, J., Liang, X., Shetty, S., & Bowden, D. (2018, September). Towards secure and smart healthcare in smart cities using blockchain. In *2018 IEEE International Smart Cities Conference (ISC2)* (pp. 1-4). IEEE.

Qi, X., Sifah, E. B., Asamoah, K. O., Gao, J., Du, X., & Guizani, M. (2017). Medshare: Trustless medical data sharing among cloud service providers via blockchain. *IEEE Access : Practical Innovations, Open Solutions*, 5(99), 14757–14767.

Queiroz, M. M., Telles, R., & Bonilla, S. H. (2019). Blockchain and supply chain management integration: A systematic review of the literature. *Supply Chain Management*, 25(2), 241–254. doi:10.1108/SCM-03-2018-0143

Radanović, I., & Likić, R. (2018). Opportunities for Use of Blockchain Technology in Medicine. Applied Health Economics and Health Policy, 16(5), 583–590. doi:10.100740258-018-0412-8

Rakic, D. (2018, March). Blockchain Technology in Healthcare. In ICT4AWE (pp. 13-20).

Ramadhani, A. M., Choi, H. R., & Kim, N. R. (2018). Blockchain Implementation in Government: A Review. *Internet E-Commerce Research, 18*(2), 35-48.

Ramani, V., Kumar, T., Bracken, A., Liyanage, M., & Yliantila, M. (2018). Secure and efficient data accessibility in blockchain based healthcare systems. *IEEE Global Communications Conference*, 206–212. 10.1109/GLOCOM.2018.8647221

Ramirez Lopez, L. J., & Beltrán Álvarez, N. (2020). *Blockchain application in the distribution chain of the COVID-19 vaccine: A designing understudy*. doi:10.31124/advance.12274844.v1

Rangi, P. K., & Aithal, P. S. (2020). A Study on Blockchain Technology as a Dominant Feature to Mitigate Reputational Risk for Indian Academic Institutions and Universities. [IJAEML]. *International Journal of Applied Engineering and Management Letters*, 4(2), 275–284.

Rathee, G., Sharma, A., Saini, H., Kumar, R., & Iqbal, R. (2019). A hybrid framework for multimedia data processing in IoT-healthcare using blockchain technology. Multimedia Tools and Applications, •••, 1–23.

Rathee, G., Sharma, A., Saini, H., Kumar, R., & Iqbal, R. (2020). A hybrid framework for multimedia data processing in IoT-healthcare using blockchain technology. *Multimedia Tools and Applications*, 79(15), 9711–9733.

Rathod, J., Gupta, A., & Patel, D. "Using Blockchain Technology for Continuing Medical Education Credits System", *Software Defined Systems (SDS) 2020 Seventh International Conference on*, pp. 214-219, 2020.

Ray, P. P., Dash, D., Salah, K., & Kumar, N. (2020). Blockchain for IoT-Based Healthcare: Background, Consensus, Platforms, and Use Cases. *IEEE Systems Journal*, 15(1), 85–94. doi:10.1109/JSYST.2020.2963840

Reisman, M. (2017). EHRs: The Challenges of Making Electronic Data Usable and Interoperable. International Journal of Pharmacy and Therapeutics, 42(9), 572–575.

Rejeb, A., Treiblmaier, H., Rejeb, K., & Zailani, S. (2021). Blockchain research in healthcare: A bibliometric review and current research trends. *Journal of Data. Information & Management,* 3(2), 109–124. doi:10.100742488-021-00046-2

Reyes, C. L. (2016). Moving beyond Bitcoin to an endogenous theory of decentralized ledger technology regulation: An initial proposal. *Vill. L. Rev.,* 61(1), 191–204.

Reyna, A., Martin, C., Chen, J., Soler, E., & Díaz, M. (2018). On blockchain and its integration with iot. Challenges & opportunities. *Future Generation Computer Systems,* 88, 173–190. doi:10.1016/j.future.2018.05.046

Rijo Jackson Tom. (2020). Suresh Sankaranarayanan, & Joel JPC Rodrigues. (2020). Agent negotiation in an IoT-fog based power distribution system for demand reduction. Sustainable Energy Technologies and Assessments, 38, 100653.

Rimba, P., Tran, A. B., Weber, I., Staples, M., Ponomarev, A., & Xu, X. (2020). Quantifying the cost of distrust: Comparing blockchain and cloud services for business process execution. Information Systems Frontiers, 22(2), 489–507.

Roman-Belmonte, J. M., De la Corte-Rodriguez, H., & Rodriguez-Merchan, E. C. (2018). How blockchain technology can change medicine. *Postgraduate Medicine,* 130(4), 420–427. doi:10.1080/00325481.2018.1472996 PMID:29727247

Saad, M., Spaulding, J., Njilla, L., Kamhoua, C., Shetty, S., Nyang, D., & Mohaisen, A. (2019, April 6). *Exploring the Attack Surface of Blockchain: A Systematic Overview.* https://arxiv.org/pdf/1904.03487

Saberi, S., Kouhizadeh, M., Sarkis, J., & Shen, L. (2019). Blockchain technology and its relationships to sustainable supply chain management. *International Journal of Production Research,* 57(7), 2117–2135. doi:10.1080/00207543.2018.1533261

Sabry, S. S., Kaittan, N. M., & Majeed, I. (2019). The road to the blockchain technology: Concept and types. *Periodicals of Engineering and Natural Sciences,* 7(4), 1821–1832. doi:10.21533/pen.v7i4.935

Sahoo, M., Samanta, S. & Sahoo, S. (2020). A Blockchain Based Model to Eliminate Drug Counterfeiting. In Machine Learning and Information Processing (pp. 213-224). Springer Publishing.

Sai Manoj, K., & Aithal, P. S. (2020). Blockchain Cyber Security Vulnerabilities and Potential Countermeasures. [IJITEE]. *International Journal of Innovative Technology and Exploring Engineering,* 9(5), 1516–1522.

Sanka, A. I., Irfan, M., Huang, I., & Cheung, R. C. (2021). A survey of breakthrough in blockchain technology: Adoptions, applications, challenges and future research. *Computer Communications,* 169, 179–201. doi:10.1016/j.comcom.2020.12.028

Sapirshtein, A., Sompolinsky, Y., & Zohar, A. (2016). Optimal selfish mining strategies in bitcoin. In *International Conference on Financial Cryptography and Data Security*. Springer.

Shae, Z., & Tsai, J. J. (2017, June). On the design of a blockchain platform for clinical trial and precision medicine. In *2017 IEEE 37th international conference on distributed computing systems (ICDCS)* (pp. 1972-1980). IEEE.

Shahnaz, A., Qamar, U., & Khalid, A. (2019). Using Blockchain for Electronic Health Records. *IEEE Access : Practical Innovations, Open Solutions*, *7*, 147782–147795. doi:10.1109/ACCESS.2019.2946373

Shala, B., Trick, U., Lehmann, A., Ghita, B., & Shiaeles, S. (2020). Blockchain and Trust for Secure End-User-Based and Decentralized IoT Service Provision. *Access IEEE*, *8*, 119961–119979.

Sharma, S. (2019, December). pubHeal-A Decentralized Platform on Health Surveillance of People. In *2019 IEEE Pune Section International Conference (PuneCon)* (pp. 1-6). IEEE.

Shi, S., He, D., Li, L., Kumar, N., Khan, M. K., & Choo, K. R. (2020). Applications of blockchain in ensuring the security and privacy of electronic health record systems: A survey. *Computers & Security*, *97*, 101–166. doi:10.1016/j.cose.2020.101966 PMID:32834254

Shoaib, M., Lim, M. K., & Wang, C. (2020). An integrated framework to prioritize blockchain-based supply chain success factors. *Industrial Management & Data Systems*, *120*(11), 2103–2131. doi:10.1108/IMDS-04-2020-0194

Shrestha, R., & Kim, S. (2019). Integration of IoT with blockchain and homomorphic encryption: Challenging issues and opportunities. In Advances in Computers, 115, 293–331. Elsevier, 2019.

Shubbar, S. (2017). *Ultrasound medical imaging systems using telemedicine and blockchain for remote monitoring of responses to neoadjuvant chemotherapy in women's breast cancer: concept and implementation* (Doctoral dissertation, Kent State University).

Shukla, R. G., Agarwal, A., & Shukla, S. (2020). Blockchain-powered smart healthcare system. In *Handbook of Research on Blockchain Technology* (pp. 245–270). Academic Press.

Sivan, R., & Zukarnain, Z. A. (2021). Security and Privacy in Cloud-Based E-Health System. *Symmetry*, *13*(5), 742.

Siyal, A. A., Junejo, A. Z., Zawish, M., Ahmed, K., Khalil, A., & Soursou, G. (2019). Applications of blockchain technology in medicine and healthcare: Challenges and future perspectives. *Cryptography*, *3*(1), 3. doi:10.3390/cryptography3010003

Sodero, A. C., Rabinovich, E., & Sinha, R. K. (2013). Drivers and outcomes of open-standard interorganizational information systems assimilation in high-technology supply chains: t. *Journal of Operations Management*, *31*(6), 330–344. doi:10.1016/j.jom.2013.07.008

Soltanisehat, L., Alizadeh, R., Hao, H., & Choo, K. K. R. (2020). Technical, Temporal, and Spatial Research Challenges and Opportunities in Blockchain-Based Healthcare: A Systematic Literature Review. *IEEE Transactions on Engineering Management*, ●●●, 1–16. doi:10.1109/TEM.2020.3013507

Soni, S., & Bhushan, B. (2019, July). A comprehensive survey on blockchain: Working, security analysis, privacy threats and potential applications. In *2019 2nd International Conference on Intelligent Computing, Instrumentation and Control Technologies (ICICICT)* (Vol. 1, pp. 922-926). IEEE.

Stafford, T. F., & Treiblmaier, H. (2020). Characteristics of a Blockchain Ecosystem for Secure and Sharable Electronic Medical Records. *IEEE Transactions on Engineering Management*, *67*(4), 1340–1362. doi:10.1109/TEM.2020.2973095

StClair, J., Ingraham, A., King, D., Marchant, M. B., McCraw, F. C., Metcalf, D., & Squeo, J. (2020). Blockchain, Interoperability, and Self-Sovereign Identity: Trust Me, It's My Data. *Blockchain in Healthcare Today*, *3*(1), 1–3.

Suite, T. Available online: Https://truffleframework.com/tutorials/configuring-visual-studio-code (accessed on 23 April 2019).

Sultana, M., Hossain, A., Laila, F., Taher, K. A., & Islam, M. N. (2020). Towards developing a secure medical image sharing system based on zero trust principles and blockchain technology. *BMC Medical Informatics and Decision Making*, *20*(1), 1–10.

Swan, M. (2015). *Blockchain: Blueprint for a new economy*. O'Reilly Media, Inc.

Szabo, N. (1996). Smart Contracts: Building Blocks for Digital Markets. Extropy. *The Journal of Transhumanist Thought*, *16*(18), 2–20.

Tanwar, S., Parekh, K., & Evans, R. (2020). Blockchain-based electronic healthcare record system for healthcare 4.0 applications. Journal of Information Security and Applications, 50, 102407.

Tapscott, D., & Vargas, R. V. (2019). Unleashing the Power of Blockchain in the Enterprise. *MIT Sloan Manag.* https://sloanreview.mit.edu/article/unleashing-the-power-of-blockchain-in-the-enterprise

Tcheng, J. E., Crowley, J., Tomes, M., Reed, T. L., Dudas, J. M., Thompson, K. P., Garratt, K. N., & Drozda, J. P. Jr. (2014). Unique device identifiers for coronary stent postmarket surveillance and research: A report from the food and drug administration medical device epidemiology network unique device identifier demonstration. *American Heart Journal*, *168*(4), 405–413.e2. doi:10.1016/j.ahj.2014.07.001 PMID:25262248

Team, F. (2018, October 22). *The Use of Blockchain in Healthcare – How Can Technology Keep Health Data Secure and Private?* Academic Press.

Team, G. T. (2019). *Global Blockchain Technology Market in the Healthcare Industry, 2018–2022*. Frost & Sullivan.

Terzi, S., Zacharaki, A., Nizamis, A., Votis, K., Ioannidis, D., Tzovaras, D., & Stamelos, I. (2019). Transforming the supply-chain management and industry logistics with blockchain smart contracts. In Y. Manolopoulos, G. A. Papadopoulos, A. Stassopoulou, I. Dionysiou, I. Kyriakides, & N. Tsapatsoulis (Eds.), *Proceedings of the 23rd pan-hellenic conference on informatics* (pp. 9–14). ACM. 10.1145/3368640.3368655

Thomas, L., & Coveney, S. (2012). *Blockchain Applications in Healthcare.* News Medical. https://www.news-medical.net/health/Blockchain-Applications-in-Healthcare.aspx

Tom, R. J., Sankaranarayanan, S., Joel, J. P. C., & Rodrigues, J. J. (2020). Agent negotiation in an iot-fog based power distribution system for demand reduction. Sustainable Energy Technology and Assessments, 38, 100653.

Tomasz GÓrski. Jakub Bednarski, "Transformation of the UML Deployment Model into a Distributed Ledger Network Configuration", *System of Systems Engineering (SoSE) 2020 IEEE 15th International Conference of*, pp. 255-260, 2020.

Treiblmaier, H. (2018). The impact of the blockchain on the supply chain: A theory-based research framework and a call for action. *Supply Chain Management, 23*(6), 545–559. doi:10.1108/SCM-01-2018-0029

Tripathi, G., Ahad, M. A., & Paiva, S. (2020, March). S2HS-A blockchain based approach for smart healthcare system. *Health Care, 8*(100391), 1–13.

Tschorsch, F., & Scheuermann, B. (2016). Bitcoin and beyond: A technical survey on decentralized digital currencies. IEEE Communications Surveys and Tutorials, 18(3), 2084–2123.

Uddin, M. A., Stranieri, A., Gondal, I., & Balasubramanian, V. (2018). Continuous patient monitoring with a patient-centric agent: A block architecture. IEEE Access : Practical Innovations, Open Solutions, 6, 32700–32726.

Uddin, M. A., Stranieri, A., Gondal, I., & Balasubramanian, V. (2020). Blockchain leveraged decentralized IoT health framework. Internet of Things, 9, 100159.

Ullah, H. S., Aslam, S., & Anrjomand, N. (2020). *Blockchain in Healthcare and Medicine: A Contemporary Research of Applications, Challenges, and Future Perspectives.* arXiv preprint arXiv:2004.06795.

Verma, M. (2021). Amalgamation of Blockchain Technology and Knowledge Management System to fetch an enhanced system in Library. IJIRT, 7(11), 474-477.

Verma, M. (2021). Emerging applications of blockchain technology. *International Research Journal of Modernization in Engineering Technology and Science, 3*(4), 1258-1260.

Verma, M. (2021). Modeling Identity Management System Based on Blockchain Technology. *International Journal of Research Publication and Reviews, 2*(4), 450-452.

Verma, M. (2021). Smart contract model for trust based agriculture using blockchain technology. International Journal of Research and Analytical Reviews, 8(2), 354-355.

Compilation of References

Vora, J., Nayyar, A., Tanwar, S., Tyagi, S., Kumar, N., Obaidat, M. S., & Rodrigues, J. J. (2018, December). BHEEM: A blockchain-based framework for securing electronic health records. In *2018 IEEE Globecom Workshops (GC Wkshps)* (pp. 1-6). IEEE.

Walter, A. (2013). *Technologietransfer zwischen Wissenschaft und Wirtschaft: Voraussetzungen für den Erfolg*. Springer-Verlag.

Wang, W., Hoang, D. T., Xiong, Z., Niyato, D., Wang, P., Hu, P., & Wen, Y. (2018). A survey on consensus mechanisms and mining management in blockchain networks. arXiv preprint arXiv:1805.02707, 1-33.

Wang, M., Duan, M., & Zhu, J. (2018). Research on the security criteria of hash functions in the blockchain. *Proceedings of the 2nd ACM Workshop on Blockchains, Cryptocurrencies, and Contracts, 1*(1), 47-55.

Wang, M., Wu, Y., Chen, B., & Evans, M. (2020). Blockchain and supply chain management: A new paradigm for supply chain integration and collaboration. *Operations and Supply Chain Management: An International Journal, 14*(1), 111–122. doi:10.31387/oscm0440290

Wang, W., Hoang, D. T., Hu, P., Xiong, Z., Niyato, D., Wang, P., & Kim, D. I. (2019). A survey on consensus mechanisms and mining strategy management in blockchain networks. *IEEE Access : Practical Innovations, Open Solutions, 7*(1), 22328–22370.

Wang, X., Zha, X., Ni, W., Liu, R. P., Guo, Y. J., Niu, X., & Zheng, K. (2019). Survey on blockchain for internet of things. *Computer Communications, 136,* 10–29. doi:10.1016/j.comcom.2019.01.006

Wanitcharakkhakul, L., & Rotchanakitumnuai, S. (2017, December). Blockchain technology acceptance in electronic medical record system. In *The 17th International Conference on Electronic Business, Dubai, UAE*. 53-58.

Weir, S. (2018). *Supply Chain Transparency*. Academic Press.

William, J. (2016). *Blockchain: The Simple Guide Everything You Need to Know*. CreateSpace. Independent Publishing Platform.

Williams, L., & Mcknight, E. (2014). The Real impact of counterfeit Medicine. *U. S. Pharmacist, 39*(6), 44–46.

Witowski, J., Choi, J., Jeon, S., Kim, D., Chung, J., Conklin, J., ... Do, S. (2021). MarkIt: A Collaborative Artificial Intelligence Annotation Platform Leveraging Blockchain for Medical Imaging Research. *Blockchain in Healthcare Today, 4*(176), 1–9.

Wong, D. R., Bhattacharya, S., & Butte, A. J. (2019). Prototype of running clinical trials in an untrustworthy environment using blockchain. *Nature Communications, 10*(1), 1–8.

Wood, G. (2014). Ethereum: A Secure Decentralised Generalised Transaction Ledger. *Ethereum Project Yellow Paper*, 1–32.

Wood., G. (2014). Ethereum: A secure decentralized generalized transaction ledger. Ethereum project yellow paper, 151(2014):1–32, 2014.

World Health Organization. (2019). Recommendations on Digital Interventions for Health System Strengthening – https://www.who.int/reproductivehealth/publications/digital=interventions-health-system-strengthening/en/

Wu, G., Zhang, H., Qiu, M., Ming, Z., Li, J., & Qin, X. (2013). A decentralized approach for mining event correlations in distributed system monitoring. *Journal of Parallel and Distributed Computing, 73*(3), 330–340.

Wust, K., & Gervais, A. (2018). *Do you need a blockchain? In 2018 crypto valley conference on blockchain technology (cvcbt)*. IEEE. doi:10.1109/CVCBT.2018.00011

Xie, J., Yu, F. R., Huang, T., Xie, R., Liu, J., Wang, C., & Liu, Y. (2018). A survey of machine learning techniques applied to software-defined networking (sdn): Research issues and challenges. IEEE Communications Surveys and Tutorials, 21(1), 393–430.

Xu, R., Chen, S., Yang, L., Chen, Y., & Chen, G. (2019, February). Decentralized autonomous imaging data processing using blockchain. In *Multimodal Biomedical Imaging XIV* (Vol. 10871, p. 108710U). International Society for Optics and Photonics.

Yaeger, K., Martini, M., Rasouli, J., & Costa, A. (2019). Emerging blockchain technology solutions for modern healthcare infrastructure. *Journal of Scientific Innovation in Medicine, 2*(1), 1. doi:10.29024/jsim.7

Yaga, D., Mell, P., Roby, N., & Scarfone, K. (2019). Blockchain technology overview. arXiv preprint arXiv:1906.11078.

Yaga, D., Mell, P., Roby, N., & Scarfone, K. (2019). Blockchain technology overview. arXivpreprint arXiv:1906.11078.

Yang, R., Wakefield, R., Lyu, S., Jayasuriya, S., Han, F., Yi, X., Yang, X., Amarasinghe, G., & Chen, S. (2020). Public and private blockchain in construction business process and information integration. Automation in Construction, 118, 103276.

Yaqoob, I., Salah, K., Jayaraman, R., & Al-Hammadi, Y. (2021). Blockchain for healthcare data management: Opportunities, challenges, and future recommendations. *Neural Computing & Applications*, •••, 1–16.

Yoon, H.-J. (2019). *Blockchain Technology and Healthcare*. National Center for Biotechnology Information, U.S. National Library of Medicine.

Yu, Y., Li, Y., Tian, J., & Liu, J. (2018). Blockchain-based solutions to security and privacy issues in the internet of things. IEEE Wireless Communications, 25(6), 12–18.

Yue, X., Wang, H., Jin, D., Li, M., & Jiang, W. (2016). Healthcare data gateways: Found healthcare intelligence on blockchain with novel privacy risk control. *Journal of Medical Systems, 40*(10), 206–218. doi:10.100710916-016-0574-6 PMID:27565509

Compilation of References

Zhang, L. (2019). Why Blockchain and IoT Are Perfect Partners. *DZone.* https://dzone.com/articles/why-blockchain-and-iot-are-perfect-partners

Zhang, F., Cecchetti, E., Croman, K., Juels, A., & Shi, E. (2016, October). Town crier: An authenticated data feed for smart contracts. *Proceedings of the 2016 ACM SIGSAC conference on computer and communications security, 1*(1), 270-282.

Zhang, P., Schmidt, D. C., White, J., & Lenz, G. (2018). Blockchain Technology Use Cases in Healthcare. In *Advances in Computers* (1st ed., Vol. 111, pp. 1–41). Elsevier Inc. doi:10.1016/bs.adcom.2018.03.006

Zheng, Z., Xie, S., Dai, H. N., & Wang, H. (2016). Blockchain challenges and opportunities: A survey. Work Pap., 2016, 2016.

Zheng, Z., Xie, S., Dai, H., Chen, X., & Wang, H. (2017). An overview of blockchain technology: Architecture, consensus, and future trends. In *Big Data (BigData Congress), 2017 IEEE International Congress on.* IEEE.

Zhou, S., Sheng, H., Ma, J., & Han, X. (2020). *Review of the Application of Blockchain Technology in Traditional Chinese Medicine Field.* doi:10.1145/3429889.3429932

Zhuang, Y., Sheets, L. R., Chen, Y. W., Shae, Z. Y., Tsai, J. J., & Shyu, C. R. (2020). A patient-centric health information exchange framework using blockchain technology. *IEEE Journal of Biomedical and Health Informatics, 24*(8), 2169–2176.

284

About the Contributors

Ganesh Chandra Deka is Deputy Director in DGT, Ministry of Skill Development and Entrepreneurship, Govt of India. His research interests include Bigdata Analytics, Blockchain Technology, Internet of Things (IoT), Cloud Computing and NoSQL Databases. He is the co-author for 4 text books in fundamentals of computer science. He has edited 19 books (6 IGI Global, USA, 7 Chapman and Hall/CRC Press, USA, 3 Springer (includes 1 Internal conference proceeding) & 3 Elsevier) on Bigdata Analytics, NoSQL Database, Internet of Things (IoT) and Blockchain Technology as of now. He has published 5 Special Issue in journals published by IGI Global. USA. He is the Chief Editor of International Journal of Computing, Communications and Networking (IJCCN) published by WARSE,India and Associated Editor of International Journal of Applied Research in Bioinformatics (IJARB), IGI Global, USA. He has authored 14 Book Chapters as of now. He has published 8 research papers in various reputed Journals (IEEE 2, Elsevier 1) and more than 47 papers in Conferences, workshops and International of IEEE & Elsevier. So far he has organized 08 IEEE International Conference as Technical Chair in India.

* * *

P. S. Aithal is Vice Chancellor of Srinivas University, Mangalore, India.

Amulya Murthy Aku is a final-year MD Scholar at KAHER's SBMK Ayurveda Mahavidyalaya. She is currently working on a thesis on oxidative stress and obesity and two departmental projects on food and nutrition in Ayurveda. She has clinical experience in Ayurvedic medicine, nutrition and food, lifestyle conditions, prevention, and yoga. She aspires to be a lifestyle consultant and researcher specialising in Ayurveda.

Muralidhar Kurni is an Assistant Professor, Department of Computer Science, School of Science, GITAM (Deemed to be University), Hyderabad, India.

Shilpa Mahajan joined NCU in 2007 and has more than 13 years of teaching experience at postgraduate and undergraduate level. She is a committed researcher in the field of Sensor Network, and has done her PhD in the area of Wireless Sensor Network at Guru Nanak Dev University, Amritsar. She specializes in Computer Networks, Cyber Security, Data Structures, Operating System and Mobile Computing. She has published 37 research papers, 25 in peer reviewed reputed International Journals and 12 in IEEE and Springer indexed Conferences. She has set up a CISCO Networking Academy and developed CISCO lab at NCU, Gurgaon in Jan 2014. She is a CISCO certified Training Instructor for CCNA module-1,2,3 and 4. She has been awarded as an Advanced Level Instructor this year. She got an appreciation from Cisco Networking Academy for 5 years active participation.

Mujeeb Mohammed is an Assistant Professor, Department of CSE, School of Technology, GITAM (Deemed to be University), Hyderabad, India.

Kamalendu Pal is with the Department of Computer Science, School of Mathematics, Computer Science and Engineering, City, University of London. Kamalendu received his BSc (Hons) degree in Physics from Calcutta University, India, Postgraduate Diploma in Computer Science from Pune, India; MSc degree in Software Systems Technology from Sheffield University, Postgraduate Diploma in Artificial Intelligence from Kingston University, MPhil degree in Computer Science from University College London, and MBA degree from the University of Hull, United Kingdom. He has published dozens of research papers in international journals and conferences. His research interests include knowledge-based systems, decision support systems, computer integrated design, software engineering, and service oriented computing. He is a member of the British Computer Society, the Institution of Engineering and Technology, and the IEEE Computer Society.

Anusha Thakur has done B.Tech in "Electronics and Instrumentation Technology" from Tumkur, Karnataka, and Master's in Business Administration (MBA) in "International Business" from University of Petroleum & Energy Studies, (UPES) Dehradun. In addition to this, she has also completed a Post-Graduation certification course in "Market Research and Data Analytics" from MICA, Ahmedabad. Anusha has also been writing few papers and chapters for journals/books in India and abroad. One of her published works is a chapter on "Market for Plant-Based Meat Alternatives" for the book "Environmental, Health, and Business Opportunities in the New Meat Alternatives Market" which has won accolades across the world. The book was considered #1 in the WORLD in the category of Vegetarian Writing. Further, the book was also announced as the national winner for Australia in the Vegetarian Writing Category. Further, she has a work experience of approximately 4 years in the

Market Research Industry. Her work primarily focuses, on the secondary research, market analysis, market sizing, interpretation, forecasting and report writing.

Manish Verma is a member of the International Association of Engineers. He is currently working as a 'Scientist-D' in Defence Research and Development Organisation. He completed his Master in Science in 2005. He has more than twenty research papers in various high-impact international journals. His research areas are distributive technologies like Blockchain, IoT and Artificial Intelligence.

Index

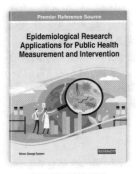
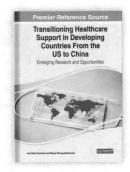
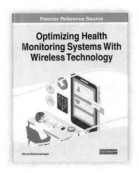
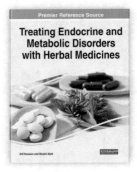
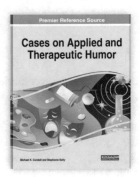
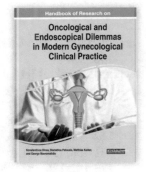
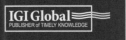

Ensure Quality Research is Introduced to the Academic Community

Become an Evaluator for IGI Global Authored Book Projects

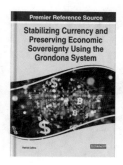
Premier Reference Source
Stabilizing Currency and Preserving Economic Sovereignty Using the Grondona System

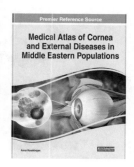
Premier Reference Source
Medical Atlas of Cornea and External Diseases in Middle Eastern Populations

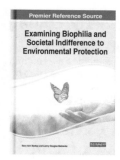
Premier Reference Source
Examining Biophilia and Societal Indifference to Environmental Protection

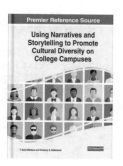
Premier Reference Source
Using Narratives and Storytelling to Promote Cultural Diversity on College Campuses

The overall success of an authored book project is dependent on quality and timely manuscript evaluations.

Applications and Inquiries may be sent to:
development@igi-global.com

Applicants must have a doctorate (or equivalent degree) as well as publishing, research, and reviewing experience. Authored Book Evaluators are appointed for one-year terms and are expected to complete at least three evaluations per term. Upon successful completion of this term, evaluators can be considered for an additional term.

If you have a colleague that may be interested in this opportunity, we encourage you to share this information with them.

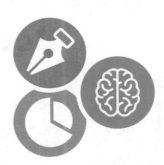
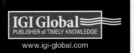

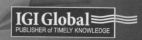

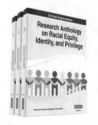
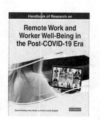
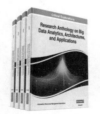
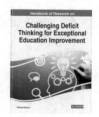

 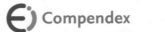
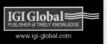

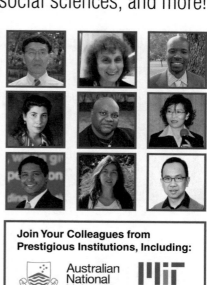
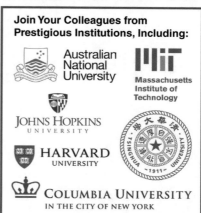

Printed in the United States
by Baker & Taylor Publisher Services